Blood, Sweat and Fears

MEDICAL PRACTITIONERS AND MEDICAL STUDENTS OF SOUTH AUSTRALIA WHO SERVED IN WORLD WAR 1

Presented to the medical staff of Flinders Medical Centre and medical students of Flinders University to commemorate the centenary of World War 1 and the contribution of South Australian medical practitioners during this war. This has been made possible by a generous grant from the Flinders Medical Centre Clinician's Special Purpose Fund and from the Army Museum of South Australia, Army Health Services Historical Research Group.

CHRISTOPHER VERCO | ANNETTE SUMMERS | TONY SWAIN | MICHAEL JELLY

First published July 2014
Reprinted November 2014

ISBN 978-0-646-92750-3

Cover Art:
Septimus Power Australia, 1878 – 1951
No 3 Australian Advance Dressing Station, Somme Front 1917, Somme
Oil on canvas 89.3 x 110.2
Gift of Dr & Mrs C Bollen 1953
Art Gallery of South Australia Adelaide.

Design and print by Openbook Howden, St Marys, South Australia 5042
www.openbookhowden.com.au

Online sales from:

yourbooksonline
www.yourbooksonline.com.au

OBH 23141

Contents

Dedication

'Blood, Sweat and Fears: Medical Practitioners and Medical Students of South Australia who served in World War 1', is dedicated to the memory of the South Australian Medical Practitioners and Medical Students who served in the Army, Navy and Flying Corps in the Great War, 1914-1918:

To commemorate those who lost their lives and to those who lost their health, faith, hope and aspirations; and

To celebrate the achievements of those who received Military or Civilian honours in recognition of their bravery under fire, their leadership and contribution to their profession and society in the aftermath of the war, and finally to those whose contributions remain unknown and unacknowledged.

"The profession of medicine and surgery must always rank as the most noble that men can adopt. The spectacle of a doctor in action among soldiers, in equal danger and with equal courage, saving life where all others are taking it, allaying pain where others are causing it, is one which must always seem glorious, whether to God or man."

Churchill Winston S., 1898, 'The Story of Malakand Field Force'.

Foreword

Australia, in August 1914, with the British Empire joined the Grand Alliance against the Central Powers in the Great War of 1914-1918. Some 416,809 Australians enlisted and of these 331,000 served overseas; 61,720 died and 155,000 were injured. Australian casualties (64.98%) were the highest in the British Empire, and then there were those Australians who also served, were injured or died with other forces making the overall total hard to calculate accurately. What can be said with certainty was that this war was the most costly conflict in terms of death and casualties.

The centenary of this conflict provides an opportunity for all Australians to reflect upon and commemorate the service and sacrifice of our servicemen and women. 'Blood, Sweat and Fears' describes a very small number of Australians who served in World War 1, namely the South Australian Medical Practitioners and Medical Students who served at home and overseas in the armed services of the Grand Alliance.

Over two hundred one page biographies have been written; these describe men and women ranging in age from 18-65 years, from Professors to Rhodes Scholars and students. A number were to join the pantheon of war heroes with significant Military decorations recognizing their bravery and leadership under fire. A number were to go on to achieve considerable professional success and leadership in Australia and Great Britain.

This book enables us to reflect on the pressures of overseas service, the impact at home of the loss of medical manpower, the devastation of those who lost family members and the challenge of injured servicemen and women reintegrating back into a community that was keen to forget war. The Army Health Services Historical Research Group, formed in Adelaide 7 years ago, through its '2014 Project' subcommittee is responsible for this book and I encourage you to read their text and join in the Public Commemoration of the lives of all Australians who served in war.

Lest We Forget

His Excellency Rear Admiral the Honourable Kevin Scarce AC CSC RANR
Governor of South Australia

Introduction

The Army Health Services Historical Research Group (AHSHRG) was formed in 2007 by Colonel Bruce Perks FANZCA, then Honorary Representative Colonel, RAAMC. The broad objective of the group, which comprised senior Australian Defence Force health officers, is to preserve the history of the Australian Defence Force Health Services relating to South Australia. The Patron of the Group is Colonel Donald D Beard AM RFD ED FRCS FRACS. A subcommittee of the AHSHRG was formed in March 2011 to undertake the '2014 Project'. The '2014 Project' sought to publish a book, by mid-2014, in which all Medical Practitioners and Medical Students with a South Australian connection, be it by birth, domicile, education or medical practice who served in the Armed Services in World War 1, each had a one page biography. Each biography was to comprise a photograph, a paragraph on pre-enlistment, service and on post war life.

Why might one wish to do this? First to honour those of our predecessors who served in WW1 some of whom have been succeeded in their chosen profession by sons, grandsons, and great grandchildren, secondly it seemed timely given the centenary of WW1, thirdly there has always been a perception that the South Australian medical profession has always 'punched above its weight' in its military service to Australia.

There is good reason to support this perception in WW1 as Colonel AG Butler DSO VD MB ChB BA reflected on the Deans of the three Australian Medical Schools of the time: *"If Anderson Stuart made the Sydney graduate the most enterprising and worldly wise, HB Allen made the Melbourne student a student for life and Joseph Verco impressed on the Adelaide School a fervour and scientific outlook and a professional standard which enabled the South Australian assembly to lead the way in the professional reaction to war needs."*

Amongst those who served 12 were decorated with the Companion of the Distinguished Service Order (DSO) and twenty with a Military Cross (MC) or Military Medal (MM); 14 received Knighthoods later in life. Sir Henry Newland CBE DSO and Sir Leonard Lindon were Presidents of the Royal Australasian College of Surgeons, Sir Charles Bickerton Blackburn KCMG OBE was the first President of the Royal Australasian College of Physicians, JS Verco the first President of what is now the Royal Australian and New Zealand College of Radiologists, and Gilbert Brown the founding President of the Australian Society of Anaesthetists.

Our title, 'Blood Sweat and Fears' is derived from the records of Leonard Darby MBChB SMO Surgeon on the HMAS *Sydney* in November 1914: Darby describes establishing two operating theatres in the stoker's bathrooms; each bathroom was 10ft x 8ft x 7ft. He describes the horrific injuries when HMAS *Sydney* was hit by shells from the *Emden; 'At one time we keeled over and the operating table with Hoy upon it took charge. It seemed as though we had been hit but it was only a sudden alteration of course"* The action over; *'Our clothes [were] saturated in blood and perspiration and altogether it had been a terrific two hours of high tension.'*

The task facing the authors was more complex than may be imagined; there was no extant list of those doctors and medical students who served at home or overseas in WW1, the Adelaide Hospital Row had disrupted the medical school so that a number of South Australians undertook their medical training interstate or overseas and, of course, a number of practitioners in South Australia had graduated from interstate and overseas in the normal course of medical training and emigration. The authors chose to be as inclusive as possible but freely acknowledge that we may well have missed some who served overseas and undoubtedly have missed many who served at home. The biographies of those who served at home should be regarded as representative of a much larger group which certainly included Honorary Majors Niesche, Harrold, Poulton, Lind,

Marten, Pulleine and Honorary Captains Cherry, Plummer, Jay, Carden and Frayne to name but a few.

Not all of our biographies have filled the desired one page. The authors have chosen to complete the rest of such pages with interesting extracts which have been taken from the diaries of Captain Harry Nott and Lieutenant Colonel John Corbin, each a South Australian who served overseas; they have also been taken from Dr Leonard Darby's report, the British Medical Journal (BMJ) and the Medical Journal of Australia (MJA). The majority of the South Australian population during WW1 would have considered themselves an integral part of the British Empire; the weekly publication of the BMJ would have provided South Australian doctors and medical students with news and views of contemporary medical practice. The MJA was published from 1914. The British Medical Association State Branches joined with the Australian Medical Association (AMA) in 1962 when the Federal AMA was formed.

The next page identifies those who have been a great help to the authors. However, it would be remiss of me not to personally acknowledge the great support received from Colonel Roger Freeman OAM RFD FRACR, who sadly died late in 2013, and Colonel Robert Likeman CSM FRANZCOG. Each is a recognized military historian and without their generous help we would not have had sufficient information to progress as rapidly as has been possible. The authors, in addition, to collecting information and writing biographies, contributions are acknowledged: Colonel Annette Summers AO RFD (rtd) has kept the database, the files and undertaken extensive typing of the manuscript, Surgeon Lieutenant Commander Tony Swain (rtd) has been our photographic sleuth and wizard and, moreover, provided most of the introductory pages and Colonel Michael Jelly RFD (rtd) brought to bear his knowledge of Medical Registration and the Medical Board in South Australia. Heartfelt thanks are due to each.

The dedication is a sincere statement of our purpose. The authors hope that you gain the same inspiration from the material we present as we have derived in preparing our text.

Christopher J Verco RFD MD FRCOG FRANZCOG
Chairman
2014 Project

Sources:

Butler AG (1943) 'Official History of the Australian Army Medical Services in the War of 1914-1918' AWM Canberra Vol. 111 'Problems and Services' p224.
Darby Leonard, 'The Post-Action Report of the Senior Medical Officer of HMAS *Sydney* after the engagement with SMS Emden, 9th November 1914'.

About the Authors

Dr Christopher J Verco RFD MD FRCOG FRANZCOG, a Senior Lecturer – Senior Consultant in Obstetrics and Gynaecology at Flinders Medical Centre and the Flinders University, graduated MBBS Adelaide (1972) and trained in Adelaide (Royal Adelaide Hospital, Adelaide Childrens Hospital, Queen Victoria Hospital) and London (The London Hospital and Hammersmith Hospital). He is a Group Captain in the RAAF; he joined the RAAF in 1967 and has remained a member since. He has served overseas in Malaysia, Bougainville and East Timor; in Australia he has served with the South Australian University Squadron, 24 Squadron and the RAAFSR. He was Hon ADC (Air) to HE the Governor of South Australia, Sir Marc Oliphant from 1973-1976, Director of Health Reserves in SA and variously NT and WA from 2001-2009 and Chairman of the Obstetrics and Gynaecology Consultative Group 2001-2012. He is a former Chairman of the Army Health Services Historical Research Group and the Chairman of the '2014 Project' Committee. He is a former President of the Australian Salaried Medical Officers Federation and of the South Australian Salaried Medical Officers Association. He was the first chairman of the Australian Clinical Casemix Committee (Commonwealth Department of Health) and of the Clinical Advisory Committee of the SA Health Commission.

Professor Annette Summers AO RFD PHD MEDST, BN DIP APP SC, is a Professorial Fellow at Flinders University, School of Nursing and Midwifery. She retired in 2006 as the Professor and Head of School of Nursing and Midwifery, University of South Australia. She also retired in 2004 from the Army Reserve at the rank of Colonel and had several postings in her military career from a junior lieutenant nurse to Matron of 3rd Forward General Hospital (now 3HSB) in her last posting she was Consultant nurse to the Surgeon General's Office with the Australian Defence Force in Canberra. Annette has a strong interest in medical military history is currently a member of the Board of the Army Museum of South Australia. Other previous boards and committee membership include ministerial appointments to the Board of the North Western Adelaide Health Service and The Queen Elizabeth Hospital. She is also the author of several professional articles and reports. Annette has been recognised for her contribution to Midwifery and Nursing education, her contribution to the ADF and community service in the Australia Day Honours of 2004 as an Officer in the Order of Australia (AO). She has also received a Reserve Forces Decoration (RFD) and a Land Command Commendation for her service to Australia in the Army Reserves and a Red Cross Award for her service to the Humanitarian Law Committee of South Australia.

Dr Michael Jelly RFD MB, BS, FRACMA, FRACGP, FCHSM is a graduate of the University of Adelaide in 1963 with higher qualifications in General Practice, Medical Administration and Health Service Executives. He started his medical career in general practice and then moved into medical administration and became the Chief Medical Officer, South Australian Health Commission/Department of Health until 2002. He was President of RACMA from 1998-2000 and a member of the Medical Board of South Australia from 1993 to 2002. He was awarded the Commonwealth Centenary Medal in 2001 and he also received the College Medallion of Royal Australasian College of Medical Administrators. He has been the author of many government reports, proposals and discussion papers. In conjunction with his medical career Dr Jelly has had a military career which spanned 60 years from a Rostrevor College cadet, to National Service and promotion to Colonel in 1989 and posting as CO of 3rd Australian General Hospital. He was appointed the Honorary Colonel RAAMC in 2012.

Dr Anthony (Tony) Swain MB BS, FANZCA, graduated from Sydney University in 1961. After Hospital residency he served 4 years Short Service Commission in the RAN. This time was shared between sea going on board HMAS *Quiberon, Melbourne* in the Strategic Reserve and HMAS *Moresby* on survey work offshore Port Hedland; and on shore at HMAS *Penguin,* Balmoral Naval Hospital. On completion of the commitment he moved to Adelaide to complete his anaesthetic training at The Queen Elizabeth Hospital and the newly formed Adelaide rotation anaesthetic training program. He spent a further 20 years in the RANR and sometime as the Principal Medical Officer HMAS *Encounter.* During these years he qualified as a Specialist Medical Officer at the RAN School of Underwater Medicine and as a member of the Undersea Medical Society of USA. He was instrumental in the establishment of the Hyperbaric Unit at the RAH. He worked as a specialist anaesthetist from 1970 in private practice and as a Visiting Medical Officer in Public Hospitals retiring in 2007. In the years 2002-2012 he was a Clinical Surveyor with the Australian Council on Healthcare Standards (ACHS). He is the currently a member of the Army Health Services Historical Research Group.

Acknowledgements

It is not possible to research and complete a book like this without being indebted to many people for their support and assistance. We are especially grateful to the late Colonel Roger Freeman OAM RFD for sharing his research with the authors as a base for this research and giving us the support to start the project. Colonel Robert Likeman CSM deserves special thanks for his generosity in sharing his own research and publications with the authors and Robert Kearney and Scott Revell for their assistance and Anne Stott for the Corbin diaries. We are also indebted to many organisations and their archivists; including the University of Adelaide. Particularly Andrew Cook for all his assistance, the University of Edinburgh, the University of Sydney, Tony Aldous Prince Alfred College, the Adelaide High School, St Peter's College, Stephen Skinner of the Royal Adelaide Hospital Heritage Office, Royal Prince Alfred Hospital museum and archives, Doug Paterson at the Army Museum of South Australia, Dr Rachel Norris for assistance with birth and death records, the Mount Gambier History Group, the Port Pirie Historical Society and many other Regional History Societies in SA, the Tunnellers Association Queensland and the National Archives of Australia. Our thanks also go to the Anzac Centenary Local Grants Committee, Hindmarsh electorate, Mr Matt Williams MP and the Department of Veteran Affairs for granting us part funding to enable this project to reach completion. The South Australian, Minister for Veterans' Affairs, the Hon Martin Hamilton-Smith MP, for a grant to assist in the reprint of this book. The generous support of Wing Commander Bruce Paix, senior consultant anaesthetist at Flinders Medical Centre is greatly appreciated.

The authors of this publication endeavoured to obtain a head and shoulder photo of the doctors and medical students as they were at their age of enlistment, and in uniform if possible. This has been a mammoth task and is reflected in poor quality in some of the 100 year old photos. In this respect the Adelaide University Archives collection of graduating classes and sporting teams has been invaluable as have the WW1 Collection's at the State Records Office and State Library. The Australian War Memorial extensive collection was fully exploited. The "Cup Book" from the Adelaide Children's Hospital was valuable for the early photos of our more senior Medical Officers. The generosity of families and time in their personal research has contributed to an almost complete catalogue of photos of that era. To the best of our ability we have recognised in the source of our photographs in the style of the citations required.

Most importantly we give special thanks to all the families and friends of the subjects of this book who have provided us with insights to their fathers, grandfathers, great grandfathers, aunts and uncles. Finally we thank the Army Health Services Historical Research Group and the Army Museum of South Australia for their support throughout the process of this project.

✝ This cross denotes that this serviceman was killed-in-action or died during World War 1.

List of Abbreviations

AAH	Australian Auxiliary Hospital
AAMC	Australian Army Medical Corps
ACFA	Australian Camel Field Ambulance
ACH	Australian Clearing Hospital
ACCS	Australian Casualty Clearing Station
ADBD	Australian Divisional Base Depot
ADMS	Assistant Director of Medical Services
ADS	Advanced Dressing Station
AFA	Australian Field Artillery
AFC	Air Force Cross, Australian Flying Corps
AGH	Australian General Hospital
AIF	Australian Imperial Force
AIR	Australian Infantry Regiment
ALH	Australian Light Horse (Brigade)
AMF	Australian Military Forces
AMO	Army Medical Officer
AN&MEF	Australian Naval and Military Expeditionary Force
ANZAC	Australian and New Zealand Army Corps
ASA	Australian Society of Anaesthetists
AWM	Australian War Memorial
Bde	Brigade
BEF	British Expeditionary Force
MB	Bachelor of Medicine
BMJ	British Medical Journal
Bn	Battalion
BSc	Bachelor of Science
BS	Bachelor of Surgery
Bty	Battery
Cantab	Cambridge
CB	Companion of the Order of the Bath
CBE	Companion of the Order of the British Empire
CCS	Casualty Clearing Station
CGS	Chief of the General Staff
MCh	Master of Surgery
CMF	Citizens Military Forces
CMG	Companion of the Order of St Michael and St George
CO	Commanding Officer
Con	Convalescent
Coy	Company
DA	Diploma of Anaesthetics
DADMS	Deputy Assistant Director of Medical Services
DCM	Distinguished Conduct Medal
DDMS	Deputy Director of Medical Services
DFC	Distinguished Flying Cross
DGAMS	Director General of Army Medical Services
Div	Division
DMS	Director of Medical Services
DNMO	Divisional Naval Medical Officer
DSM	Distinguished Service Medal
DSO	Distinguished Service Order
Dub	Dublin
Ed/Edin	Edinburgh
ED	Efficiency Decoration
FCRA	Fellow of the Australasian College of Radiologists
FdAmb	Field Ambulance
FFARACS	Fellow of the Faculty of Anaesthetists Royal Australasian College of Surgeons
FFR	Fellow of the Faculty of Radiologists
FRACMA	Fellow of the Royal Australasian College of Medical Administrators
FRACP	Fellow of the Royal Australasian College of Physicians
FRACS	Fellow of the Royal Australasian College of Surgeons
FRCOG	Fellow of the Royal College of Obstetricians and Gynaecologists
FRCS	Fellow of the Royal College of Surgeons
FRCS(Ed)	Fellow of the Royal College of Surgeons Edinburgh

FRCSI	Fellow of the Royal College of Surgeons Ireland
FRS (Ed)	Fellow of the Royal Society of Edinburgh
GH	General Hospital
GHQ	General Headquarters
Glas	Glasgow
GMO	Government Medical Officer
GOC	General Officer Commanding
HMAHS	His Majesty's Australian Hospital Ship
HMAT	His Majesty's Australian Transport
HMS	His Majesty's Ship
HMAS	His Majesty's Australian Ship
HMT	His Majesty's Transport
HQ	Headquarters
Inf	Infantry
KBE	Knight Commander of the Order of the British Empire
KCMG	Knight Commander of the Order of St Michael and St George
KIA	Killed in Action
KStJ	Knight of the Order of St John
LFPS	Licentiate of the Faculty of Physicians and Surgeons
LRCP	Licentiate of the Royal College of Physicians
LGH	London General Hospital
LH	Light Horse
LHFA	Light Horse Field Ambulance
LHQ	Land Headquarters
LHR	Light Horse Regiment
LM	Licentiate in Midwifery
LRCP	Licentiate of the Royal College of Physicians
LRCS	Licentiate of the Royal College of Surgeons
LSA	Licentiate of the Society of Apothecaries
MC	Military Cross
MD	Military District
MD	Doctor of Medicine
MDS	Main Dressing Station
MEF	Mediterranean Expeditionary Force
MID	Mentioned in Despatches
MJA	Medical Journal of Australia
MM	Military Medal
MO	Medical Officer
MR	Mounted Rifles
MRCS	Member of the Royal College of Surgeons
MS	Master of Surgery
MT	Motor Transport
Mtd Div	Mounted Division
Mtd Inf	Mounted Infantry
NCO	Non Commissioned Officer
OBE	Officer of the Order of the British Empire
OC	Officer Commanding
Oxon	Oxford
P&O	Peninsular and Oriental Steam Navigation Company
PDMS	Principal Director of Medical Services
PMO	Principal Medical Officer
Pnr	Pioneer
POW	Prisoner of War
QM	Quartermaster
QSM	Queen's South Africa Medal
RAAF	Royal Australian Air Force
RAF	Royal Air Force
RAAMC	Royal Australian Army Medical Corps
RAMC	Royal Army Medical Corps
RAP	Regimental Aid Post
RAN	Royal Australian Navy
RANBT	RAN Bridging Train
Regt	Regiment
RFC	Royal Flying Corps
RMO	Regimental Medical Officer
RSL	Returned Servicemen's League
Sig	Signals
Sqn	Squadron
TB	Tuberculosis
TD	Territorial Decoration
Tp	Troop
Tpr	Trooper
Trg	Training
VC	Victoria Cross
VD	Volunteer Decoration
VDC	Volunteer Defence Corps
WWDS	Walking Wounded Dressing Station

Australia's Military Defence Preparedness

One of the first acts of the new Australian Commonwealth Parliament after Federation in 1901 was to establish a Commonwealth Department of Defence. A general order of 30th July 1902, promulgated the change from the State to the Federal organization of the Military Forces of Australia, which proposed that *"The whole of the existing Army Medical Services of each State will be dealt with as one Corps and will be styled the Australian Army Medical Corps."* This was to comprise of:-

(a) Permanent Army Medical Corp (nucleus only).

(b) Militia Army Medical Corps.

(c) Volunteer Army Medical Corps.

(d) Reserve of Officers.

(e) Army Nursing Service Reserve.

The civilian hospitals of the States were to be used as general hospitals, and the medical and surgical staffs of hospitals were requested to give their service. The various colonial military forces had been absorbed into an Australian Army by the beginning of 1903.

The Defence Act of 1909 provided for a program of universal training and this was introduced in 1911. All males of 18-26 years were liable for military training in peace time and for service within Australia in time of war. The medical profession in Australia were concerned with the arrangements for the medical examination of trainees. Provision for this work was made by establishing part-time "area medical officers," paid at the rate of £60 per annum; medical officers of the existing militia were given preference over civilian doctors. The duty of the area medical officer was to examine all the boys within his area at 13 years of age and assess their fitness for military service, and to re-assess annually the trainees as senior cadets who were 14 to 18 years of age, and those in the citizen force who were 18 to 26 of age. All findings, together with weight, height, and chest measurement, were recorded on statistical cards. The medical profession, on the whole, undertook their duty on a patriotic basis rather than a financial basis, and voluntarily staffed the medical units. Six months after commencement of the new senior cadet training (31st December. 1911) the total registrations in training areas numbered 155,122. Of these 105,133 had been medically examined, and 93.2% passed as fit. Of 33,767 junior cadets examined, 97.3% were certified as fit. At the outbreak of World War I, the medical personnel in the Permanent Force numbered four AAMC Officers and 29 Other Ranks, and in the Militia and Citizen Forces 183 AAMC Officers and 1649 Other Ranks.

The Commonwealth Government pledged Australia's whole hearted support to Great Britain when war broke out in 1914, and recruited a force of volunteers for overseas service with the Australian Naval and Military Expeditionary Force (AN&MEF) and the Australian Imperial Force (AIF). Altogether Australia raised and maintained five Infantry Divisions, the greater part of two Cavalry Divisions (including Corps cavalry on the Western Front), a Flying Corps of four combat squadrons and numerous small units. Some 416,809 men and women, including about 2,500 nurses (who were not part of the Army but a service to the Army) volunteered for service with the Australian Imperial Force.

Sources:
http://www.defence.gov.au/Health/about/docs/RAAMC.html
http://static.awm.gov.au/images/collection/pdf/RCDIG1069901—1-.PDF

Australia's Naval Defence Preparedness

The Commonwealth assumed overall responsibility for the State Naval Forces at Federation, at which time their strength numbered 1684. However, with Federal policy primarily relying on the Royal Navy to provide naval defence needs, the State-based forces languished with few resources and declining numbers. As part of the 1903 Naval Agreement, the Royal Navy was required to establish training facilities for a Royal Naval Reserve (Australasian Branch) numbering some 33 officers and 700 ratings. The State Naval Brigades continued to exist as separate organisations until 1907 when they were disbanded and the Commonwealth Naval Militia was formed. This remained until 1911 when all reserve training in Australia became subject to the provisions of the Commonwealth Defence Acts of 1909-10, and a Universal Training Scheme. The Scheme provided for six years elementary training for boys under military age followed by seven years intensive training as adult members of the Citizen Navy.

The Naval Militia thereafter became the Citizen Naval Forces with members placed in one of two categories. Reservists under 18 years of age and liable for compulsory training became the Commonwealth Naval Reserve (Obligatory), while those older than 18, and hence not liable for compulsory service, became the Commonwealth Naval Reserve (Militia). The Commonwealth Naval Forces became the Royal Australian Navy (RAN) from 5 October 1911 and the Reserves became the Royal Australian Naval Reserves (O) and the Royal Australian Naval Reserves (M) respectively. The 1903 Naval Agreement expired in July 1913, and the Australian element of the Royal Naval Reserve was transferred to Commonwealth control and renamed the Royal Australian Naval Reserve (Sea-going). This Reserve mainly comprised professional civilian seamen and was confined to officers.

The first force raised for overseas service WWI was the Australian Naval and Military Expeditionary Force (AN & MEF). The Director of Naval Reserves, on 11 August 1914, reported that he could raise a naval contingent of 500 men. Advertisements in the press called for volunteers from time-expired seamen belonging to the Naval Reserves of Great Britain or Australia. Australia's first naval casualty of WWI, Able Seaman Bill Williams, fell during the AN&MEF's assault in German New Guinea on 11 September. Whilst tending to Williams, Captain BCA Pockley AAMC was killed and was the first Australian medical casualty of WW1. Lieutenant Thomas Bond, RANR, was awarded the DSO, for his bravery during the same action, the first Australian decorated during the War.

The 1st Royal Australian Naval Bridging Train (RANBT), an engineer unit, was formed from surplus reserve manpower in February 1915. The unit retained naval ranks and ratings but organised along Army lines. The RANBT served at Gallipoli and the Suez Canal before being disbanded in July 1917. Meanwhile, in January 1917, a naval reorganisation resulted in the RANR (Sea-going) being renamed the RANR, while the RANR (O) and (M) became the Royal Australian Naval Brigade. Several trawlers were commissioned at Sydney with crews from the recently established 'Minesweeping Section' of the RAN Brigade in October 1917. The trawlers were used to sweep for mines laid off the south-east coast of Australia by the German raider Wolf.

Sources:

http://www.navy.gov.au/join-navy/reserves/brief-history-royal-australian-naval-reserve

http://www.montevideomaru.info/Montevideo/html/Early%20Rabaul.htm

http://www.anaspides.net/military/bitapaka_war_cemetry_png.html

The University of Adelaide

The University of Adelaide sent a request to the families of their students, in 1916, to ask if their sons or daughters were serving in the war. Below is a copy of the letter sent the families and a poignant letter from the mother of Reginald Blockley Lucas, who was not aware that her son had been killed.

now 11th F. Ambulance
in France

The University of Adelaide.

Address:
Box 498 G.P.O.

UNIVERSITY GRADUATES & STUDENTS AND THE WAR.

MEMO.

We are endeavouring to make our list of men who have enlisted, and who are at the front or in camp, as complete as possible in time for the Commemoration which will be held on the 13th inst.

I shall be very much obliged if you will kindly give me what information you can in regard to Dr G. Wien-Smith as to where he is, whether he has been wounded, and what rank he holds, also any further particulars that will be of interest.

Will you kindly let me have your reply by Friday next and oblige,

Yours faithfully,

CHAS. R. HODGE,
Registrar.

4th December, 1916.

Northgate St
Millswood
6th Dec. 1916

Dear Mr Hodge,

I have just received your request for particulars about my son Dr R. B. Lucas, & am pleased to tell what I know.—

He was Captain in the R.A.M.C & attached to the 7th Norfolk Regiment as he went to England in ~~March~~ February 1915 & joined there, — he was in camp at Eastbourne for a month, & since that time has been serving in France, at first in a Hospital in Rouen, then in a Field Hospital & later with the Regiment, living much in the trenches; but I am sorry to say he was reported as missing since 3rd July, & it was supposed he was an unwounded prisoner, but three weeks ago I had a cable that he was wounded & a prisoner, but up to now we have no later news, so the want of further information is causing me grave anxiety.—

Trusting I have not wearied you with too long details,

Yours truly,
Ellen Lucas.

4th Military District

South Australia and Broken Hill were proclaimed the 4th Military District (4MD) by WW1. During WW1 4MD consisted of the following units: Head Quarters at Keswick Barracks, 7AGH at Keswick, 17AAH at Torrens Park and Mitcham Camp.

Mitcham Camp

The first 4MD camp was established on Hawker's Estate at Morphettville with accommodation for 3,000 men including 3 FdAmb Coy. The camp had a measles outbreak and was overcrowded by 1st November 1914. It was decided that half the force and the 4 FdAmb Coy should be moved undercover to Mr. Tait's property at Ascot Park by the 21st November 1914. By the end of March 1915 Ascot Park was considered quite unsuitable as a winter camp, and a camp was established at Mitcham. The South Australian Government purchased the Grange Farm estate of William Tennant Mortlock on 22nd June 1915. It consisted of 298 acres and cost £20,193.13.9 ($40,386.38). This tented and training area and embarkation depot for SA was bounded by Goodwood Road, Grange Road, View St, Winnall St, and Springbank Rd with close proximity to Mitcham Railway Station for access to the 7 AGH at Keswick, as well the departure by sea from Port Adelaide and Melbourne. The Army occupied the site from 1st April 1915 until 30th January 1920. After the war it was established as the suburb of Colonel Light Gardens.

7 Australian General Hospital Keswick

As the numbers of enlistments and wounded military personnel returning to Australia grew, the field ambulances were supplemented by the creation of the 7th Australian General Hospital (AGH). At Keswick Barracks, buildings were allocated for 7AGH on the northern side facing Anzac Highway in July 1915. It is likely that the adjacent Wayville Showgrounds accommodated part of 7 AGH as the allocated structure, built in 1913, was not suitable to accommodate ward patients. It is also believed that some of the stables at Keswick were cleaned and used for patients. The Commanding Officer, 7AGH, was Lieutenant Colonel Richard S Rogers and the Principal Medical Officer (PMO) of 4MD was Lieutenant Colonel Herbert Henry Ernest Russell.

17 Australian Auxiliary Hospital Torrens Park

Robert Barr Smith of Torrens Park, Mitcham offered the Commonwealth Defence Department his home and grounds for the use of wounded soldiers in May 1915. He also offered to defray the costs for any alterations needed to convert it to its new purpose. The 17 AAH was established at Torrens Park (now Scotch College) on the 13th January 1916 under the command of the PMO, Lieutenant Colonel Russell. It was to be used to accommodate the sick and wounded members of the AIF who had returned from active service and required medical and nursing care during their convalescence. When it opened in January 1916 it had accommodation for 127 patients and this soon increased to 239. Over 1000 soldiers passed through 17 AAH between January 1916 and June 1917. The more serious cases were admitted to the 7 AGH. 17 AAH was transferred to Angas College, North Adelaide on the 17th May 1918 and closed on 30th April 1919. Torrens Park later was upgraded to the status of a general hospital and became 12 AGH Torrens Park; this was a 220 bed hospital catering mainly for orthopaedic patients.

Sources:

Last Peter, 1994. The Repat. A biography of Repatriation General Hospital (Daw Park) and a history of repatriation services in South Australia

Mitcham Heritage Research Centre Torrens Park Estate; Preis and Oborn 1991.

Hospital Ships

Hospital Ships

During the War, sea transport posed great problems for Australia, and the trafficking of casualties through the Mediterranean and around the Cape called for special arrangements. In spite of the development of hospitals in forward and semi-forward areas, many ships were needed to carry patients from the Middle East to Great Britain and back to Australia. These ships were known as "white" ships or "black" ships in the military vernacular of the day; "white" ships were brought under the protection of the International Conventions and were comprised of fully equipped floating hospitals like the *Karoola* and the *Kanowna,* and more temporary "hospital carriers" which could transport and deal with the less serious casualties. The "black" ships were sea ambulance transport, carrying large numbers of ill and convalescents; these sailed without Red Cross protection. Fast "black" ships could brave a solitary journey. All of the patients who returned to Australia by these various forms of sea transport arrived safely to their destination. There were many transport and hospital ships like the following:-

HMAHS *Karoola*

7,391 tons. Requisitioned on 9th May 1915. HMAS *Karoola* boarded with troops and general cargo and departed for Egypt on 25th June 1915. After disembarking troops proceeded to England where the ship was converted into a hospital ship with accommodation for 463 patients. For the next three years HMAS *Karoola* transported sick and wounded between Egypt, England and Australia.

HMAHS *Kanowna*

6,042 tons. Requisitioned as a transport ship in Townsville, Queensland, on 8 August 1914 and embarked troops of the AN&MEF for New Guinea. Commonwealth control ended 21 August 1914 but was requisitioned again for Europe on 1st June 1915. HMAS *Kanowna* then proceeded to England where she was converted into a hospital ship with accommodation for 452 patients. For the next three years she transported sick and wounded between England and Australia. After the war, on 18th February 1929, *Kanowna* was shipwrecked when it ran into rocks between Sydney and Melbourne near Cleft Island, south of Wilson's Promontory.

HMAT *Kyarra*

Requisitioned on 6 November 1914 and converted into a hospital ship for the purpose of transporting Australian medical units to Egypt. The hull was painted white with a large red cross on the side. However, in March 1915, HMAT *Kyarra* was converted into a troop transport.

Sources:
Medical Services of the RAN and RAAF, AWM Series 5, Medical, 491.
http://www.auspostalhistory.com/articles/1949.php

The Army Medical Chain of Evacuation

Regimental Aid Post (RAP)

Medical treatment was to start as soon as feasible, and as near to the front line as possible, for this reason RAPs were set up with a medical officer, orderlies (medics) and stretcher bearers. The RAP was situated a few metres behind the front line; wounded men were either to make their own way or be carried, usually by a member of his own unit. The RAP had no holding capacity. The casualty was treated and returned to duty in the line or if more severely wounded or sick evacuated from the front, via hand carriage, wheeled stretchers, or walk, if able, to the advanced dressing station.

Field Ambulance (FdAmb)

The Field ambulance was the most forward of the AAMC units and the first line of more definitive treatment and documentation. The FdAmb controlled the forward sections of the evacuation chain and comprised of several different sections consisting of: **Advanced Dressing Stations, Collecting Posts, Relay Posts and Main Dressing Station (ADS, CP, RP, and MDS).** The ADS was normally set up 400 yards behind the RAP but this distance could change with the variability of the situation. There was at least one, but normally two, ADS set up by the FdAmb and a MDS sited roughly one mile further back. In WW1 Collecting Posts and Relay Posts were established to avoid congestion. This meant there were teams of AAMC stretcher bearers, strung out over miles of ground unpassable by motor or horsed transport, who shuttled between the posts and passing the wounded on to the next team. The ADS did not usually have a holding capacity but this could change depending on the circumstances.

Casualty Clearing Station (CCS)

The Casualty Clearing Stations were to facilitate movement of casualties from the battlefield to the hospitals and usually situated about midway between the front line and the Base Area. A typical CCS could hold 1,000 casualties at any time, and each would admit 15-300 cases, in rotation. The CCS need approximately half a square mile of land to be established. It was staffed by Medical Officers, Dentist, a Pathologist, and up to 100 other non-medical personnel attached. A specialised surgical team could be brought forward if needed. Each CCS would carry its own marquees and wooden huts so as to create medical and surgical wards, kitchens, sanitation, dispensary, operating theatres, medical stores, surgical stores, incineration plant, ablution blocks, mortuary, and sleeping accommodation for staff.

Australian Stationary Hospital (ASH)

Australia deployed two Stationary Hospitals in WW1 1ASH and 2ASH, they were smaller than general hospitals and equipped for fieldwork and placed closer to the front. 1ASH was formed in South Australia and was deployed in Egypt, Lemnos and England. 2ASH was formed in Western Australia and deployed in Egypt, Gallipoli, Sinai, and Palestine.

Australian General Hospital (AGH), Australian Auxiliary Hospitals (AAH)

Australia had several general hospitals and auxiliary hospitals either deployed overseas or within Australia. These were large base hospitals with 250, 500 or 1000 beds. They also generally administered a number of auxiliary hospitals. The 1st, 2nd, 3rd, 10th and 14th AGH served overseas and the others were based in Australia. They were placed on or near lines of transport to facilitate movement of casualties to the ports for either onward movement to England or repatriation to Australia. Large buildings such as hotels or existing hospitals were requisitioned for their use but some were huts and constructed on open ground. The general hospitals were mainly in the Head Quarters area and had complete X-Ray departments, laboratories, operating theatres and wards etc.

Sources:
http://www.ramcww1.com/chain_of_evacuation.pp
http://www.1914-1918.net/wounded.htm
http://www.anzacday.org.au/digging/hospitals.html
http://www.aif.adfa.edu.au:8888/Medical.html
http://en.wikipedia.org/wiki/List_of_Australian_Army_medical_units_in_World_War_I

The Adelaide Hospital Row

The University of Adelaide medical school commenced on 17th March 1885. Clinical instruction was provided by the honorary medical staff in the wards of the Adelaide Hospital, which at this time had 185 beds and was the only public hospital in Adelaide and ultimately under the control of the Government. Therefore the Government, the Medical School, the Adelaide Hospital, the Board and its staff were inextricably linked.

The dispute that occurred and affected many of the doctors who enlisted during World War One began when the Board of the Adelaide Hospital, in a climate of cost saving, when advertising the vacant position, decided to decrease the Superintendent of Nurses' annual salary from £120 to £100 pounds in 1894. The intention of the Board was to re-employ a Miss Thackthwaite, a much respected nurse, who had been previously at the Adelaide Hospital but had moved to another Colony in 1891. Miss Thackhwaite refused the position due to the reduction of salary. The position was then offered to a Miss MacLeod who was, at the time, the Superintendent of the night nurses. This now left Miss MacLeod's position vacant and the Board resolved to fill the position from their current staff. The Medical Superintendent, Dr Perks, was asked to find a suitable staff member. Dr Perks recommended a junior charge nurse, Miss Gordon. This was supported by Miss MacLeod and other staff members. However this was resented by other more senior charge nurses and they put their protest to the Board. The appointment could not be finalised until it received Government approval. It then transpired that Miss Gordon was related to the South Australian Chief Secretary. The Premier of South Australia, Mr Kingston, took the matter in hand and after some investigation and delay Miss Gordon was confirmed in the position. During this time there were several forceful and public protests led by a junior charge nurse Miss Hawkins, who felt she should have been offered the Night Superintendent position and a probationer nurse Miss (Margaret) Graham who had just finished her 3 year probation and was about to be appointed as a charge nurse. Miss Hawkins was dismissed and Miss Graham whose probationary term had expired was now considered ineligible for employment. The affair became news in the press and the two nurses were portrayed as being 'martyrs to a rightful cause'. The Board's management of the situation was called into question and, as a result of the publicity, the Government decided on a Royal Commission to investigate the matter. The Royal Commission found that the Board's decision to appoint Miss MacLeod was made in 'good faith and without undue influence'. However, it also found that the two nurses were justified in protesting but should have used better judgement in the way they protested. The Commission recommended that they be reinstated.

At the same time the honorary medical staff had met and unanimously passed a resolution supporting Dr Perks and the Board. The honorary medical staff believed that the nurses should be disciplined and not reinstated. They opined that reinstatement of the nurses lessened the ability of the Board and hospital management to manage the hospital and control staff and that the previous harmonious relationship between management and staff within the hospital would be eroded. This resulted in a stand-off between the Board and the Government. Dr Perks resigned and found a position elsewhere. Miss Hawkins returned to the hospital despite much protest from the medical and other administrative staff. She subsequently took 6 months leave. The Government informed the Board that their positions would not be renewed in March 1896 and that Miss Graham would be reinstated to the hospital at that time. Both Miss MacLeod and Miss Gordon resigned in February 1896 finding the situation in the hospital intolerable. The new Board was appointed in March 1896 and a meeting of the honorary medical and surgical staff voted unanimously to resign. This effectively closed the University of Adelaide's medical school.

A deadlock ensued; the Government were inflexible about the reinstatement of the nurse and the staff would not work in an environment of disorganisation and lack of discipline. The vacant positions were advertised but brought little interest from other local medical practitioners, so the Government sought to fill the positions from England. This dispute had far reaching consequences for medicine in South Australia. Medical students and potential medical students were forced to study in Melbourne, Sydney or overseas, replacement doctors were labelled 'strike breakers' and endured much criticism from the established medical fraternity, and many of the students never returned to practice in South Australia. The Medical School reopened in March 1901 with its first graduate's in 1902 and by 1906 there were 60 undergraduates enrolled.

'The Adelaide Hospital, Adelaide, South Australia, A short Account of the Circumstances which led to the Resignation of the Honorary Staff', BMA SA, WK Thomas & Co, Grenfell Street, 1906

University of Adelaide Graduates

MB BS

from 1910 to 1918

1910

Black EC
Corry SL
Delprat Lica
Everard JE
Goode RA
Jones E Britten *
Moulden OM
Yeatman C

1911

Boer AO
Dolling CE
Donnelly TH
Drew CF
Hains IC
Harvey GA
Kneebone JLeM *
Moffat May J
Muirhead LG
Pitcher CF
Stoddart HWD
Thomas EB
Russell EAH
Wilton AC

1912

Baker RA
Dunstone HE
Florey Hilda J
McEwin K
Rennie HCC *
Tassie LG
Wells JC

1913

Close WJW
Davey LL
Holder SE
Le Messurier FN
Lucas RB
Mayo JC
Nott HC
Penny HJ
Powell H
Verco JS *

1914

Beard JRSG
Cockburn P
Gardner JF
George Mildred M
Godfrey KC
Guymer EA
Haste RA BSc (1911)
Hayward LA
Smith WL
Steele KN
Strachan JCP
Turner CT
Wall FL
Wibberley BW BSc (1911)
Williams AE

1915

Ashby IE
Barlow DL
Birch JB
Guymer AH
Jose IB
Kenihan RL
Kollosche (Dunstan)HF
Love JA
Phillips WJE
Rice PW *
Sweeney JG
Wien-Smith G
Wyllie HA

1916

Abbott NBG
Black GH
Burden CB
Burnell GH
Plotz OA
Shipway GS
Southwood AR

1917

Bean AR
Beare FH
Broadbent EE
Cairns HWB *
Davies HW
Gault AK
Gillen JB
Hall NB
Kendrew GH
Lendon GA
Moore BF
O'Neill S
Rolland JA
Symons EL
Webb JN
Webb WFS

1918

Cilento RW * (Shared)
Collins WK
Bollen KW
Gurner C
Grant RLT * (Shared)
Keipert LJ
Linn LW
McGlew Phyllis D
McNeil Ian (John)
Messent PS
Pomroy HR
Wallmann DK
Wilson LA

* Everard Scholar

Medals Issued to Australians in World War 1

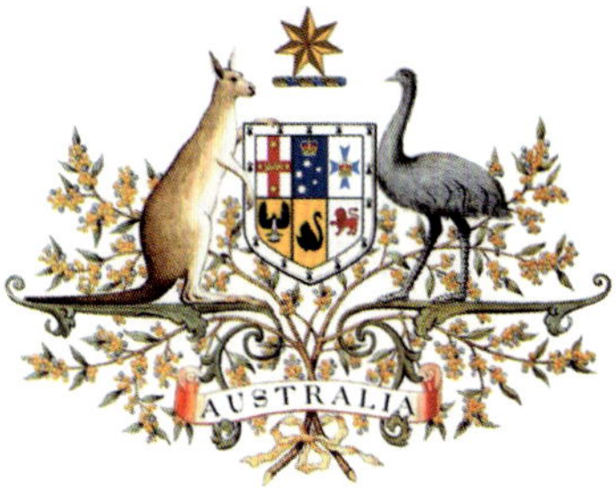

- In 1914 the Australian population was 4,870,000.
- South Australia's population was 441,690.
- Total enlistments from August 1914-November 1918 was 416,809.
- Total number who embarked was 331,781.
- Total number of casualties was 215,585, of these
- Total number who died was 59,342.

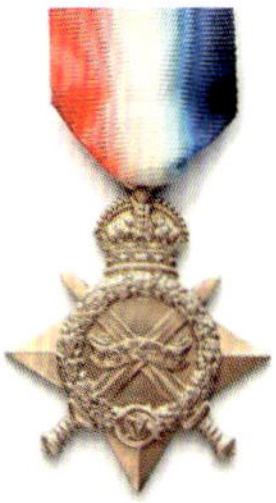

The 1914–15 Star was authorised in 1918 and was issued for service in specified theatres of war between 5 August 1914 and 31 December 1915. A recipient of the 1914 Star could not also be awarded the 1914–15 Star.

82,000 issued.

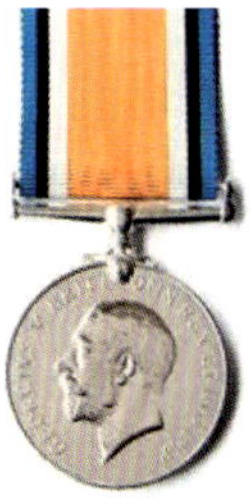

The British War Medal was issued for service in a theatre of war between 5 August 1914 and 11 November 1918. Those eligible included members of women's organisations; persons on the staffs of military hospitals and members of recognised organisations who handled sick and wounded; and members of other duly recognised or other authorised organisations as specified in medal regulations. The qualification period was later extended to cover post-war mine clearance and service in Russia during 1919 and 1920.

338,000 issued.

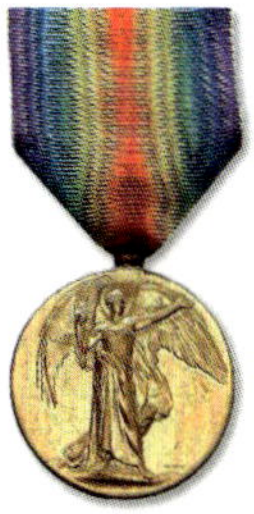

The Victory Medal was authorised in 1919 to commemorate the victory of the Allied Forces over the Central Powers. Each of the Allied nations issued a 'Victory Medal' to their own nationals with all of these having the figure of Victory on the obverse as a common feature. Australians were awarded the medal issued by Great Britain. 336,000 issued.

A member mentioned in despatches (MID) for service during World War 1 wears a bronze spray of oak leaves on the Victory Medal ribbon. Only one emblem is worn no matter how many times a member may have been 'mentioned'. When a ribbon alone is worn a slightly smaller oak leaf is worn as a ribbon emblem.

Medals to Australians in World War 1

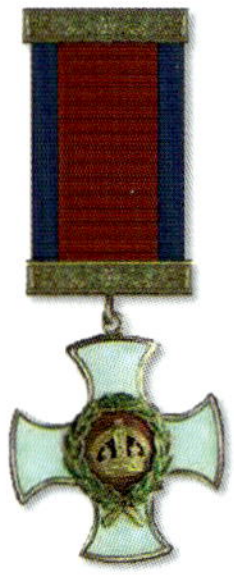

The Distinguished Service Order (DSO)

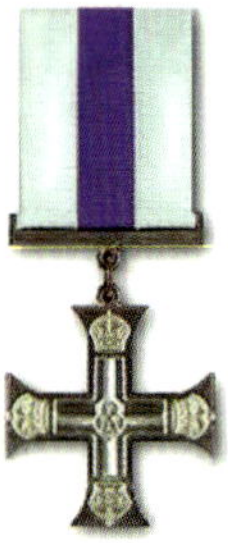

Military Cross

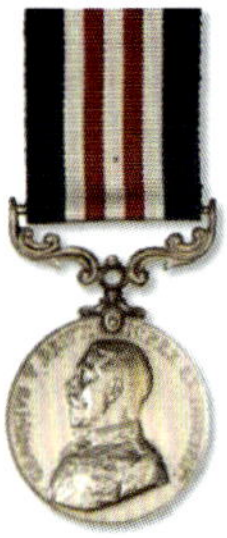

Military Medal

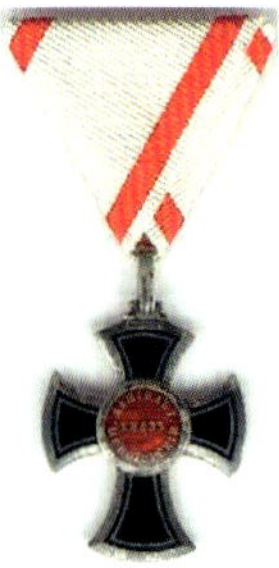

Order of Prince Danilo 1
of Montenegro

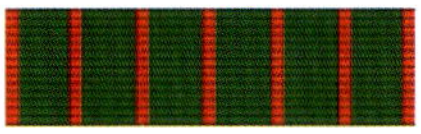

The French Croix de Guerre
1914-1918 Ribbon

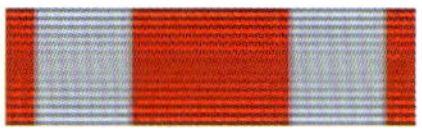

Star of Serbia
Ribbon

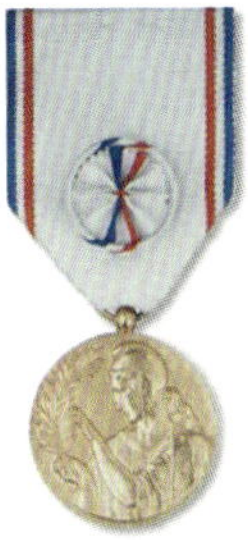

Medaille de la Reconnaissance Francaise

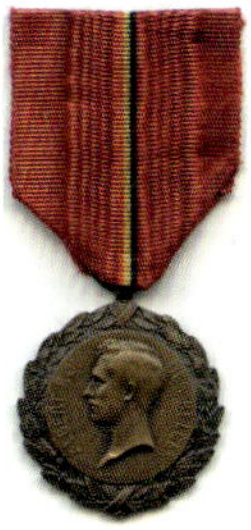

Medaille du Roi Albert

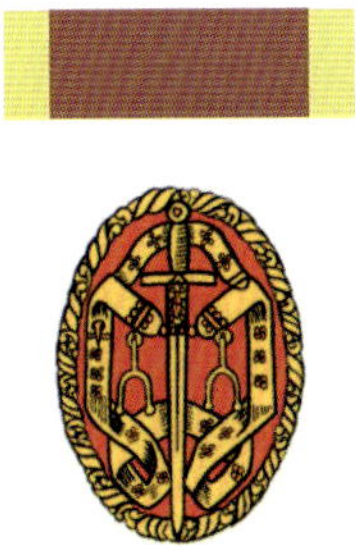

Knight Bachelor Ribbon and Crest

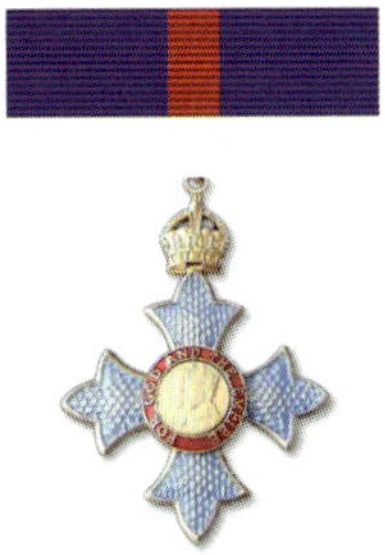

The Order of British Empire

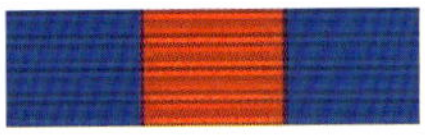

The Order of St Michael
and St George
Ribbon

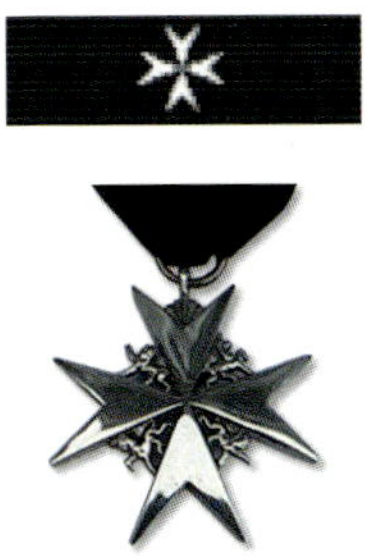

The Order of St John of
Jerusalem

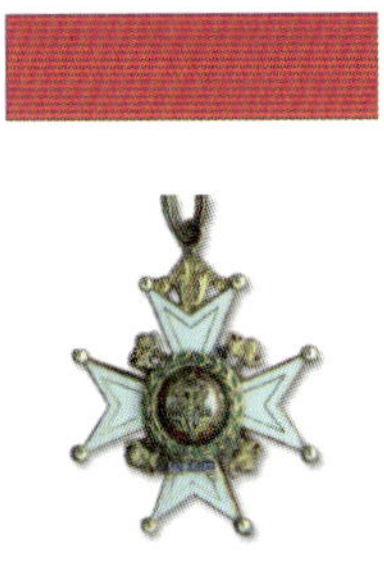

The Order of the Bath

ABBOTT Nigel Basil Gresley

MB BS

1891 - 1978

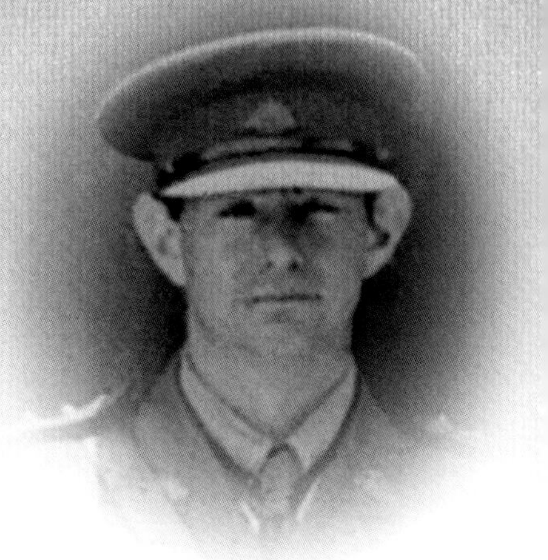

Nigel Basil Gresley Abbott was born in San Francisco on the 4th May 1891 the son of Dr Charles T Abbott, of Tasmania, and Susanna Evelyn, nee Beitsch. His father had left Australia in 1883 and returned to Sandy Bay, Tasmania after the 18th May 1906 San Francisco earthquake. He reported that his wife was in poor health and his sons were still in trauma from the shock of the event. He later received a Letter from Congress on behalf of the President and Congress of America for his contribution to the relief of the population after the disaster. Later the family moved to SA to live in Woodside. Abbott studied and graduated from Adelaide University in 1916 with MB BS, under the New Regulations. Abbott's father moved to Clunes, Victoria after Abbott's enlistment in the AAMC.

Abbott enlisted in the AIF in July 1916 with the rank of captain. He was 25 years old and single, 5ft 10ins tall, weighing 11st 2 lbs. He was described as being of medium complexion, brown eyes and dark brown hair. His prior medical experience was 3 months as an Acting House Surgeon at the Adelaide Hospital and 8 days as a House Surgeon at Broken Hill. He indicated that his previous military experience was, in 1909, a lieutenant on probation in the Commonwealth Military Cadet Corps. He stated he was proficient in Latin and French and could ride. He was recommended for General Duties. He departed from Port Adelaide on the 4th November 1916 in HMAT *Bakara* for Egypt where, on arrival, he was appointed to the 2ASH. Over the next 2 years he moved between the 2nd, 5th and 6th Field Ambulances, the Medical School at Moascar, Ismailia and lastly the 31st General Hospital at Abbassia near Cairo. He embarked from Port Said in *Ormonde* for London on 24th February 1919 on duty for further post graduate study. On 21st June 1919 Abbott, married Bessie Drury Alcock aged 25 years at the Holy Trinity Church, Lyons Tower, Hertford. Together with a large contingent of the AAMC he sailed from England in HMAT *Wahene* on 14th December 1919 to Melbourne with his appointment terminated in Adelaide on 29th January 1920. Abbott was issued with the British War Medal and the Victory Medal.

After the war, at the home of his father Dr C T Abbott at Clunes his wife Bessie, on the 29th February 1920, gave birth to a son. He came to the attention of the newspapers in 1936 when he opposed the Hobart council in building the new Southport Bush Nursing Hospital. The family then returned to Hobart where he began a long and successful career as a private medical practitioner. He was also the Hobart city medical officer and the chief port quarantine officer. He was the founder of the College of General Practioners in Tasmania. His younger sibling Charles Abbott MP was Attorney General of South Australia from 1944 to 1946. Nigel Basil Gresley Abbott died in Hobart on 30th October 1978.

Sources:

Photo edited, AWM D0953.
Family notes in Adelaide
Ancestry.com
The Mercury Hobart 11 August 1936
The Mercury Hobart 1 Nov 1978
Biographical Register 1788-1939
http://ncb.anu.edu.au/sites/default/files/documents/A%20
Biographical%20Register%2017881939%20Vol%201%20A-K.pdf

ARNOLD Edwin (Weidenbach)

MB BS

1881 - 1944

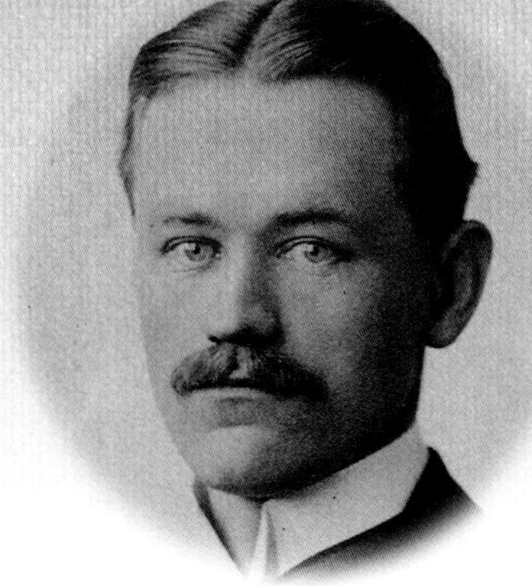

Arnold Edwin Weidenbach was born on December 22nd 1881 second son of Edwin Weidenbach and Minna, nee Beardmann. Their marriage, on 15th March 1879 at the Registry Office, Adelaide produced 8 children. His grandfather, Moritz, migrated to South Australia with his brothers in the 1840s. His parents were Australian born, his father Edwin, was born "in a valley at the back of Glen Osmond while his grandfather, Moritz, was away on the goldfields in Victoria." Moritz and his brothers were successful at Ballarat. The extended Weidenbach family of the 1840s had extensive experience in hotels, property and vineyards in Adelaide, Glen Osmond and Moonta. Arnold was educated at Adelaide University graduating MB BS in 1907 He married Martha Flecker aged 25, on 7th June 1911 at St Saviour Church, Glen Osmond; they lived at Nairne. On enlistment in the AIF his name is Arnold Edwin Weidenbach; he changed his name to Edwin Arnold by Statutory Declaration on 30th August 1919 at Keswick Adelaide.

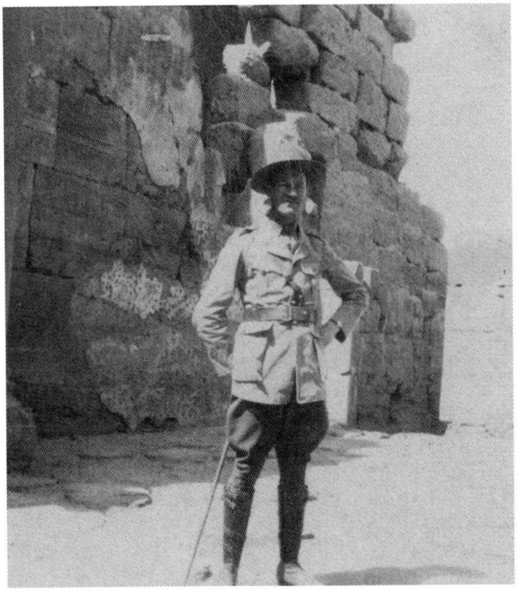

Arnold enlisted in the AIF on 23rd July 1915 at Adelaide, aged 33 years. He was 5ft 8ins, 10st 11lbs, and was commissioned in the AAMC. His wife was named as his next of kin. He embarked in *Orontes* on the 6th August 1915, allocated to the 1st AGH in Egypt. There he spent most of his time in considerable distress with sub-acute osteoarthritis until invalided to the 4th MD Adelaide, onboard RSS *Borda* on 16th September 1916. His appointment was terminated on 30th November 1916. Edwin was issued with the 1914-15 Star, British War Medal and the Victory Medal.

Arnold had a house and surgery at Fullarton Rd, Glenunga, SA, beside what is now the Arkaba Hotel building, the same house in which Dr Norman Robertson Bennett had a practice from 1936-1970. He conducted his general practice there until moving to 11 Church Rd, Mitcham in 1926. During the depression patients sometimes gave Arnold their bankbooks as payment. Money was so short two children were sent to Melbourne to live with an uncle, and Arnold did locum work around the SA country areas which included Port Pirie. His interests outside medicine were ancient Egypt and gardening. He was brought up by his grandmother and uncle, Max Weidenbach, a famous German Egyptologist and artist who left him many precious items of antiquity now in the South Australian Museum. He was happy to go to Egypt in WW1, as he was able to see all the things he had learnt about as a child. "he had a boa constrictor skin going around the wall of the surgery, and according to my uncle John, a mummies head in a glass box which when you lifted the lid smelt" He had a large garden at Mitcham; only the original house on a normal sized block now exists. Edwin Arnold died in Mitcham on 11th July 1944; he was survived by his wife, three sons and a daughter.

Sources:

http://recordsearch.naa.gov.au/scripts/Imagine.asp?B=3035965

Photos and family story Louise Sanders (grandniece).

BAKER Ralph Alderton

MB BS

1889 - 1943

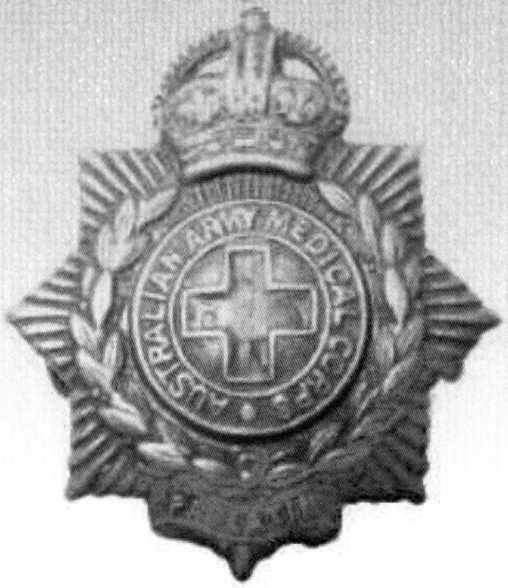

Ralph Alderton Baker was born on the 18th of May 1889 at Medindie, South Australia. He was educated at St Peter's College and studied medicine at the University of Adelaide graduating MB BS in 1912. He then gained experience as a House Surgeon at the Adelaide Hospital for 12 months in 1913. He proceeded to Ardrossan on the York Peninsula as a General Practitioner. Ralph married Emma Maud Cora Burfitt Riley prior to enlistment in the AIF.

Baker enlisted in the AIF on 16th May 1916 with the rank of Captain in the AAMC. He was 27 years old 5ft 7ins tall and weighed 150lbs. He had fair hair, blue eyes and no previous Military experience. His wife of Dequetteville Terrace, Adelaide was named as next of kin with WW Baker, Egmont Terrace Lower Mitcham as an alternative address. Baker embarked from Sydney for Egypt in HMAT *Katuna* on 26th June 1916. He was attached to the 1 LH Training Regiment in Egypt. His time there was as a RMO to Regiments, the 14 AGH, and in the 1 and 3 LH FdAmb. He also had detached duty in the 1 LH FdAmb of the British Army in September 1918 as a temporary captain. He saw duty at Mustapha, Abbassia, Moascar and the Medical School. It was during this latter part of the war that he contracted malaria and was admitted to the 14th AGH then to the HT *Kantara* and finally on board *Port Sydney* on the 5th March 1919 departed Egypt for Melbourne. From Melbourne he was transferred to 4MD Adelaide on 22nd April 1919 where his appointment was terminated on 12th June 1919. Ralph Baker was issued the British War Medal and the Victory Medal

Baker had three daughters between 1920 and 1924, born in Adelaide and in Barmera. Baker, living in Kensington Gardens, subsequently divorced his wife who was living on South Terrace, Adelaide on the grounds of her habitual drunkenness and neglect of domestic duties. He later married Johanna from NSW. He enlisted again in the Army during WW2 from Maryborough, Queensland on 18th August 1942 and his wife Johanna Baker was named as next of kin. Ralph Alderton Baker died in Maryborough Queensland on the 9th August 1943.

Sources:
http://recordsearch.naa.gov.au/NameSearch/Interface/ItemDetail.aspx?Barcode=3009955.
The Advertiser of 11th December 1935
Courier Mail Brisbane 11th August 1945
Ancestry.com

The Army Ration

The attention of the public has been called to the diet on which our soldiers in Gallipoli are subsisting... There is no question about the difficulty of catering for a large and widely distributed army...We hear of the substitution of a certain amount of bully beef by tinned tongue and of a proportion of the army biscuit by dates...it is useless to supply the equivalent of 4,000 or 5,000 calories to the men unless the heat units can be utilized. The picture has been drawn of bleeding gums, sore mouths and painful teeth caused by the mechanical properties of the renowned biscuit...When strong, healthy men suffer from persistent diarrhoea, when the medical officers find that formed stools disappear from the latrines, when the sameness of the diet and its unpalatable character palls to such an extent on all the men that an average loss weight of 28 pounds results, surely the War Office should exercise some ingenuity in the matter of rations... There are promises of better things for the men at the front. Let these promises be realized, in order that the brave boys may be given a chance and the Empire an opportunity of a glorious emergence from the Eastern problem.

MJA, 30th October 1915, p.421

BALLINGER Claude Joseph

Medical Student

1898 - 1982

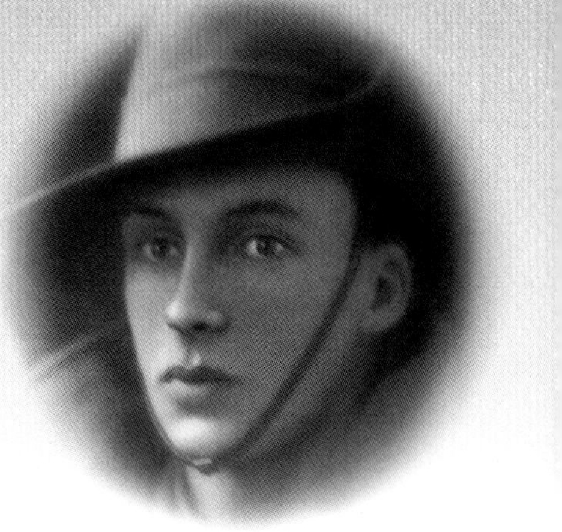

Claude Joseph Ballinger was born in Clare, South Australia on 9th January 1898. He was the son of William Ballinger and his second wife, Victoria Adelaide, nee Fryar; she was a teacher, and sister of his first wife. He was educated at Naracoorte District High School and Adelaide High School. He did well at his secondary schooling, winning a government Exhibition scholarship and the Tennyson Medal for English Literature. He commenced a medical course but after one year decided to enlist in the AIF. He had been with the senior cadets for 4 years and 2 years with the AAMC.

Ballinger enlisted as a private in the AIF on 11th July 1918 and on 29th July 1918. At that time he was 5ft 8ins tall and weighed 135lbs, he was described as having a medium complexion, light grey eyes and dark brown hair. His father William of Wolseley South Australia was named next of kin. He was allotted to the 5th General Reinforcements and was later posted to the 27th Battalion. Ballinger left for England on 14th November 1918. He contracted influenza on the journey and on disembarkation on 18th January 1919 was said to have pleurisy and he was admitted to the Military Hospital at Tillworth. He later contracted mumps and was sent to a Quarantine Hospital. Some records indicate that he contracted tuberculosis. He developed a pleural effusion and was admitted to 1AGH on 31st March 1919. This eventually led to Ballinger losing one lung. On discharge from hospital he was said to be unfit for further service and was returned to Australia on the Hospital Ship *Wandilla*. He disembarked in 4MD on 16th May 1919. His enlistment was terminated on 16th June 1919. He was issued with the British War Medal.

Ballinger resumed his medical studies at the University of Adelaide but obviously struggled with progress and did not pass the fifth year on two occasions. He went to New Guinea as a medical scientist and then to England to further his medical studies. However the climate affected his lung condition and he returned to Australia and abandoned his medical studies. He gained a position with FH Faulding, with his medical knowledge, in Perth, Western Australia. He left Fauldings to join GP Pharmaceuticals eventually becoming managing director of the company in Sydney until his retirement in 1957. Ballinger married Gertrude June Bastian on 29 June 1942 in New South Wales. They moved back to South Australia in 1972 because of the climate. Claude Joseph Ballinger died on 22nd September 1982 in Adelaide. He is buried in the North Road Cemetery. He is still survived by his wife who resides in North Adelaide.

Sources:

http://recordsearch.naa.gov.au/NameSearch/Interface/ItemDetail.aspx?Barcode=3047670
The Adelaide Advertiser Newspaper
John Ballinger, family records.
Biographical Index of South Australians 1836-1885
Personal Record University of Adelaide Archives
http://histfam.familysearch.org/getperson.php?personID=I149051&tree=SouthAustralia

BARLOW Douglas Lewis

MC ED MD FRACP

1894 - 1950

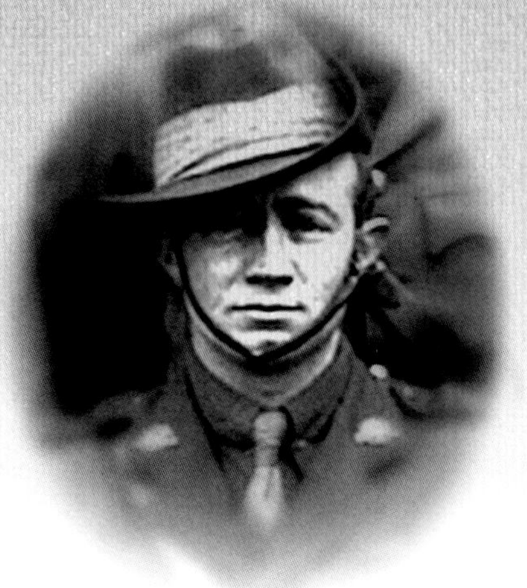

Douglas Lewis Barlow, the second son of Arthur William Barlow, retailer, was born in Gawler on the 18th June 1894. He was educated locally and then at Prince Alfred College. He had a brilliant scholastic career and was dux of the school in 1910, winning the Elder and Longbottom scholarships and top place in the State higher public school examination. He studied medicine at the University of Adelaide and graduated with first class honours in 1915. He was a house surgeon at the Adelaide Hospital and had 3 years' experience with the Senior Cadet Militia and 2 years as a private in the 31st AMC. He lived next door to the Bollens at 9 Fitzroy Terrace, Prospect, SA.

Barlow enlisted in the AIF on 19th October 1915 and applied for a commission in the AMC. On enlistment he was 21 years old, 5ft 9ins tall, weighed 10st 7lbs. His father, of Fitzroy Terrace, was named as his next of kin. Barlow embarked for England in the *Karoola* from Melbourne on 27th May 1916 and was transferred to the 1 AAH, Harefield, England; then to the 2 FdAmb and within a month to the 7th Australian Inf Battalion in France. He was awarded the Military Cross on 26th November 1917 at Ypres, *'For conspicuous gallantry and devotion to duty during an attack. He advanced with the battalion, established his aid post, and dressed the wounded and assisted in their removal under constant shelling. Owing to casualties among bearers he was cut off from the ambulance clearing post for several hours, and it was mainly owing to his exertions that the wounded received attention and shelter during this period.'* After leave breaks in England and Paris, he was gassed by the enemy on 4th September 1918. It was a mild exposure but he was managed via the AAMC evacuation through CCS, No 32 Stationary Hospital and the 2 AGH. He was discharged to duty to the Australian Division 10 Bn on 15th September 1918. There he was considered fit to travel and embarked to Australia in *Demosthenes* arriving at the 4 MD, Adelaide on 28th February 1919. A Medical Board in March found him not fit for General Duties for another 6 months due to his history of being gassed, asthma, weight loss and general debility. His Service was terminated on 8th April 1919. He was issued with the British War Medal and the Victory Medal

After the War he continued to serve in the citizen forces. He was awarded the Efficiency Decoration and promoted to lieutenant-colonel in 1935. During the Second World War he was a consultant to the Army with the rank of Colonel. He received his MD in 1922 for his thesis on Asthma, Hay Fever and Allied Conditions. He held several honorary positions as a pathologist and bacteriologist at the Adelaide Children's Hospital, Adelaide Hospital and Adelaide University. He was active in medical politics especially regarding allergy and vaccines. During WW2 he started the first private pathology service in SA which, after his untimely death in 1950, Dr Eugene McLachlan continued. Douglas Lewis Barlow died on the 4th December 1950 at the time he lived and practiced on Portrush Road. He was survived by wife Mora and their three children; a daughter and a son who became doctors, and a son who became an engineer.

Sources:
http://recordsearch.naa.gov.au/NameSearch/Interface/ItemDetail.aspx?Barcode=3049568.
MJA, 1.1951.; Photo: AWM E01814
Commonwealth Gazette no 137, August 1918

BEAN Alan Reid

MB BS

1895 - 1958

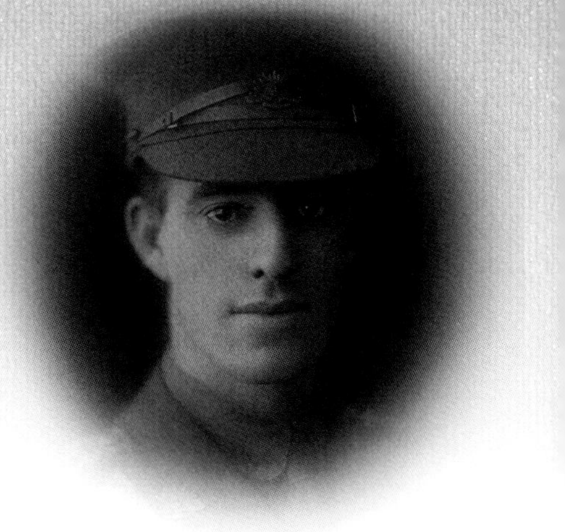

Alan Reid Bean was born on the 9th March 1895 at Moonee Ponds, Victoria. His parents moved to Kalgoorlie, Western Australia. There are records of his marks at the Kalgoorlie Central State School. He was later educated at Scotch College, Cranbourne, Western Australia. He studied medicine at the University of Adelaide and graduated in 1917. The Chancellor, in presenting the degrees, congratulated the candidates, and particularly the medical graduates who, he stated, had all volunteered for active service. He then became a RMO at the Adelaide Children's Hospital.

Bean enlisted in Adelaide on 14th February 1918; he stated he had 7 months prior service in the AAMC Reserve. He was single living at the home of his Mother, Mrs G A Bean, at 10 Lanor Ave, Goodwood Park. He was 23 years, 5ft 11ins, 136 lbs, auburn hair, fair complexion and grey eyes. He embarked on the 23rd March 1918 via the 2 MD Melbourne from Sydney in HMAT *Persic* as a captain AAMC reinforcements. From here his deployments in the north of France included 13 FdAmb, 12 FdAmb, 48 Bn, 46 Bn and 2 AGH. His appointment in the AIF was terminated on the 19th June 1920. Bean was issued with the British War Medal and the Victory Medal.

Bean went to the Sheffield Infirmary to work for one year with Sir Ernest Finch after the war. He returned to Adelaide, but footloose, he travelled to Perth with his sister, first to Brookton for 6 months, then to Bruce Rock, 250 km east of Perth, in the wheat belt. Here he stayed 8 years and helped build a Hospital. He married Alison Stuart daughter of Graham Stuart on the 9th November 1965, and they had two sons and a daughter. Education was soon considered critical and in 1930 the family moved to Fremantle. Here he did locum work and another son was born. Later that year he was appointed Medical Officer at the Fremantle Prison and was the Fremantle Police Doctor. He also purchased, and worked for many years, in private practice close to the Fremantle Hospital. The family lived in the Prison Doctor's Residence. He held these positions at his death on the 21st March 1958.

Sources:
http://recordsearch.naa.gov.au/NameSearch/Interface/ItemDetail.aspx?Barcode=3061045....
Personal correspondence from granddaughter.
NLA.
Photo SLSA: GRG26_5_4_01422
The Advertiser 27 July 1916

The Medical Needs of the Army

A battalion medical officer who considers that he does his full duty to his battalion ...by giving two hours a day to routine duties, is lamentably lacking in the understanding of what is expected from him. What about the lectures on sanitation...How many men has he inoculated...What is the state of his chiropodist department, and what is the state of the feet of his men...What is the state of the men's teeth...Is he telling his men how to avoid vermin, or...how to rid themselves of pests...Does he know every officer and man in the battalion... Is he present at gymnastic exercises...looking out for those upon whom the strain is telling unduly... What care is he taking to see that the men's food, ablution, and conservancy arrangements are as they should be...Is he quite certain that his men who are billeted are living in such sanitary conditions as to ensure freedom from disease? ... The battalion medical officer is the most important individual in the medical organization.

BMJ, 20th March 1915, p. 511

BEARD Jack Roland Stanley Grose

MC MB BS FRCS FRACS FRCOG

1890 - 1975

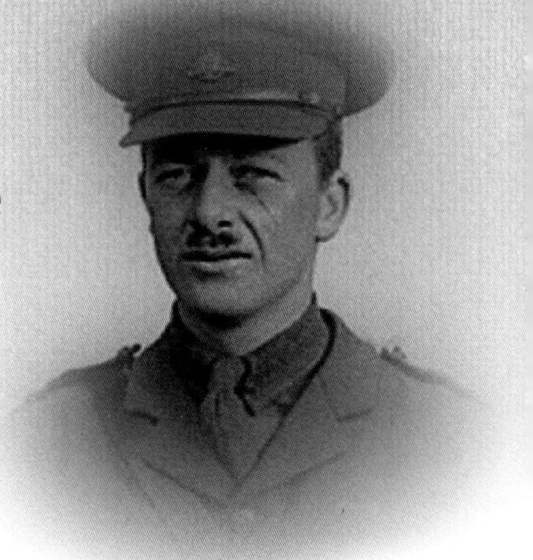

Jack Roland Stanley (Roland John) Beard was born on the 4th October 1890 at Norwood, son of Charles Robert Beard and Emily Jane, nee Bennett, the youngest of nine children. He was always known as Jack. He was educated with private tuition and studied medicine at the University of Adelaide graduating in 1914. He then was a medical officer at the Adelaide Hospital.

Beard joined the AAMC on the 19th of May 1915. He was 24 years old single, 5ft 8ins tall, 10st 7lbs. He gave his widowed sister Olive, Mrs A W Hart c/o S R Page, Milne Terrace Moonta as his next of kin. He was commissioned in late June and sailed for the Middle East expecting to be posted to 2 AGH, but on arrival was posted to the Otago Inf Bn on Gallipoli. However, on 20th August, whilst still on the ship by Gallipoli, he suffered an acute attack of cholecystitis and was taken to Mudros in September and from there to 3 LGH in England with acute cholecystitis. He underwent surgery for gall stones in England, and was attached to 1 AAH at Harefield until March when a Medical Board declared him fit to return to Egypt. He was posted to 15 FdAmb, and went to France with the unit. During the Somme battles he had short attachments to 25 Howitzer Bde (Fromelles) and to 30 Bn. (Somme). He was transferred to 14 FdAmb in January 1917, and again had several detachments to infantry Battalions. Beard was awarded the Military Cross for gallantry at Bullecourt in May 1917. *The RAP was situated in a place subject to heavy enfilading artillery fire. On May 10th the RAP was blown in and he himself buried. Though badly shaken he refused to leave his post even for a short rest. On May 11th a stretcher case was being taken away when the enemy opened up a barrage and two of the stretcher bearers were wounded. Capt Beard at once ran out and brought in these two men without waiting for the barrage to cease.* Before going to the Somme Beard was billeted in a family chateau (which was also a farm) and there met the 16 year old daughter, Andree. The family used the cellars during raids and Beard cared for wounded soldiers assisted by Andree. She was very helpful over the time of the battles and they became very close, so close, he told her family that he would marry her after the War. He was told to come back in 3 years as she was only 16. Beard continued to serve with 53 Bn until the end of 1917 and was promoted Major in August. In March 1918 he took over command of 5 San Section, and later in the year was A/DDMS of 5 Div. relieving DADMS on leave. He embarked HT *Pakeha* as SMO for Australia 6th October 1919 and on arrival in Adelaide in November 1919 he resided with his sister at 77 Hill St, North Adelaide. His appointment was terminated on 26th January 1920. He was issued with the 1914-15 Star, the British War Medal and the Victory Medal.

After being discharged Beard returned to England and spent the next five years studying in the UK. During this time he went to France to meet Andree, the girl from the cellar; they had continued a written correspondence with each other. They married on 15th November 1921 in Daours, Picardie, France. Her widowed mother supported them whilst he was studying in England and Andree took the baby to the family chateau whilst he studied. They returned to Australia and Beard became senior gynaecologist at the Royal Adelaide Hospital in 1941, and an Obstetrician at the Queen Victoria Hospital. He was also assistant to the Professor of Midwifery and Gynaecology in Birmingham, England. Jack Roland Stanley Beard of 1 Edwin Avenue, Collinswood died 1st January 1975, aged 84. He was survived by his wife and son Dr Roland Beard, an obstetrician and gynaecologist.

Sources:
http://recordsearch.naa.gov.au/NameSearch/Interface/ItemDetail.aspx?Barcode=3061722
Likeman R, Gallipoli Doctors, Slouch Hat Publications, Melbourne Aust., 2010
Donald Beard family notes.
Photo: AWM E01672-1
Daily Herald Adelaide 24 March 1910

BEARE Frank Howard

CBE ED MD FRACP

1895 - 1955

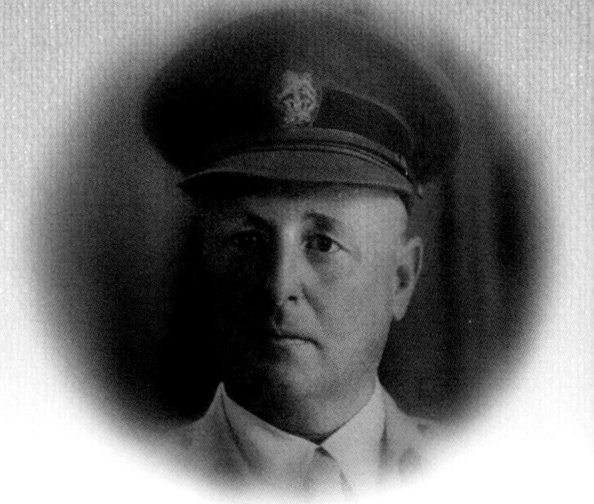

Frank Howard Beare was born on Mauritius on 20th January 1895 the eldest son of Mr and Mrs Charles Beare. His ancestor Mr Thomas Hudson Beare and his family were one of the first families to settle in South Australia. They came to South Australia on the Duke of York and arrived in Kangaroo Island on 29th July 1836, some 6 months before the proclamation of South Australia. Beare was educated at Queen's School, Adelaide where he excelled in study and cricket. After matriculation he began medicine at Adelaide University in 1912 and graduated with Honours in 1917.

Beare enlisted in the AAMC on the 7th August 1917 with 3 months experience at the Adelaide Children's Hospital, and with previous military militia experience in the 31 AAMC 78th Inf. He was a single 22 year old, 5ft 7ins tall, 11st 7lbs, could ride and spoke French. He embarked from Melbourne for England on the 9th November 1917. He proceeded to France in May 1918 to the 5th, 6th, 7th Australian FdAmb, and 20th Bn and towards the end of November the Gas School. After the Armistice he stayed in England as a RMO at the Essex County Hospital, Colchester, with his appointment terminated on 18th April 1920. He was issued with the British War Medal and the Victory Medal.

Beare was house surgeon at the Adelaide Hospital on returning home in 1920 and soon completed an MD with his study gastro-enteritis in children. He entered general practice at Mile End in 1922 and married Beatrice Field in 1923. Subsequently he was joined by Dr E F West (later one of the pioneer orthopaedic surgeons of Adelaide) and returned to England in 1930 for further studies as a physician. On his return in 1932 he was a founding fellow of the RACP. This career was followed by senior appointments at the RAH through to his retirement in 1955. Other medical related interests were the Mareeba Babies' Hospital and the Royal British Nursing Association. He retained his interests in Military affairs; a lieutenant colonel in the Militia, DDMS at Keswick then joined the 2nd AIF in 1939 aged 44 years and eventually became ADMS of the 6th Division, Northern Territory, 7th Division and the CO of the 2/2nd AGH. He was appointed CBE and awarded the ED. After the war he resumed practice and was a lecturer and examiner at the University of Adelaide. He is recorded as a trusted and loyal, a true friend, a trifle hot tempered, quick to recover his composure and bore no malice. He was a man of strong principles and he upheld tenaciously that which he believed to be right and proper. He was a good physician and teacher, singularly happy in his domestic life and had 3 sons. Frank Howard Beare died on the 9th October 1955.

Sources:
http://recordsearch.naa.gov.au/NameSearch/Interface/ItemDetail.aspx?Barcode=306166
MJA. 3rd Dec 1955 p957-8.
Photo RAH Digital Collection.

Amputations at Base Hospitals in France

The toxaemia is so fatal as to be unparalleled. Within a few hours of the onset of physical signs of gas, extensive gangrene may develop in the wound, and life will hang upon the slender thread of an immediate and rapid amputation, with the minimum of shock.....When infection becomes general, on auscultation, gas may often be heard circulating in the heart, like the sound of a boiling kettle.....A general infection is usually fatal from cardiac failure or gas embolism. After death not only the damaged limb but the entire body, including the great veins, liver, etc., may be distended with gas.

BMJ, 1st April 1916, p. 479

BENNETT Norman Robertson

MB BS

1894 - 1957

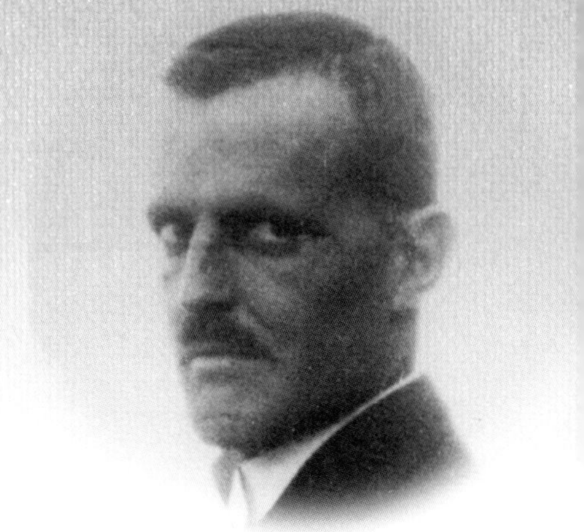

Norman Robertson Bennett (known as NR) was born in Adelaide on 8th February 1894, the third son of Arthur Barkly Bennett, an ironmonger's assistant working in Port Adelaide, of Burlington St, Nth Walkerville. He won a Scholarship at Sturt St School and was an Honours student at Adelaide High School. He began his study of medicine at the University of Adelaide in 1912.

Bennett enlisted in the AIF, on the 21st August 1914 at Fort Largs. He was 20 years old and a 2nd year medical student with previous experience as a Senior Cadet for 2 years. He was single, 6ft tall, and weighed 164lbs. He was posted to B Sect 3 FdAmb from 28th August 1914 as a Lance Corporal. Bennett embarked from Adelaide on the 20th October 1914 and with the Unit moved to the Gallipoli Peninsular. At Anzac on the 3rd September 1915 he was wounded with shrapnel. His wound included a compound fracture of the R occipital bone. He was transferred to Mudros and the 19 General Hospital at Alexandria. Subsequently he was invalided to Australia in November 1915. A decision by the DGMS on the 15th December 1915 and noted by the Principle Medical Officer, 4MD, Lieutenant Colonel Russell that Bennett *"will not be accepted for Service with the AIF so long as remains as a Medical Student at any University of the Commonwealth of Australia"*. He was discharged at the 4 MD as a lance corporal on the 14th February 1916 as medically unfit. Bennett applied to re-join the AIF on the 19th June 1918 aged 24 years, and still a medical student; citing his previous 18 months with the 3 FdAmb in Gallipoli. He passed his physical examination with normal vision despite some visual loss after the removal of the bullet from his skull in 1915. However, he was not called up for duty due to the "cessation of hostilities." He qualified in medicine at Adelaide University in December 1919 with MB BS. He was issued with the 1914-15 Star, the British War Medal and the Victory Medal.

Bennett married Gweneth Willimott on the 3rd December 1921 and had three sons. During the years 1924-1926 he had a small practice in Cleve later moving to a larger house and practice in Port Lincoln with Donald MacDonald Steele. Bennett took an active interest in the social and medical politics of the area notably the Hospital, the Bowling and Racing Clubs; he loved fishing and bird watching. The family lived there until 1936 when they returned to Adelaide for the education of the boys at St Peter's College and his new employment with the Repatriation Department. By 1937 he had established his own practice at 19 Fullarton Rd and was there for 20 years. His sons graduated MB BS at Adelaide University and worked with their father in Fullarton Rd next to the Arkaba Hotel. Norman Robertson Bennett died on 15th January 1957 and was survived by his wife until 1970 and his three sons.

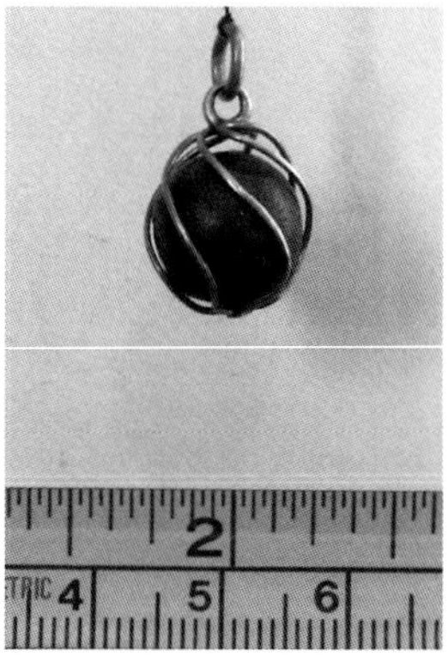

*"The bullet that was removed after he was shot at Gallipoli.
I remember him asking me to put my finger in the hole in his head! Not something to ever forget.
James Bennett Dilke SK Canada S0G 1C0"*

Sources:
http://recordsearch.naa.gov.au/scripts/Imagine.asp?B=3073071;
Photo from Family taken 1924.
Family notes from Helen Bennett.

BENSON Alexander Vigors

MD (Brux), MRCS (Eng), LRCP (Lond)

1869 - 1939

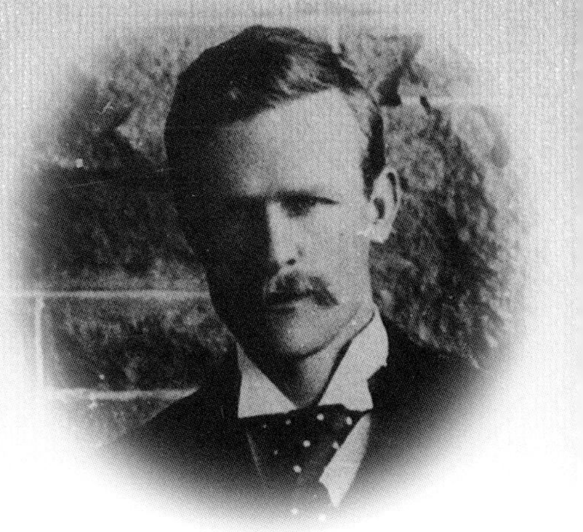

Alexander (Alick) Vigors Benson was born on the 18th May 1869, Kensington, South Australia of a family of eight sons and a daughter. His father Dr John Benson died at the age of 36 years. He was educated at St. Peter's College. He dispensed (pharmacy) at the Adelaide Hospital on leaving school and he acted as dispenser for several years at the Mount Gambier Hospital. Whilst there he was prominent in sporting circles, especially football. He was President of the Mount Gambier Football Association, and Captain of the Mount Gambier Football Club. He travelled to England and studied medicine at London University and then to Brussels where he studied for the MD degree. He married Jane Flett, a daughter of the late Mr Andrew Loutit, manager of the National Bank at Mount Gambier for many years, in 1906. He was registered to practice in Adelaide in December 1904 and had a successful practice at Port Adelaide until 1920.

Benson joined the AIF on the 16th July 1917 when he was 48 years old. He had experience with the 50 AAMC, 77 Bn and had various Camp appointments, He was described as 5ft 8ins, weighed 147lbs with fair hair and blue eyes. His next of kin was named as his wife Jane Flett Benson of Buller Terrace, Alberton South Australia. He had previously been a Medical Assistant to the Transcontinental Railway camps, Mount Gambier Hospital South Australia and 2 years work in Ear Nose and Throat surgery at The London Hospital. On the 7th September 1917 he embarked from Melbourne in Reinforcements for the 14 AGH, Egypt then to Mosscar and other camp and hospital duties in Egypt. He was hospitalised in June 1918 with general debility, however he returned to duty after one month. He was promoted major in September 1918 and finally, after the end of hostilities, was invalided and returned to Australia on the 15th November 1918. His appointment was terminated on the 15th February 1919. He was considered to be recovered and the prior conditions were due to and aggravated by Military Service. He was issued with the British War Medal and the Victory Medal.

Benson shared rooms with Dr Henry Newland on North Terrace, Adelaide from 1920 (who described him as a "beloved physician"). He served a term as President of the SA Branch of the BMA. A lover of horses, Benson raced several, the best of which was Princess Aides. He was President of the Port Adelaide Football Club for several years. He had been an active member of the committee of the Port Adelaide Club since he was first elected in 1909, except during his temporary absence from Australia. He was appointed chairman in 1915, and had filled that position with credit. He was a strong advocate of the movement for the licensing of bookmakers and the establishment of a school for apprentices, and did much valuable work in the interests of racing. It was noted his health had been failing for some time in 1938, and for the last few months in 1939 he had been confined to his room. He died on the 24th December 1939 whilst living at Audley House, 32 Prospect Road, Prospect South Australia. He was survived by his wife Jane. Mr W. B. Carr (chairman of the S.A.J.C.) described Dr. Benson as one of the pillars of the turf.

Sources:
http://recordsearch.naa.gov.au/scripts/Imagine.asp?B=3074118
NLA
Photo SLSA.B15841
Newland HS, MJA; February 17 1940 p 251
The Register 9th Dec 1904

Water Famine

Our winter rains have been a failure – not only in Adelaide but throughout the State–hence the harvest is one of the worst of recent years...At Christmas 1913, we were careful with our water; since September we have been prohibited from using it to water our gardens; now we are advised to take shower baths only – this in a country where the temperature may reach 115° [F] in the shade.

BMJ, 16th January 1915, p. 137

BETTS Lionel Oxborrow

OBE MCh (Orth) MB FRACS

1886 - 1943

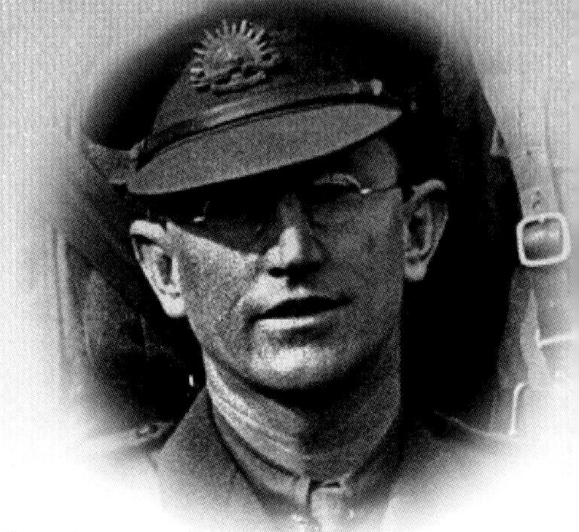

Lionel Oxborrow Betts was born at Streaky Bay on 27th April 1886, son of William Henry and Elizabeth Betts. He was educated at Way College, Greenhill Rd, Wayville and studied medicine at the University of Adelaide where he graduated in 1907. Betts played cover point in the SA Lacrosse team against Victoria in 1908. He practiced in Maitland until he enlisted. He married Miss Beatrice Mills, eldest daughter of Mr. and Mrs. S. Mills of Beetaloo.

Betts enlisted in the AAMC on 13th November 1914 as a Captain. He was 28 years, 5ft 10ins tall, 154lbs, blue eyes with fair hair. His wife was noted as next of kin. Betts embarked in HMAT *Karroo* from Melbourne on 11th Feb 1915 and was posted to 9th LH Regt and served in Egypt, Gallipoli and the desert campaigns. He was invalided to Australia for 8 months in 1916 due to a paratyphoid B infection. He once again embarked from Australia on 14th August 1916 in *Itria* returning to duty. He was promoted to Major on the 11th November 1916. He saw service in the No.2 Aust Command Depot, Weymouth, England in 1918 and then in France at Boulogne with the 13 FdAmb, 52 Bn, 49 Bn in Boulogne and Wimmereux which formed one of the chief hospital areas. Betts was appointed OBE on 3rd June 1919. He was promoted to Lieutenant Colonel in March 1919. Betts returned to Australia on the *Davanha* to 4MD Adelaide on 20th June 1919 with his service terminated on 19th August 1919. He was issued with the 1914-15 Star, British War Medal and Victory Medal.

Betts took up general medical practice at Semaphore Road, Semaphore until 1926, when he went to Liverpool to study orthopaedics under Sir Robert Jones, gaining the Robert Jones Medal. He became one of the pioneers of orthopaedic surgery in Adelaide on his return in 1928, and for many years worked at Escourt House at Semaphore South. It was in this period that he became attached to the Port Adelaide Rowing Club; he was its Patron from 1923-1930. A boat bearing his name was launched by the Club in 1924. He unveiled the Memorial Clock Tower on the foreshore at Semaphore on the 24th May 1925 when he was president of the local RSL Sub Branch. Betts was a keen stud stock master, and his Ryeland and Corriedale sheep studs were widely known. His Talungabee Ryeland flock, founded in 1932, was regarded as one of the best in Australia. Championship honours and many class prizes were gained by his rams and ewes at the Adelaide, Sydney, and Melbourne shows. The Corriedale flock was established in 1929, and although not so prominent in the interstate show rings, the type and quality of the sheep have been highly regarded in South Australia. During WW2 he was placed on the active reserve list AAMC 4MD. Betts was living at, Kings Grove, Tranmere in 1942. Lionel Oxborrow Betts died on 19th January 1943 aged 56 years; he was survived by his wife and son Dr WJ Betts and daughter Mrs J Cohn. After his death a memorial fund was established under the Chairmanship of the Lord Mayor to erect a sun playroom for children at Escourt house.

Sources:

http://recordsearch.naa.gov.au/NameSearch/Interface/ItemDetail.aspx?Barcode=3085768

Photo AWM No?

MJA: June 24th 1944 Obituary p.595.

Escourt Hughes J., A history of the Royal Hospital

Adelaide Advertiser 21st January 1943

BICKLE Leonard Watkins

FRCS(Ed) LRCP (Lond)

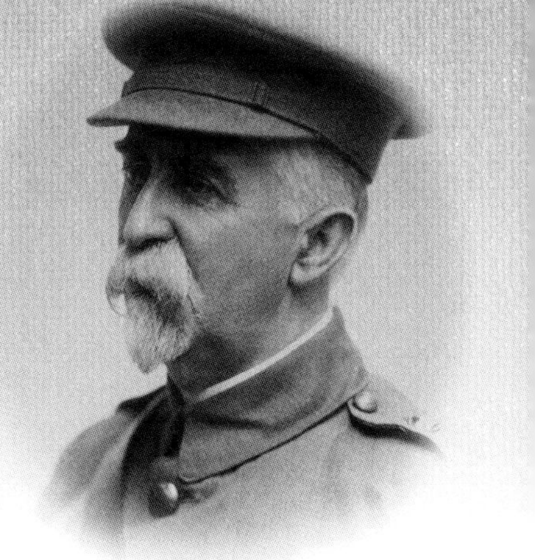

1857 - 1921

Leonard Watkins Bickle was born at St Leonards, Sussex, England on 10th September 1857. He studied at St Thomas' Hospital in London and in 1881 he obtained the conjoint diplomas of the Royal Colleges of Physicians and Surgeons. He practiced at St Thomas' Hospital for three years and was appointed to the resident staff of Queen Charlotte's Hospital, London. Bickle immigrated to South Australia in 1884 and settled in Gawler where he practised for two years. He took up a practice in Mount Barker in 1886. He moved to Adelaide in 1897 and was attached to the Adelaide Hospital and continued in private practice. Bickle obtained a commission in the South Australian militia on the 29th April 1897. He rose to the rank of Major. He attended the Indian medical congress in Calcutta and whilst he was there he was commissioned by the South Australian government to investigate the sanitation in hospitals in 1910. He retired in 1912 with the rank of Honorary Lieutenant Colonel in the Australian Army Medical Corps. He retired from practice in 1913.

Bickle volunteered for active service in WW1 and was accepted as a lieutenant colonel in the Army Medical Corps of the AIF on 2 November 1915. He is described as a widower, 58 years old, 5ft 7ins in height, fit with good eyesight. His next of kin is recorded as his son, Neil Stoneman Bickle, who was in the Royal Navy. Bickle was assigned to duty on various transport ships to the Middle East and England. These included the *Demosthenes,* the *Marathon,* the *Wirilda,* the *Themistocles* and the hospital ship *Kanowna.* During his war service he had frequent discussions about his pay, as although given the rank of lieutenant colonel he was paid as a captain; this was amended during his service to a Major's pay. Bickle's appointment with the AIF was terminated on the 30th November 1916. He was issued with the 1914-15 Star, the British War Medal and the Victory Medal. The 1914-15 Star was the subject of a long running dispute with the military after his discharge. Although awarded in 1915 he was asked to return it as was deemed by Base Records to be *'eligible* [for the 1914-15 Star] *a Medical Officer must have either, been on the strength of a recognised Hospital ship, or else have actually landed and taken on the establishment of a unit in a theatre of war.'* Despite the fact that he was the medical officer on many transport ships to the Middle East during those two years. Bickle continued to argue with the military over recognition of his substantive rank of lieutenant colonel which was eventually accepted.

Leonard Watkins Bickle never returned to Adelaide but remained in Sydney, where he was involved with one or two commercial concerns. He had a very large circle of friends in almost every state of the Commonwealth. *"In his practice he attached great importance to the pharmacological activities of drugs and combination drugs and was very successful in the treatment of minor conditions which are so important to the patients and which are frequently neglected by modern practitioners."* Leonard Watkins Bickle's health deteriorated in 1920 and he died on the 28th June 1921. He was survived by his son Neil; his wife and daughter had predeceased him.

Sources:
http://recordsearch.naa.gov.au/NameSearch/InterfaceItem Detailaspx?Barcode=3080497
MJA; 13 August 1921, p 120,
NLA
Photo, AWM H19220

BIRCH John Bright

MC MB BS FRCS(Ed)

1890 - 1975

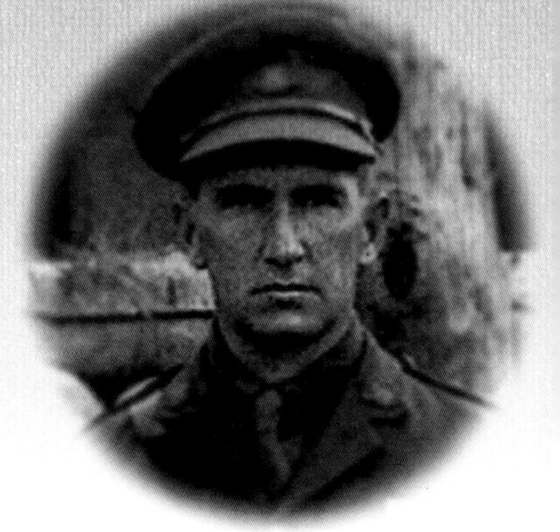

John Bright Birch was born on the 1st December 1890 at Glenelg, South Australia, the son of John William Birch. He was educated by private tuition at Semaphore, South Australia. He studied medicine at the University of Adelaide where he graduated in 1915.

Birch enlisted in the AIF and was commissioned in September 1915. He was single, 25 years old, 5ft 9ins tall weighed 150lbs, medium complexion, blue eyes and brown hair. His father of Park Terrace, Eastwood South Australia was named next of kin. He embarked for the Middle East in December for General Duties. He was assigned to 4 FdAmb on arrival, only to be reassigned to 12 FdAmb two weeks later. He went to France with the unit in June 1916, and 29th December 1916 was awarded the Military Cross for *conspicuous service rendered* at Pozières between July and September when the FdAmb was heavily engaged. He was ill whilst on leave in December in England, and on his return to France in January was kept at 1 AGH for two months before he was allowed to rejoin 12 Fd Amb. He had a brief detachment to 46 Bn during May 1917, and from August to December served as RMO of 51 Bn. He was posted to 3AGH at Abbeville in February 1918, and in September 1918 he was promoted to Major and sent to the POW cage as MO for a month. After the Armistice he was transferred to 14 FdAmb until March 1919. He was granted study leave for six months and completed a residency at the Queen's Hospital, Birmingham. He was repatriated in November 1919 with his appointment terminated on the 7th March 1920. He was issued with the British War Medal and the Victory Medal.

Birch entered general practice in South Australia on his return. He worked at various locations including Unley and Renmark. During World War I, the corner of Urrbrae Ave and Ferguson Ave, Myrtle Bank became a Repatriation Hospital for tuberculosis and although much of the property has been subdivided the house and its garden remain as part of the War Veterans' Home. The Duke and Duchess of Gloucester were met by Dr. J. Birch during a visit to the Hospital in May 1927. He was at 99 Fullerton Rd, Unley by 1932. He was Commanding Officer of 3 FdAmb at Keswick in 1932-33. In 1933 he decided to specialize in surgery, and went to Scotland to obtain his surgical fellowship. On his return to Australia he worked first at Richmond NSW, and then settled at Tweed Heads where he also became the GMO. During WW2 he moved to Sydney. He later returned to South Australia. John Bright Birch died in Adelaide in 1975.

Sources:

http://recordsearch.naa.gov.au/scripts/Imagine.asp?B=3084044.
NLA
The Register Adelaide 19 Dec 1910
The Register Adelaide 15 Oct 1915
Likeman R, From the Tropics to the Desert, Slouch Hat Publications 2012.
Photo AWM, E02567

The Price of Patriotism

The news of the first engagement of the Australian Forces... brought home to the whole of the Commonwealth the real meaning of war....the sacrifice, no doubt, has to be made, and the nation owes a debt of gratitude to the six brave men who lost their lives during the operations of the occupation of New Britain by the Australian troops. The medical profession has sustained an especial loss of a field surgeon in the death of Captain Pockley, who...was prepared to risk his life in the attempt to bring aid to those who were sick or wounded...considerable losses among the [Australian] Army Medical Corps must be expected....through them we may expect to obtain the most vivid accounts of the gruesome horrors of war.

MJA, 9th September 1914, p. 277.

BLACK Eustace Couper

MB BS BA

1886 - 1971

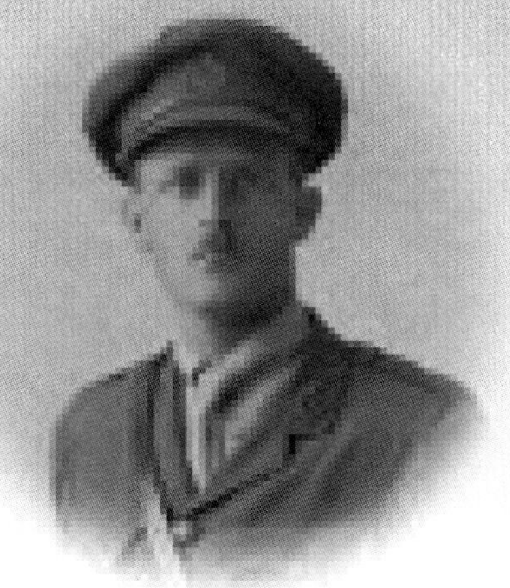

Eustace Couper Black was born on 28th February 1886 at Adelaide, the son of eminent South Australian Botanist John McConnell Black, author of the Flora of South Australia and the original published papers on Aboriginal languages. He was educated at Norwood and Rose Park Primary Schools and Prince Alfred College. He studied medicine at the University of Adelaide graduating in 1910. Following a year as Resident Medical Officer at the Royal Adelaide Hospital he worked briefly in North Queensland at the Mungana Hospital.

Black travelled to England early in 1912 to study as a fellow of the RCS at Paddington Green and Middlesex Hospitals; however, prior to completion joined the RAMC the day following declaration of war in 1914. He was in the retreat from Mons and thus an "old contemptible". He served in France from 1914 to 1917, initially as RMO to 13th Battalion of the Royal Scots, then 7th Battalion Royal Scots, No 2 General Hospital, Le Havre, 2nd/3rd Ghurkha Rifles (at Flanders), Meerut Division, the 1st Battalion Highland Light Infantry and finally the 1st Battalion Cameroonians. Black was promoted to the rank of Captain in 1915. In 1917 he was appointed Medical Officer in charge of troops in HM Transport *Anglo-Egyptian* to Dar-Es-Salaam and then served as CO of the field ambulance service in Portuguese and German, East Africa.

Black married Julia Dixon at Barrow-in-Furness, Lancashire on 27th March, 1917. Upon discharge he returned to Australia and set up practice in Spalding, SA, being for many years the only doctor covering a large rural area. He subsequently practiced at Tranmere and was Medical Officer for the South Australian railways from 1940 to 1950. He held an appointment as a lecturer at the University of Adelaide and worked as an Anaesthetist at the Royal Adelaide and Adelaide Children's Hospitals from 1929 until April 1971. He was a member of the Royal Society, the Anthropological Society, the Royal Geographical Society of South Australia, a life member of the AMA, was active in legacy and the Old Contemptible Society. At the age of 71 Black completed a Bachelor of Arts in Anthropology. He developed a passion and interest in Aboriginal archaeology and anthropology. He participated in the Board of Anthropological Research expeditions to the Granites in 1936, Nepabunna in 1937 and Ooldea in 1939, assisting with the recording of anthropometric data and blood testing. He recorded numerous Aboriginal campsites, stone arrangements and other archaeological sites in the Fleurieu Peninsula, Kangaroo Island, River Murray, Coorong, South-East, Mid-North, York Peninsula, Broken Hill and areas along the Upper Murray and Darling Rivers, either in association with the Anthropological Society of South Australia or during family holidays from 1940 to 1970. During the 1940s Black carried out the major detailed survey of Aboriginal sacred trees along the Finniss River and in the late 1960s surveys of sacred trees and Aboriginal sites in the Chowilla area. In 1966 he assisted in archaeological excavations at Lake Robe and in 1967 at Koonalda Cave on the Nullarbor Plain. His other interests included early Australian Exploration, Medical History and Philately, discovering the first Australian stamp forgery in 1949. His wife passed away in 1970. Eustace Couper Black died on 12th November 1971 and was survived by his three children, Jack, Roger and Molly.

Sources:

Quentin Couper Black, (grandson).

http://www.samuseum.sa.gov.au/collections/information-resources/archives/black-dr-eustace-couper-aa-31

BLACK Geoffrey Howard Barham

MB BS FRACS DOMS

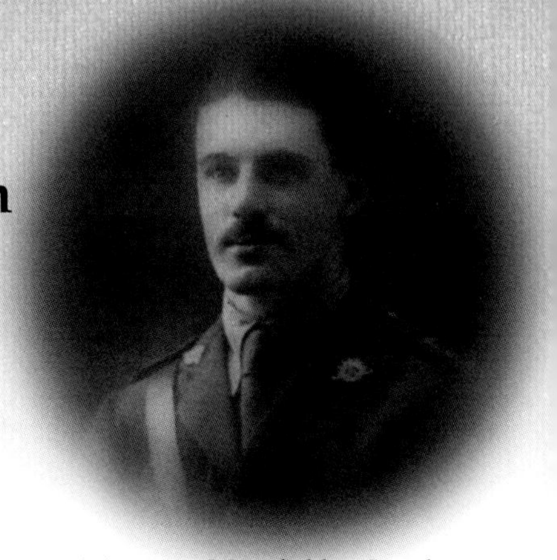

1893 - 1956

Geoffrey Howard Barham Black was born at Burnside on 14th September 1893 son of Alfred Barham Black and Jessie Howard, nee Clark. He was educated at Mrs Hübbe's Private School at Knightsbridge (1900-1904) and, in 1905, went to St Peter's College where he won a University Bursary for Medicine at the University of Adelaide. He graduated MB BS with 2nd Class Honours in 1916. At the University he had been awarded a Rifles shooting Blue, rowed and played cricket. Black with Kyle Gault, Hugh Cairns and Albert Ray Southwood attempted to enlist soon after the outbreak of WW1 but were encouraged to complete their course.

He enlisted as a captain in the AAMC on 8th August 1916. He was single, 23 years old of average build, 175 cm tall and weighed 69 kg and living at 26 Stanley St, North Adelaide. He disembarked in Devonport, England on 28th December 1916 then immediately went to France. There he served with the 1 AGH, 1 Bn, 1 FdAmb, 1 Fd Arty in which he was gassed at Passchendaele on 28th Oct 1917. He was evacuated via the 3 FdAmb and then to 3rd London General Hospital at Wandsworth and returned to Duty on 29th January 1918. He was transferred to 3 AAH Dartford within weeks with "toxic jaundice". After recovery he returned to France now with the 3 FdAmb and 3 AGH. He was posted to AIF HQ London on 4th Nov 1918 and then granted leave and undertook post graduate study as an RMO at Queens' Hospital, Birmingham. After a year's study he embarked for Australia aboard *Nestor* on 1st November 1919. His AIF appointment was terminated on 2nd January 1920. He was issued with the British War and the Victory Medals.

Black continued his medical career on returning home to Adelaide as a specialist with prior General Practice experience. He began at the Adelaide Children's Hospital in 1920 and then to a General Practice in Snowtown, Hindmarsh. Black married Catherine Gilmore Reid at the St Peter's College Chapel on 16th February 1925. He travelled to England to undertake Ophthalmology training at Moorfields, London, and Bristol in 1930-31. He returned to Adelaide and started a Specialist Ophthalmological Practice at 206 Nth Terrace, Adelaide from 1932. At the same time continued with honorary appointments at the Adelaide Hospital, the Adelaide Children's Hospital and the Queen's Home until 1953. He was also a contributor to the connection of rubella and congenital ocular defects in the newborn. Black continued to serve in the Inter War Service Militia from 10th January 1927; promoted to Major 1st October 1934. He also served in WW2 as DADMS and CO 3 FdAmb and promoted lieutenant colonel on the Reserve of Officers from 2nd March 1942. It is a family understanding that his command of the 3 FdAmb was terminated as he was deemed unfit to go overseas following his WW1 gassing. He was replaced by Lieutenant Colonel Stannus Gunning. It was a bitter blow to Black, exacerbated by the subsequent receipt of a white feather in the mail. Black would then wear his uniform at every opportunity even when consulting to show that he had not shirked his responsibility. The family lived at 25 Northgate St, Unley Park. He played tennis until his death, was a good bridge player and a superb inventive furniture craftsman. Geoffrey Howard Barham Black died in Adelaide on 13th January 1956, survived by his wife; two daughters, Elizabeth and Nancy, sons James (Barry) and twins Andrew and Robert.

Sources:
Photo; SRSA GRG2G/5/4, Packet 2400
AWM/NAA barcodes 3086872 WW1 and S213049 WW2,
Personal correspondence from GPCAPT RBB Black (son).
MJA 1943, 2:201, 1944, 1:409, and 1946, 2:889.

BLACKBURN Sir Charles Bickerton

KCMG OBE MD BA FRCP FRACP

1874 - 1972

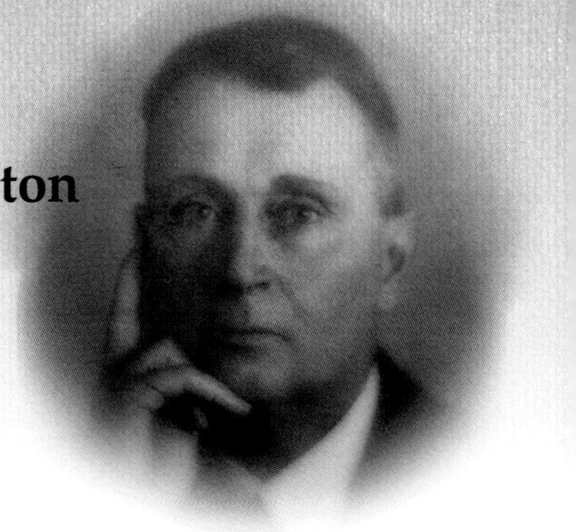

Charles Bickerton Blackburn was born at Greenhithe Kent, the second son of Rev. Thomas Blackburn. Charles was seven years old when his father moved to Hawaii as the Acting Anglican Dean of Honolulu (1881-1882). A year later Thomas Blackburn moved to South Australia and became an Anglican Priest in Port Lincoln. Blackburn's mother died in 1885 and his father later remarried. One of Charles' half-brothers was Brigadier Arthur Seaforth Blackburn VC, CMG, CBE, ED. His father moved to Adelaide in 1886 where he became Rector of St. Margaret's, Woodville. Blackburn's initial education had been at home but in 1886 he attended St Peter's College, Adelaide and was a prefect in 1890. He was the recipient of the Short Scholarship for classics to the University of Adelaide where he gained his BA degree in 1893. Blackburn went on to study medicine at the University of Adelaide while working three nights a week as librarian at the Woodville Institute for £25 a year. He had to go to Sydney University in 1896 to complete his degree, when he was a successful 3rd year undergraduate, due to the 'Adelaide Hospital Row'. Charles graduated in 1899, top of his class. He obtained his MD 4 years later in 1903. He became the Medical Superintendent within 3 years of graduating at the Royal Prince Alfred Hospital, then became an assistant Physician in 1903 and a Consultant in 1911. He married Vera Louise Le Patourel on 3rd of August 1910 and they had 2 sons.

Blackburn enlisted in the AAMC on the 14th August 1916, in Sydney as a 42 year old, married medical practitioner and named his wife Vera Louise of 12 Macleay St, Potts Point as his next of kin. He was posted to the 14 AGH in Egypt with the rank of lieutenant colonel. During 1918 he was regularly detached to the AIF Headquarters whilst serving with the 14 AGH. He was twice mentioned in despatches by General Allenby and was appointed an OBE in 1919. Blackburn returned to Australia in March 1919 with his appointment terminated on the 2nd June 1919. He was issued with the British War Medal and the Victory Medal with Oak Leaves.

Blackburn remained on the reserve of officers, and in 1924, chaired the Commonwealth Royal Commission on the assessment of war service disabilities. He served as lieutenant colonel in WW2 at the 113th Australian General Hospital, Concord. Blackburn was committed to the University of Sydney. He was elected to its Senate in 1919, lectured part time until 1934 and was Dean of Medicine in 1932-35. He became Deputy Chancellor in 1939 and Chancellor in 1941. He was the founding president of the Royal Australasian College of Physicians and was appointed KCMG in 1960. Outside the university and his profession Blackburn served on the council of the Australian Red Cross Society. He took great pride in his vegetable and flower growing, and was a keen beach and trout fisherman and weekend golfer until his nineties and still liked to win. Charles Bickerton Blackburn died on 20th July 1972 at the age of 98 years. He was survived by one of his sons, Charles Ruthven Bickerton Blackburn.

Sources:

Photo: RPAH Museum and Archives, as Medical Superintendent.
http://recordsearch.naa.gov.au/NameSearch/Interface/ItemDetail.aspx?Barcode=3088003
C. R. B. Blackburn, 'Blackburn, Sir Charles Bickerton (1874–1972)', Australian Dictionary of Biography, National Centre of Biography, Australian National University, http://adb.anu.edu.au/biography/blackburn-sir-charles-bickerton-5257/text8859.

BOLLEN Christopher

MD (Toronto)

1866 - 1952

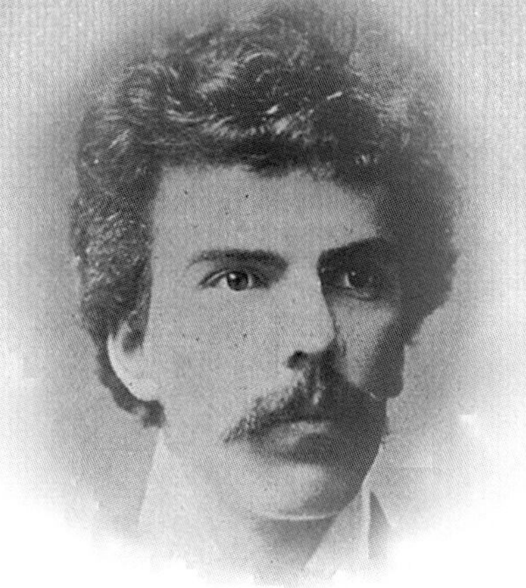

Christopher Bollen was born at Mt Barker on the 29th July 1866, son of Dr George Bollen and his wife Rebecca, nee Steer who were married in Brighton, Sussex in 1847. George Bollen, a cooper by trade, immigrated to South Australia in 1854; he developed an interest in medicine, and in 1872 went to Chicago Illinois to obtain a medical diploma. Dr. George Bollen was the health officer for City of Port Adelaide, appointed in 1898 and for several years chairman of the Institute Library Committee. He became a well-known doctor in SA, with a particular commitment to homeopathy, and was Mayor of Adelaide in 1882. Christopher Bollen was educated at Prince Alfred College and, in May 1888, graduated as MB at Toronto University, Canada. He then returned to Adelaide. Three years later he gained doctorates of medicine at Toronto and the University of Adelaide in 1894. Christopher Bollen set up practice in Fitzroy Terrace, Prospect and was appointed Health Officer for the Port Adelaide Municipality in 1905.

He applied for a Commission in the AIF on the 16th July 1915 at Adelaide. He had previous experience in the AAMC and with a commission in the Commonwealth Military Forces in 1909. He 49 years old, 5ft 10ins, 9st 4lbs, with his wife Helen of Woodville, named as his next of kin. He was posted as a major to the 8 FdAmb as OC, C Coy. Throughout 1916 he was overseas in attachments in Egypt and France with the 15 and 8 FdAmb, and temporary command of the 4th Division Sanitary Section. He returned to Australia in December and his appointment terminated on the 8th February 1917 at the rank of lieutenant colonel. He was issued with the 1914-15 Star, the British War Medal and the Victory Medal.

Bollen practised continuously as physician and surgeon in the Port Adelaide and Woodville districts for more than 64 years. It is said that he was the first doctor in South Australia to drive a car. At the age of 81, he was involved in a minor car crash, which perhaps convinced him that he should give up driving. During his last 30 years he also consulted at his rooms on North Terrace. Always a quiet and retiring man, Bollen had few interests outside his profession. He lived at 8 Fitzroy Terrace, Prospect. He maintained that medicine was his hobby as well as his calling, and consulted until within 10 days of his death. Christopher Bollen died on the 12th September 1952 at the age of 86 and reported to be the oldest practicing physician in Australia at the time. He was survived by his second wife and two daughters, Mrs Alec Bagot and Miss Helen Bollen. Two of Bollen's brothers were doctors, Dr Frederick Bollen, who became a Fellow of the Royal College of Surgeons, and Dr Percival Bollen whose son Dr Kenneth Willoughby Bollen also served in WW1.

Sources:

http://recordsearch.naa.gov.au/scripts/Imagine.asp?B=3096413.
Likeman R. "'No Time for Regret: Doctors of the Western Front, In Press, Rosenberg Press, 2013.
NLA
Local History; City of Port Adelaide Enfield
Photo, Pt Adelaide, about 1902

BOLLEN Kenneth Willoughby

MB BS

1896 - 1972

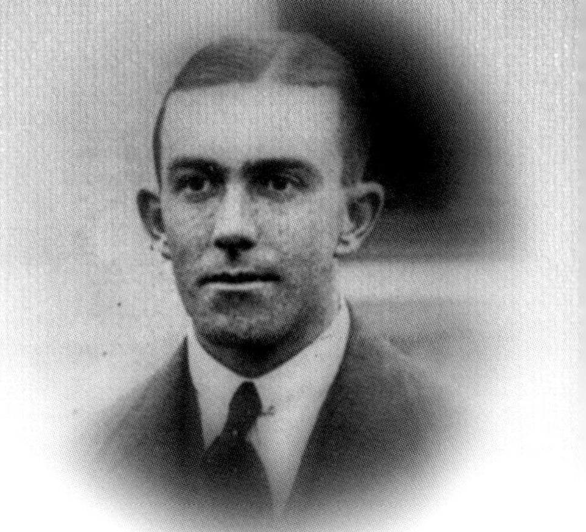

Kenneth Willoughby Bollen was born on the 26th February 1896, son of Dr Percival and Elizabeth Ellen, nee Willoughby of Semaphore. He was educated at Prince Alfred College and studied medicine at the University of Adelaide graduating in 1918. He attempted to enlist in the AIF whilst he was a final year student in June 1918. He had previous experience for four years as a Senior Cadet. He was found fit but was not called up for duty and advised to complete his studies that year but was maintained at B Company Mitcham AIF Camp until the 18th November when he was discharged. He graduated on the 26th November 1918.

After graduation, Bollen reapplied for enlistment. He was 22 years old, single, 5ft 9ins tall, weighed 145lbs, of fair complexion brown eyes, brown hair with several scars. He embarked at Port Adelaide on the 14th January 1919 on the HMAT *Boonah* for England with a few hours notice and disembarked at Tilbury on the 28th March 1919. He was then attached for duty with the Parkhouse extension on the 3rd April 1919. He marched out to Lewes Detention Barracks on 16th July 1919. He was informed that he could not be released from duty until the Detention Barracks were closed. He also performed duty at 1st ADH, Belford from 1st May -16th July 1919. Bollen's records state that he completed 1 year 152 days in the AIF. His discharge was post-dated in February 1920 to be 28th April 1920 so that he could undertake a post graduate course in America. He provided evidence of letters from Dr Thomas S Cullen, Senior Gynaecologist of John Hopkins Hospital, Baltimore to support his request.

Bollen practised for many years in Semaphore after the war and certainly until the 1950s. He married Kathleen Maime Beaver on the 27th January 1926. He was well known and respected in that area. His rooms were on the north side of Semaphore Rd. and he used the Wolverton Hospital (later Le Fevre Hospital). Kenneth Willoughby Bollen died on the 30th May 1972. He was survived by his wife.

Sources:
The Boonah Tragedy Ian Darroch. ISBN 0 86445 169 5.
NAA barcode: 3098543
Photo: 1918 Class Adelaide University Series/Report no.: 1151196
The Adelaide Advertiser 12 December 1913
Ancestry.com

The Medical Contingents

The first contingent after many delays, sailed from Western Australia – twenty-five troopships were required to convey the Australian divisions and the New Zealand contingents. Accompanying them are many of the best of the medical profession, and many of them have sunk their rank in order to be allowed to serve. The veteran of the Sudan and Boer wars, Surgeon General WDC Williams CB, Colonel Charles Ryan of Plevna fame…have gone, also Major JW Barrett CMG and a host of others. Sir Alexander MacCormick is in England. From this State [South Australia] we have sent or are sending Lieutenant Colonel Ramsay Smith (the City Coroner) who has been appointed to the charge of a base hospital of over 500 beds; Professor Watson, who goes as consulting surgeon, Majors Powell, Simpson-Newland, Jermyn, Corbin, TG Wilson, Major Goldsmith (who served in Montenegro two years ago), Captains Le Messurier, JS Verco, Cavenagh-Mainwaring, Pitcher, Meikle, Nott, Jeffries, Fry (ex-Rhodes Scholar), and Bells [Betts]. Altogether two months ago it was announced that 200 medical men were leaving Australia, as well as 3000 of other ranks in the medical service, and 100 nursing sisters. Major Strangman has gone to the "tropics," possibly New Guinea, with a contingent from South Australia.

BMJ, 16th January 1915, p. 137

BRITTEN JONES Sir Edmund

MA (Oxon) MB BS FRCP FRACP

1888 - 1953

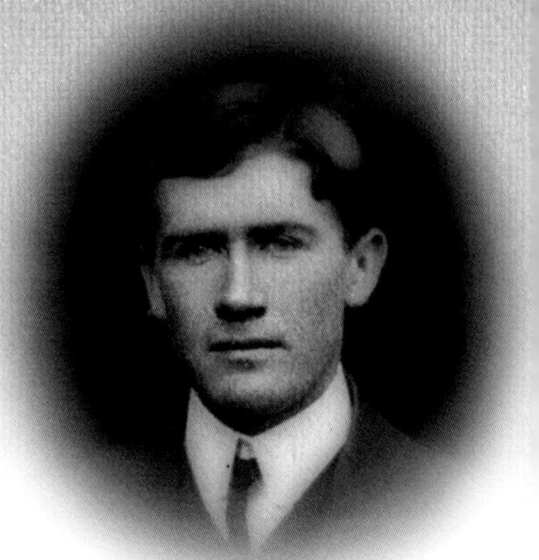

Edmund (Teddy) Britten Jones was born in Adelaide, the son of Edward Britten Jones, the South Australian Government Valuator, and his wife Mary. He was educated initially at St Dominic's Priory in North Adelaide and, from 1899-1905, at Christian Brothers College in Adelaide. He excelled academically and at most sports. He studied medicine at the University of Adelaide and graduated in 1910 at the top of the class winning the Everard Scholarship. At the university he played tennis, cricket and competed in athletics; he was awarded a Blue for cricket. He also played league football for North Adelaide. He was the South Australian Rhodes Scholar in 1912 and, at Magdalen College, was awarded First class honours in Physiology.

Britten Jones joined the RAMC in 1914 shortly after the outbreak of the war. He was to serve in the RAMC for the next 6 years. Much of this service was in India where he rose to the rank of lieutenant colonel. He married Hilda, daughter of Francis Fisher, an Adelaide barrister, in Bombay, India in 1915. They moved to Bangalore where in 1918 their son Richard was born.

He returned to South Australia in 1920. Initially he entered practice in Penola SA (where his daughter Peggie was born) before moving to general practice in Henley Beach (where his daughter Jocelyn was born). He lived at 343 Seaview Road and the consulting rooms, which were attached to the house, were entered from Marlborough Street. He was the doctor at Estcourt House, Tennyson, which was supported by the James Brown Memorial Trust. Estcourt House accommodated blind and other disabled adults and children with joint tuberculosis. He was responsible, from 1921, for the long term convalescence of children with rheumatic fever. He travelled to England in 1926 and took the MRCP and was awarded the MA (Oxon). He returned to South Australia and was appointed Honorary Physician for Children at the Queen Victoria Hospital in 1927 and Honorary Physician at the Adelaide Children's Hospital in 1929. He was president of the SA Branch BMA 1927-1929 having previously been the honorary medical secretary. He was a private doctor to His Excellency the Governor of South Australia and a doctor on call for the Archbishop Room at Calvary Hospital in North Adelaide. Britten Jones re-joined the Army in WW2 and served as a lieutenant colonel in Kantara in the Middle East as Officer Commanding Medical of 2/2 AGH and was Mentioned in Despatches. Britten Jones and Hilda were enthusiastic sports persons and greatly enjoyed their membership of the Royal Adelaide Golf Club. He also was a keen enthusiast for horseracing and, in time, owned his own racing horses; sadly to report only moderately successful. He was knighted for service to Medicine in 1953 and received his knighthood from the young Queen Elizabeth 11 at Buckingham Palace in the Coronation Year. Later that year he died at his home in North Adelaide just short of his 65th birthday.

Sources

Cassidy, R., (2007) "Sir Edmund Britten Jones MBBS (Adel) MA (Oxon) MRCP FRACP FRCP"
Henley & Grange Historical Society Journal 28
Photo; Adelaide University Archives. 1910 graduates

BROADBENT Eric Elihu

MB BS

1893 - 1971

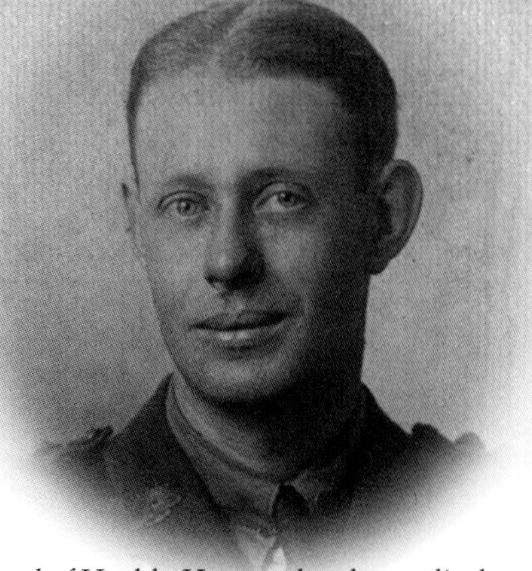

Eric Elihu Broadbent was born on the 13th June 1893 at Burnside son of Elihu Broadbent and Eliza Jane, nee Thorn. He was educated at Adelaide High School and studied medicine at the University of Adelaide graduating in 1917. He married Dorothy Mary Windle, at Peterborough, on the 12th October 1917.

Broadbent volunteered for the AIF after graduation and enlisted on the 3rd December 1917. He was 24 years old, with no previous military experience. He was described as 5ft 10ins tall, 154lbs, and he could ride. His wife, of 34 Gloucester Street, Prospect, was named as his next of kin. He sailed on the *Nestor* on 28th February 1918 after a month's service at the 7AGH Keswick for General Duties. After general training in England he proceeded to France on the 15th August 1918 to Le Havre and Rouen at the 1st AGH. After a minor hospitalisation with dysentery he returned to duty to the 1st and 3rd Australian Div. 9 FdAmb with the 33 Bn and returned to England April 1919. He returned to Australia at the end of hostilities with his appointment terminated on the 13th September 1919. He was issued with the British War Medal and the Victory Medal.

Broadbent moved to Bordertown after discharge and was in general practice there until 1939. He took an interest in jersey cattle and was the Officer of Health to the Local Board of Health. He was also the medical officer at the Tatiara Hospital, and President of the RSL branch. He was instrumental in the building of the local War Memorial Hospital at Bordertown, and clerk of scales at the Bordertown Racing Club. At a farewell to Broadbent and his wife by 300 of the local people he, *...was presented with a roll-top oak desk, a veneer occasional table, and a cheque. Miss Erica Broadbent was given a fountain pen and pencil. Mrs. Broadbent was previously bidden farewell by the Methodist and Anglican churches and croquet club. Dr. and Mrs. Broadbent will live at Crafers (S.A.) before they leave for England for a holiday.* He later became the first registrar at the 105 Australian Military Hospital, Daw Park, which after 1947 become Repatriation General Hospital, Daw Park. Eric Elihu Broadbent died on the 28th April 1971 and was survived by his wife who died on the 12th March 1979. A daughter, Erica Dorothy, died in a car accident in Hong Kong in the early 1950s.

Sources:
http://recordsearch.naa.gov.au/scripts/Imagine.asp?B=3125697
NLA
Photo PAC collection.
Likeman R. No Time for Regrets: Australian Doctors of the Western Front, in press, Rosenberg Press 2013

The AAMC

For many months responsible and irresponsible critics have raised their voices to point out the defects of the Australian Army Medical Corps. The critics have emphasised what appeared to them to be the wastage of energy, the wrong application of material and the want of prominence given to the functions in which they were most interested. The authorities have apparently not been moved by the vapouring's of these malcontents....without exception these young men had proved themselves to be "extremely good and capable, not only at their professional work, but by their adaptability and by their willingness to go wherever ordered without demur." In the early stages of the war there were admittedly defects in the organization in the Australian Army Medical Corps directly traceable to unsuitable material...We may therefore assume that we have the very best material for the machine in these young men, who have completed their studies rapidly in order to do their duty to their country.

MJA, 25th November 1916, p. 455

BROWN Edgar Jabez

MB BS (Melb) FRACS DPH (Cantab)

1875 - 1964

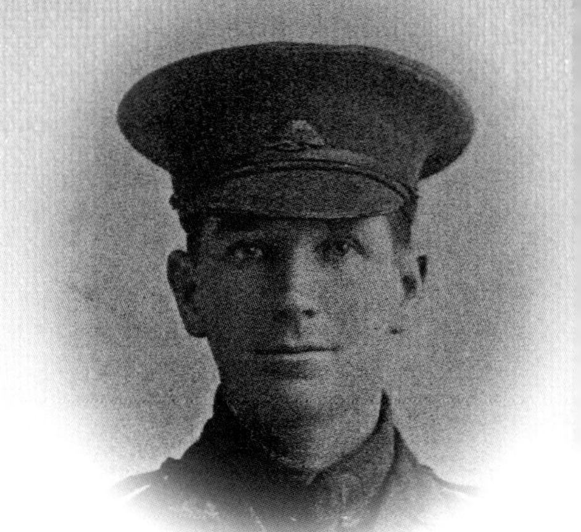

Edgar Jabez Brown was born on the 5th May 1875 at Mintaro, South Australia. The thirteenth of fifteen children, he was born to early pioneer settlers James Brown and his wife Sophia Jane, nee Torr. Brown was educated at Stanley Grammar School, Watervale, Prince Alfred and Way Colleges in Adelaide and at the Melbourne University. He enrolled in medicine in 1897, graduating in 1902. He travelled to England in 1907 where he completed his Diploma of Public Health at Cambridge University. Brown worked at the Great Northern Hospital, Moorfields Royal London Ophthalmic Hospital, and Southampton Free Eye Hospital and completed extensive training in massage. He also studied in Vienna. He commenced practice as an Eye, Ear, Nose, and Throat surgeon in Adelaide on his return to Australia in 1910. He was appointed Deputy Chairman of the Adelaide Hospital Board, and an Official Visitor to the Parkside Mental Hospital, and for a short time Temporary Deputy Inspector General of Hospitals. He married a young widow, Annie Louise Anderson in 1915. She was born at Strathalbyn in 1877, daughter of Sir John Gordon, politician and judge. She is better known as Louise Brown the novelist (1877-1955). They lived at 212 Brougham Place, North Adelaide.

Brown was commissioned in the AAMC as a major in October 1915. He was 40 years old, an ophthalmologist and married; his postal address was 3 North Terrace, Adelaide. He was 5ft 10ins, 12 stone, with near normal vision. He sailed from Adelaide for the Middle East later in the month with reinforcements for 1 AGH. During the months he spent in Cairo he consulted both at Heliopolis and Luna Park. Brown went to France with the hospital in March 1916. During the winter he developed severe sinusitis and was evacuated to 3 LGH in December 1916. He was discharged in January 1917 and sent to 3 AGH which was at that time still in Brighton, Sussex. He was transferred to 3 AAH in March, as 3 AGH was now packing up for its move to Abbeville in the Somme area of France. Brown re-joined 1 AGH at Rouen in May 1917, and served until December when a medical board recommended his return to Australia. He was however allowed to remain in England, and was posted to 1 AAH in December 1917. He was promoted temporary lieutenant colonel in November 1918 and in January 1919 attached to AIF HQ in London. He returned to Australia in May 1919 to the 4 MD with his appointment terminated on the 18th August 1919 due to the "Cessation of Hostilities" He was issued with the 1914-15 Star, the British War Medal and the Victory Medal

Brown resumed his practice at 172 North Terrace Adelaide. His appointments included the following:- Senior Surgeon and Consulting Surgeon, Nose and Throat Department, Adelaide Children's Hospital, Assistant Surgeon, Nose and Throat Department, Adelaide Hospital. Occasionally he joined his peers in a game of golf at Mount Osmond and Kooyonga Golf Clubs. He bred bulldogs in his spare time, some winning awards. He also participated as a 'ring steward' for the South Australian Bulldog Club and there was The Dr Edgar Brown Trophy. Brown travelled widely in Europe and the Far East. He and his wife were prominent members of the social scene in Adelaide. Edgar Jabez Brown died on the 10th November in 1964 and was buried alongside his wife, who predeceased him, at the North Road Cemetery, Nailsworth, South Australia. Dr William Jethro Brown (1868-1930), Professor of Law at Adelaide University from 1906-16, was his older brother.

Sources:
http://recordsearch.naa.gov.au/scripts/Imagine.asp?B=1795757
NLA,
The Argus Melbourne 25 Dec 1897
The Argus Melbourne 12 Dec 1955
Likeman R., From Tropics to the Desert, Slouch Hat Publications Port Melbourne 2012.
Photo: Family collection
Family personal interview.

BROWN Gilbert

CBE MB ChB FFARACS DA OStJ

1883 - 1960

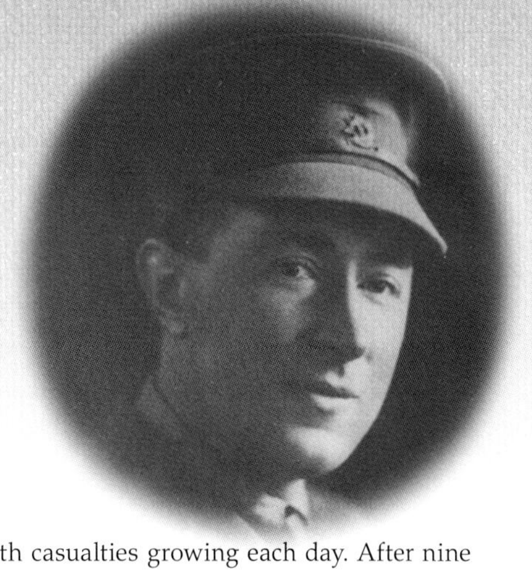

Gilbert Brown was born in Wigan, Lancashire England on 14th August 1883. He graduated with MB ChB, University of Liverpool, in 1908. This was followed by terms as a House Surgeon and Physician at the Royal Infirmary, Liverpool, House Surgeon at the Hospital for Women and SMO at the Children's Infirmary, Liverpool. He migrated to Australia in 1912, first joining a practice as surgeon to the medical group at Snowtown. He married Dr Marie Simpson, a medical graduate from London University, in 1914. They lived at 31 Watson Ave, Rose Park. When war broke out in 1914 he continued with the General Practice whilst all other members of the practice enlisted and by 1918 he was able to enlist.

Brown enlisted in the AIF on 15th July 1918. He was described as 5ft 10ins weighed 185lbs, chest 34-40ins, of fair complexion with brown eyes and brown hair. He could ride, spoke some French and had 4 years previous service with the voluntary engineers. He was recommended for general duties on 11th September 1918 and sailed in HMAT *Boonah* from Port Adelaide on 22nd October 1918 bound for the England via Fremantle and South Africa; she was the last Australian troop ship to leave Australia in WW1. Carrying about 1200 AIF soldiers, she arrived in Durban, South Africa just three days after the armistice was signed and on hearing the news, made arrangements to return home promptly. Before her departure however, local stevedores from the Spanish 'flu stricken city of Durban were used to load and unload supplies from the ship and in the course of doing so infected soldiers who were billeted in crowded conditions throughout the ship. By the time the ship had arrived back at Fremantle on 12th December, more than 300 cases had been reported and Commonwealth immigration authorities initially refused to allow the soldiers to disembark. Meanwhile, on board ship, where most of the men remained, conditions were said to be deplorable. Public outrage grew against the refusal of the immigration authorities to allow all of the soldiers ashore with casualties growing each day. After nine days of acrimony, and despite breaking quarantine regulations, the ship was ordered to depart for Adelaide, presumably to defuse the situation, and the sick disembarked at the Quarantine Station just north of Adelaide. No further deaths occurred and the remaining men returned home. A total of twenty-seven soldiers and four nurses at Woodman Point, Western Australia died of influenza during the crisis. His appointment was terminated in September 1919.

On return to Adelaide Brown and his wife moved to Walkerville Terrace, Gilberton where they both practised. Brown was a pioneer of modern anaesthesia in Australia with appointments at Adelaide Children's Hospital, the Adelaide Hospital and the Repatriation Hospital when it was at Keswick. From the beginning of this career he kept records of all the anaesthetics that he had undertaken with comments on the procedures. All his records were bound in annual volumes and have been retained. His influence of the progress of anaesthesia in South Australia was profound. He was the first president of the Australian Society of Anaesthetists (ASA). His wife Marie died on 21st November 1949. He was appointed CBE in 1953 and also Officer Brother of the Venerable Order of St John of Jerusalem. Gilbert Brown died on 6th January 1960 and was survived by his son Ian.

The Gilbert Brown Award, by the ASA and Gilbert Brown Prize by the Australian and New Zealand College of Anaesthetists are given annually in his memory.

Sources:

Photo; Brown Family collection; SLV
Darroch I., 'The Boonah Tragedy', ISBN 0 86445
http://recordsearch.naa.gov.au/scripts/Imagine.asp?B=1797126;
Gwen Wilson Fifty Years, ASA 1934-1984,
Hughes J E, A History of the Royal Adelaide Hospital 1967
http://www.austehc.unimelb.edu.au/guides/brow/provlist.htm

BROWNE John Walter

MB BCh BA

1873 - 1948

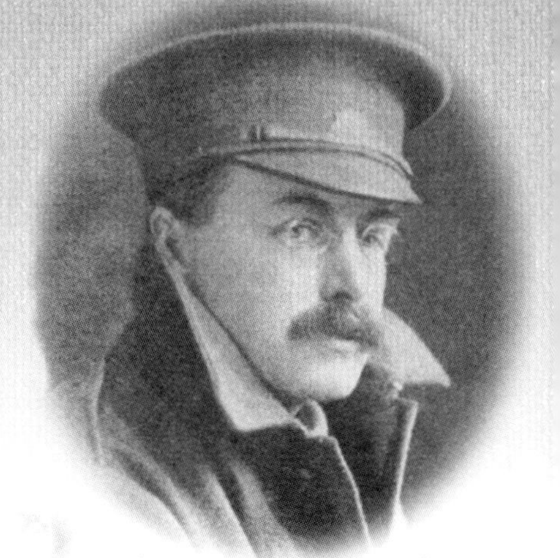

John Walter Browne was born on the 7th June 1873. He was educated in Belfast and completed his residency at Nottingham Children's Hospital and the Royal Victoria Hospital, Bournemouth. He then immigrated to Australia, and, on the 6th April 1904, married Melicent Dove, the daughter of Archdeacon Dove at St Andrews Church, Walkerville SA. However he did not register as a medical practitioner in SA until 1905. Browne developed a special interest in chest diseases, and became Medical Superintendent of the Kalyra Sanatorium at Belair in the Mt Lofty Ranges; the first sanatorium to be established in South Australia. He was appointed later an assistant physician in infectious diseases at the Adelaide Hospital. He was commissioned in the AMF in November 1913 and posted as RMO of 78th INF Regt (Adelaide Rifles).

Browne volunteered for the AIF in October 1915 and was granted the rank of major. He was 42 years old, 5ft 8ins tall, just over 10st in weight, eye sight corrected from 6/60 to 6/6 with glasses. He could ride and had a fair knowledge of French. His wife was named as his next of kin and they lived in Hutt Street, Adelaide. He was classified as a senior specialist in diseases of the chest for hospital duty. Browne embarked for the Middle East in November 1915 with 2 ACCS, and went on to France with the unit in April 1916. Following short attachments to 1 AGH and 2 FdAmb he was formally posted to 1 AGH in Rouen in September 1916. He returned to Australia in October 1917 on duty as Ship Staff and in November he was "Struck off Strength", but continued to serve with Home Forces until July 1918. He was issued with the 1914-15 Star, the British War Medal and the Victory Medal.

Browne's expertise in the treatment of tuberculosis was recognised and he became an Honorary Clinician, TB Clinic at the Adelaide Hospital, and he had rooms at 8 North Terrace, Adelaide. Throughout the 1920s and 1930s the names of Dr and Mrs J Walter Brown appear frequently in the Adelaide press in the company of prominent couples at social functions at Government House and Society Balls. Their son, Georges, was at Cambridge University in 1928 as an Arts undergraduate in the company with other undergraduates from South Australia including the sons of Steele Scott, Bonython, Parsons, Downer, Hawker and Birks. John Walter Browne died on 13th November 1948; he had lived at 2 South Esplanade, Somerton SA. He was survived by his wife Melicent and his son.

Sources:

http://recordsearch.naa.gov.au/scripts/Imagine.asp?B=3131325
NLA.
Likeman R., From the Tropics to the Desert, Slouch Hat Publications 2012
The Adelaide Advertiser 15 Dec 1908
The Adelaide Advertiser 20 Dec 1913
Photo, 1920-22;

The Profession

Meanwhile it would naturally be thought that those who for various reasons were unable to go the front would be reaping a rich harvest whilst the ranks of the profession are so depleted. Curiously enough, this does not seem to have been the case. Ever since August work has been slack. But the cause of this does not seem to be so much the war as the drought [in South Australia] from which we have suffered, and which at the time of writing seems to have broken up.

BMJ, 3rd July 1915, p. 32

BROWNELL Herbert Percival

DSO MB BS (Melb)

1889 - 1937

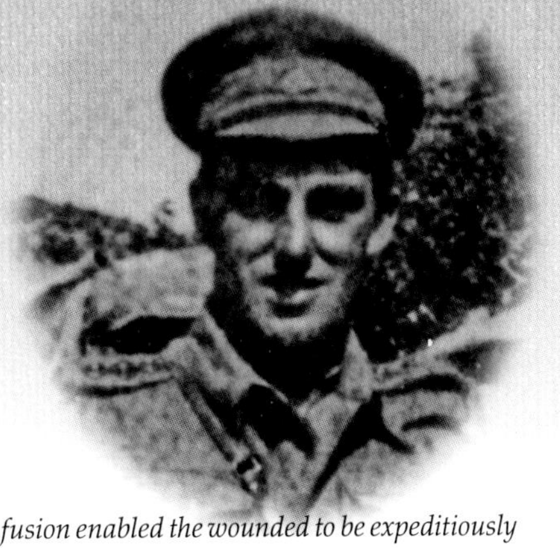

Herbert Percival Brownell (Val) was born on the 12th November 1889 in Hobart, Tasmania where his father William was a draper. He was the eldest of three boys and two girls. William Brownell (1862-1916) was a member of the Tasmanian Parliament from 1903-09. Brownell was educated in Hobart and at Scotch College, Melbourne where he served in the Senior Cadets and for two years in the Infantry Militia while a student. He studied medicine at Melbourne University and graduated in 1915.

Brownell first enlisted in the AIF on 22nd March 1915. He was 5ft 6ins and weighed 12st. His father of Newtown, Tasmania was named as his next of kin. He was commissioned as a Captain and posted to B Section, 7 FdAmb. He embarked from Sydney on the *Clan McEwan* and went with his unit to Gallipoli in September He was injured with a gunshot wound to the chest on 4th November 1915 but was returned to duty 8 days later. The Unit returned to Egypt then to France in March 1916. In May he was posted to 27 Bn then on to the Somme in July. He was promoted to major in April 1917. Brownell was twice recommended for the Military Cross. The first was for his actions at Messines when under heavy fire he attended wounded men, spending two hours in a difficult position preventing Lieutenant HB Walker bleeding to death. This was followed on 4th-6th August at Pozières, when he worked for 30 hours attending to wounded under shell fire. Nevertheless the award of MC was not made. The Bn took part in the attack on Malt Trench in March and in May in the Second Battle of Bullecourt. Brownell was again recommended for the MC but was awarded a DSO on 2nd June 1917. The citation read: *For conspicuous gallantry and devotion to duty whilst attending to the wounded under heavy fire. His coolness in organising matters amidst the greatest confusion enabled the wounded to be expeditiously treated, and he personally treated some hundreds of cases under heavy shell fire.* He also was Mentioned in Despatches. Brownell was posted back to 7 FdAmb in July 1917; in October 1917 he returned to Australia for 'family reasons'. These reasons are not specified in his records, but seem to have included marrying Mary Salier Ferguson, which he did on the 7th September 1918. He did not return to active service. His appointment was terminated in Australia on the 31st March 1918 and he then re-enlisted on the 3rd July 1918. His wife was then named as his next of kin and her address given as Kensington Gardens, South Australia. He again had his appointment terminated on the 5th February 1919. He was issued with the 1914-1915 Star, the British War medal and the Victory Medal with Oak Leaves.

Back in Australia Val Brownell worked first at Broken Hill, then as a GP at Norwood, and finally on North Terrace in Adelaide. He was involved with the SA Branch of the BMA, Legacy, "Toc H", Horsemanship and Yachting. It was said that his outstanding traits were his courage both moral and physical. He inspired affection as well as respect. He was Commanding Officer of 3 FdAmb from 1926-27 and A/Director of Hygiene of 4 MD from 1927-30. He was Commanding Officer of 6 FdAmb from 1930-35. Herbert Percival Brownell died on the 26th April 1937, survived by his widow and three sons.

Sources:

http://recordsearch.naa.gov.au/scripts/Imagine.asp?B=3131862; Photo, AWM P00046.035.

Likeman R., Gallipoli Doctors: Slouch Hat Publications Melbourne Aust. 2010.

MJA: June 19th 1937, p. 973

BROWNING Denby de Courcey

MB BS (Melb)

1884 - 1942

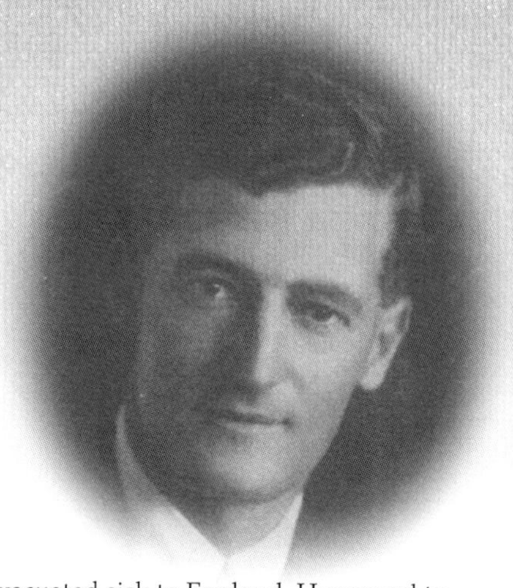

Denby de Courcey (Den) Browning was born on the 28th June 1884 in Carlton, Victoria, the son of William Browning and his wife Elizabeth Alice, nee Hutchinson. He was educated at Carlton College and Queen's College, where he won a Blue for football. He studied medicine at Melbourne University and graduated in 1911. After graduation he moved to South Australia and entered general practice at Ardrossan. The Ardrossan Vigilance Committee, on the 16th May 1913, met and discussed the necessity for a cottage hospital. They eventually secured the services of Browning who was elected to the first Board of Management for the hospital, which was completed on 31st May 1914 and was opened for business by Browning. The first nursing sister was Miss Edie Burt. When Browning enlisted for the War he left the Hospital unattended. His sister Alice was furious as she had left Melbourne to housekeep for him. However she met and married W H Cane whose father, C G R Cane, was a prominent member of the local council and also instrumental in the building of the new Hospital. Browning was also a member of the Ardrossan Cricket Club and made 84 in a game against Balaklava (the Preston Cricket Club) on the 22nd January 1915.

Browning was commissioned on the 26th March 1915, and posted to 4 LHFA. He was 30 years old, single, with previous experience in the Junior Cadets. He was 6ft, 161lbs, 35-38ins chest with normal vision. He embarked from Adelaide on board HMAT *Borda* on the 23rd June 1915. He embarked with Samuel Roy Burston and Walter John Westcott Close. When the unit was disbanded in Egypt, Browning was first posted to 2 AGH, then in March 1916 to 46 Bn as RMO. He served with the Bn in France until September when he was posted to 12 FdAmb. He also had a short attachment to 4 FdAmb, but in December 1916 he was evacuated sick to England. He proved to have pulmonary tuberculosis, and after a few months at 3 AAH at Dartford he was returned to Australia in September 1917 into the 4 MD. Whilst at the AAH he was promoted to Major to date from 27th April 1917. His appointment was terminated on the 9th October 1917. He was issued with the 1914-1915 Star, the British War Medal and the Victory Medal.

He resumed his practice at Ardrossan where another doctor had arrived and, in 1918, moved to Maitland on the Yorke Peninsula, later to Blackwood and then North Terrace, Adelaide. His wife was from Sydney and the family moved to Burwood, NSW in the height of the depression in 1929, where his wife Elizabeth died on the 6th April 1936 leaving him a widower with two children. He re-married on the 10th July 1937 at St. Jude's, Randwick to Constance Geraldine Saunders, of Adelaide. Browning became an honorary physician at the Western Suburbs Hospital in Sydney. Denby de Courcey Browning died on the 20th December 1942 when he was living at 27 Belmore Street, Burwood. Newspaper tributes were posted from the wide family and the members of the Burwood Bowling Club. He was survived by his wife Constance Geraldine Browning and children Thomas Oakley (1920-98) and Elizabeth. During WW2 Dr Thomas Oakley Browning was a Sgt in the 2/18 Bn, and a Prisoner of War in Changi Prison and an eminent scientist at the Waite Institute, Adelaide.

Sources:

NLA Trove, Ardrossan Museum,

Personal notes from Niece, Barbara Parsons, Ocean Grove, Victoria.

Photo, Ardrossan Community Hospital Inc.

http://recordsearch.naa.gov.au/scripts/Imagine.asp?B=3131960

BRUMMITT Elliott Arthur
MB ChB (Edin)

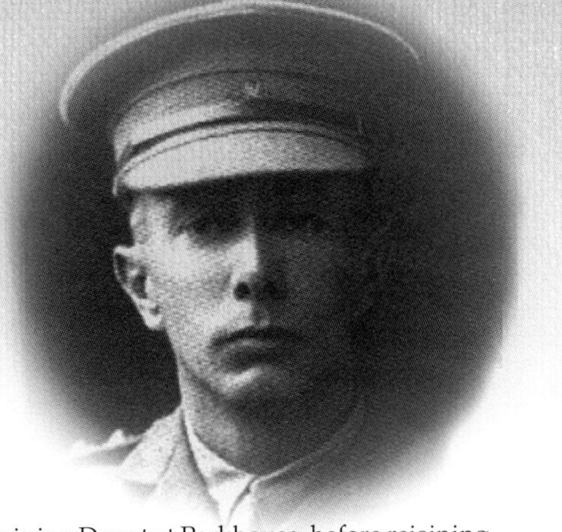

1880 - 1934

Elliott Arthur Brummitt was born on the 9th April 1880 at Burra, South Australia. He was the eldest son of Dr Robert Brummitt who had immigrated to South Australia 1877 and Jane, nee Roach, daughter of a local mill owner. He had a very happy and unconstrained boyhood; one day, he, with another boy, Essington Lewis, the future industrialist and wartime director of munitions, offered him 5s 3d to accompany him on their ponies while they drove a herd of cattle 20 miles in the blazing sun. He was educated at Prince Alfred College where he was in the first eighteen for 3 years and excelled as a gymnast. He studied medicine at the University of Adelaide where he had difficulty getting past the first 2 years. Family lore maintains that there was some animosity between Brummitt's father and Professor Archibald Watson so after these failures Brummitt was sent to United Kingdom where he graduated from Edinburgh University in 1908. After training in Scotland, he commenced work at the Adelaide Children's Hospital in 1909 and joined his father in his practice in Medindie, Gilberton and North Adelaide.

Brummitt enlisted in the AIF on 4th May 1915 He was 36 years old, single, and his mother of Medindie, Adelaide was named as his next of kin. He was 5ft 8ins, 10st 10lbs. He embarked from Melbourne on the 17th June 1915 for Egypt with the reinforcements for the 1 AGH. He was transferred on arrival to 1 Division Reserve Park as RMO, and joined them on Lemnos on the 3rd August 1915. Back in Egypt in 1916 he was posted to the Div Train of the newly raised 5th Div, but after a month was transferred to the *Karoola* which was returning to Australia. On arrival in Adelaide he was retained on the staff of 4 MD at the request of DGMS. This was a compassionate posting as his father had suffered a stroke. He managed to re-embark in December 1916, and spent 4 months at the AAMC Training Depot at Parkhouse, before rejoining 1 AGH at Rouen in August 1917, with promotion to major. He was posted in September to 11 FdAmb and remained with them until the end of the war. He was twice Mentioned in Despatches, and recommended for an OBE; *he has earned the respect of all owing to his single-minded and efficient care of the sick and wounded soldiers. He has been on occasions ready to sacrifice himself for the patient.* However, he was not appointed. Brummitt returned to Australia in January 1919 as SMO on the *Berrima* with his appointment terminated on the 13th April 1919 from the 4 MD. Brummitt was issued with the 1914-15 Star, the British War Medal and the Victory Medal with Oak Leaves.

He was physically intact and mentally well, after his return to Adelaide, although he never went to Church again. He resumed work at his father's practice with extensive consulting and maternity work load, beginning with 15-20 house calls per day. At the age of 49 years, when he appeared to be a confirmed bachelor, he met 33 year old Bertha (Bon) Kay, daughter of Mr and Mrs RH Kay of Marryatville, SA. They were married in January 1930 and had two sons Robert and Peter. Elliott Arthur Brummitt died, within a week of getting an infected finger, of septicaemia on 5th June 1934 when he was 54 years old. He was survived by his wife and two sons.

Sources:
http://recordsearch.naa.gov.au/scripts/Imagine.asp?B=3132864
Likeman R., "Gallipoli Doctors', Slouch Hat Publications Melbourne Australia 2010.
Personal letter from son Dr Robert Brummitt of Adelaide.
Photo: PAC Collection

† BURDEN Clive Britten

MB BS

1891 - 1917

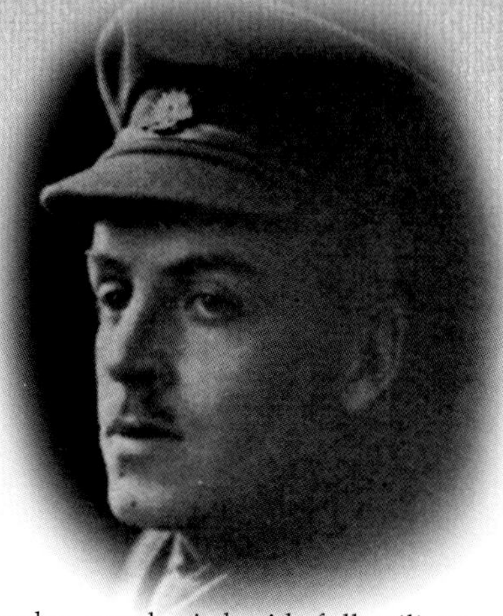

Clive Britten Burden was the son of John B Burden of 'Beaumaris' at Henley Beach the founding pharmacist of Burden the Chemist with Pharmacies at 48 King William Street and at Henley Beach. Clive was a nephew of Dr Frank Burden, of the Esplanade at Henley Beach, who had been a missionary in China. The celebrated South Australian philanthropist Sir Charles Goode was Burden's great uncle. He was educated at Prince Alfred College and studied medicine at the University of Adelaide where he was one of several medical graduates whose course had been accelerated at the University in 1916

Burden joined the AAMC on 7th July 1916 at which time he was 6' tall and weighed 13 stone 6lbs. He embarked overseas on 23rd October 1916 on the transport *Port Melbourne* arriving in Devonport on the 28th December 1916. After spending some time in camp at Salisbury Plain he was taken on strength of 1 AGH on the 15th January 1917 in France. From this he went to a Divisional Field Ambulance under Major Kenneth Fry, with whom he spent a month in the trenches. He contracted measles, and was invalided to England to 3rd London General Hospital, Wandsworth, with a pyrexia of unknown origin on the 29th April 1917. While still weak from this illness, he was on day leave on the platform of the underground near Victoria Station where he fainted and fell before an incoming train. He was taken to St George's Hospital, Hyde Park Corner where he underwent amputation of both legs and his left arm. He died at 4.15pm on the 8th May 1917. A coronial enquiry returned a verdict of accidental death. His own disappointment at this unfortunate closing of a career which he embarked upon with great enthusiasm is expressed in his own comment, *"Is it not rotten luck that, after being for months in France, this silly thing should happen to me? I fainted and fell, because I felt weak and ill."*

Clive Britten Burden was buried with full military honours at Brookwood Cemetery. A service, prior to the interment, by Chaplain A. White of AIF Headquarters in London was held in the chapel at the cemetery. The Firing Party, band and mourners were from the 3rd (Reserve) Bn, The London Regiment stationed at Blackdown, Farnborough. The polished oak coffin was draped with the Australian Flag and covered with several lovely floral tributes. The coffin was borne to the graveside by members of the AIF Headquarters staff and four of his brother officers; these were Major Verco and Captains Steele, Haste and Craig. Colonel Hayward, CO 1 AAH Harefield was also present as were Captain Burden's relatives; Sir Charles Goode (great Uncle), Mrs Swinstead (aunt), Miss Swinstead (cousin) both from London and Miss ED Proud (cousin) of Blackwood in South Australia. Burden's grave in Brookwood Cemetery is located in the Australian Military Burial Ground and is grave number 179247. The photograph of the grave was transmitted to the family in Adelaide and provided great comfort to Mrs Burden who was widowed in 1922. Burden's family received his medals which comprised the British War Medal and Victory Medal.

Sources:
http://recordsearch.naa.gov.au/scripts/Imagine.asp?B=3166929
PAC Chronicle No. 119 of August 1917,
Photo from the PAC collection

BURNARD Renfrey Gershom

MB BS MRCP MRACP

1882 - 1971

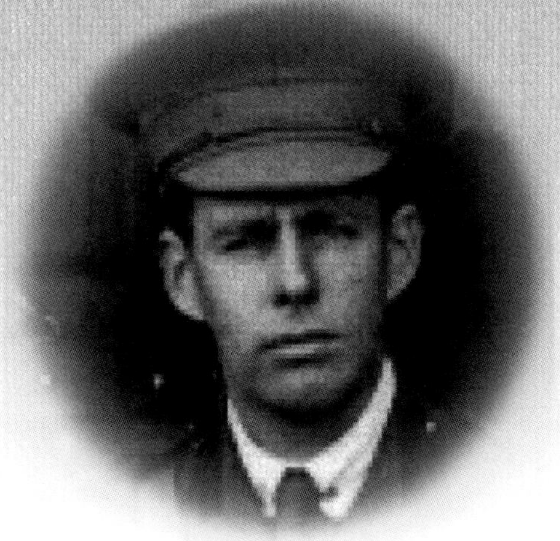

Renfrey Gershom Burnard was born in Unley, South Australia on 23rd July 1882. He was the son of a schoolmaster Richard Thomas Burnard and his wife Alice Hardy, nee Hanton. He was educated at Prince Alfred College and studied medicine at the University of Adelaide, graduating in 1904. Whilst still a student Renfrey was called to give evidence to the Court of Enquiry investigating the conduct of Dr Ramsay Smith as City Coroner in 1903. He was appointed the resident pathologist at the Adelaide Hospital in 1906, and then entered general practice at Naracoorte SA. He married Selina Victoria De Garis, from Mount Gambier, at Kent Town, South Australia in 1907. They had four children, three daughters and a son. His younger sister Eulalie was one of the University of Adelaide's first female graduates, and married one of their fellow students, Dean Dawson. Eulalie tragically died in 1907.

Burnard volunteered for the AIF on the 14th August 1916. He was a 34 year old, married medical practitioner of Naracoorte with previous experience in the AAMC Reserve. He sailed from Adelaide in January 1917. He disembarked at Devonport in March 1917, and was sent to France in April. He reported to 2 AGH at Wimereux, with instructions for detachment to the RAMC. However he developed a severe upper respiratory tract infection and was sent back to England to recuperate. He was posted supernumerary to 7 FdAmb in July 1917. He was employed as a relieving RMO within the Division, and he was attached to many units in the next two years. During this time he was involved in saving the life of Private Tom Playford, who was to become the longest serving Premier of South Australia. Burnard became Tom Playford's friend and chess opponent. He was gassed on the 31st October 1917, and sent back to England to convalesce at Cobham Hall. He recommenced his round of attachments in February 1918 which continued until October, at which time he was definitively posted to 1 Sanitary Sect. Burnard returned to England in April 1919, and sailed for Australia the following month with his appointment terminated on the 9th August 1919. Burnard was issued with the British War Medal and the Victory Medal.

Burnard resumed his practice at Naracoorte; in 1929 he moved to a western suburban practice in Adelaide. He also worked as an anaesthetist at the Adelaide Hospital. He wanted to undertake further studies in medicine but was unable to until 1937 after the Depression, when he gained his MRCP. During WW2 he maintained some military duties in the Reserve. He had a good tenor voice and enjoyed singing. He was a keen churchman and very generous to those less fortunate especially during the Depression. Renfrey Gershom Burnard died on 4th September 1971 in Adelaide at the age of 89. He was survived by his four children.

Sources:
http://recordsearch.naa.gov.au/scripts/Imagine.asp?B=3171368
NLA
The Adelaide Advertiser 12 Sept 1903
The Adelaide Advertiser 11 Feb 1905
The Adelaide Advertiser 12 Jan 1906
Burnard R. DeG, RACP College Roll: Burnard, Renfrey Gershom; http://www.mundia.com/au/Person/11823875/-380097672

University of Sydney and the War

... the University of Sydney, dealing with the proposals under consideration by the legislature... with the speeding up of the medical course...and the issuing of degrees...within a shorter period than prescribed, for the purpose of joining the [Australian] Army Medical Service...The Faculty of Medicine has had under careful consideration the suggestion that a preliminary qualification should be granted...and that afterward return to the University to complete their qualifications...

MJA, 7th August 1915, p.136

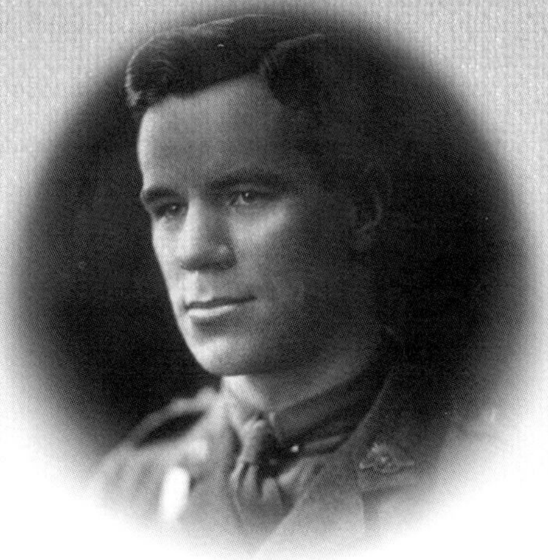

BURNELL Glen Howard

MD FRCS(Ed) FRACS

1890 - 1954

Glen Howard Burnell was born at Grange South Australia, the son of an accountant Arthur Burnell and his wife Sarah Ann, nee Norman. He was educated at Sturt Street Public School, Adelaide High School and studied medicine at the University of Adelaide graduating in 1916. After graduation he completed his residency at Broken Hill Hospital NSW. Burnell had been diagnosed with tuberculosis in 1911, but was declared clear of the disease in 1912.

Burnell enlisted in the AIF 7th September 1917. He was 27 years old, 6ft tall, and weighed 12st 4lbs. His father of East Terrace, Kensington Gardens was named as his next of kin. He was commissioned as a Captain and posted to No 1 Australian Hospital Ship *Karoola* to take immediate effect. He had a small haemoptysis early in 1917, but was again declared clear. Lieutenant Colonel Wilson was informed of the situation, and was prepared to take Burnell as a Transport Officer. However the condition deteriorated again, and Burnell did not embark. He was discharged from the AIF in January 1918 with his AIF service terminated on the 5th February 1918. He was not issued any medals.

After discharge he worked at the Broken Hill Hospital and, in 1920 was Acting Surgeon Superintendent. His MD thesis was on the control of diphtheria. He moved to Queensland and in 1921 became Director of the Anti Hookworm Campaign in Queensland Schools. He then went to Scotland for formal surgical training with FRCS (Ed) in 1929. On his return he was appointed an honorary assistant surgeon at the Adelaide Hospital. He was Vice-President of the South Australian Branch of the BMA from 1935-36. He was also a member of the council of the Institute of Medical and Veterinary Science, of the Medical Board of South Australia, and of the Nurses Board. Mary and Glen Burnell were host to Harry Daly at their home, 88 Hutt Street on January 26th 1950, and there held discussions with Ivan Jose, also visiting Gilbert Brown in Hospital at the time. This led to the formulation for a membership and fellowship by examination, of the Faulty of Anaesthetists RACS. Burnell studied throughout his life and became proficient in Italian. He retired from the Adelaide at the age of 60 years in 1950. It was said that, *"His medical career exemplifies the victory of great mind and strong personality over a succession of severe bodily handicaps".* Glen Howard Burnell died in Adelaide on the 26th August 1954 and cremated in Adelaide. He was survived by his wife Mary. Mary Burnell became the first female, President of the ASA (1953-54), and Dean of the FFARACS (1966). The Burnell-Jose and Postgraduate Medical Foundation Visiting Professorship is named by the South Australian Regional Committee of the College in honour of the late Dr Mary Burnell, and the late Sir Ivan Jose.

Sources:
NAA: 2455, barcode 3171382
The Advertiser Adelaide 22 Dec 1902
The Register Adelaide 11 Dec 1920
The News Adelaide 26 August 1954
Photo: from son Harry Burnell, Medindie
Obituary, BMJ 11 December 1954
Obituary, MJA, November 6th 1954 p.764
http://europepmc.org/articles/PMC2080322/pdf/brmedj03628-0074.pdf
Wilson Gwen, 'Fifty Years, the Australian Society of Anaesthetists', 1934-1984.

BURSTON Sir Samuel Roy

KBE CB KOStJ DSO VD MB BS FRCP(Ed) FRACP

1888 - 1960

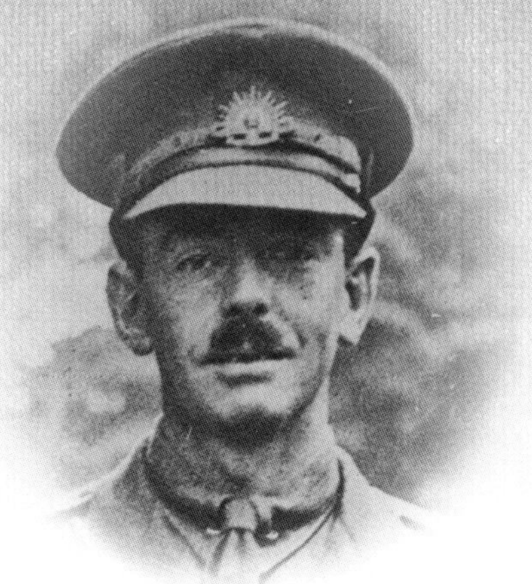

Samuel Roy Burston was born in Melbourne on the 21st March 1888, the fourth of seven children to James Burston, a soldier and businessman who served as Lord Mayor of Melbourne from 1908 to 1910, and his wife Marianne, nee McBean. He graduated from the University of Melbourne MB BS in 1910. After graduation he worked at the Adelaide Children's Hospital in 1911 and in 1912 he served in the Northern Territory as a medical inspector of Aborigines with the Aboriginal Protection Board. He returned to Adelaide where he married Helen Elizabeth Culross on the 16th April 1913 in St Michael's Anglican Church, Mitcham. He took up general practice in Mile End, South Australia. Burston was also at the Adelaide Hospital and the Adelaide Children's Hospital.

Burston enlisted in Adelaide on the 26th March 1915 as a 27 year old and his wife was named as his next of kin. He was 6ft 2ins tall, 12st 7lbs, with previous military service of 5 years as a Bugler in the Victorian Military Forces Militia and 2½ years as Captain AAMC reserve. He could ride a horse and had a speaking knowledge of French. He was appointed Major in 4 LH FdAmb and embarked for Egypt on the 26th June 1915 to join the MEF at Gallipoli on the 4th September 1915. After 6 weeks he was admitted to the ANZAC Hospital with enteric fever, transferred to Egypt and then to England to the 3 Army Hospital for further treatment. After 11 months he resumed duty to France with the 11 FdAmb on the 24th November 1916. He was transferred to be the SMO, Australian General Base Depot and then promoted to lieutenant colonel in October 1917. Further postings were as CO 1 Aust Con Depot, and DDMS, Le Havre in August in 1918. He was Mentioned in Dispatches and, in 1917 awarded the DSO for supervision of an ADS during a prolonged gas attack. After the cease fire in November he became, as temporary colonel, and Assistant DMS, at the AIF Depots, UK. He returned to Australia on duty on the *Orsova* with his wife and 2 children on the 22nd November 1919 with his appointment terminated on the 7th March 1920. He was issued with the 1914-15 Star, the British War Medal and the Victory Medal with Oak leaves. He was appointed CBE in March 1920.

Burston was reappointed to the staff of the Adelaide Children's Hospital and the Adelaide Hospital on returning to Adelaide in 1919; he also began lecturing at the University of Adelaide. He became a Fellow of the Royal College of Physicians of Edinburgh, and then the Royal Australasian College of Physicians in the 1930s. Colonel Burston officially joined the 2nd AIF on the 13th October 1939, as Deputy Director of Medical Services (DDMS); he was promoted to Brigadier, and promoted to Major General on the 16th February 1941. Burston became DGMS at GHQ Australia on the 8th May 1942, which soon became Land Headquarters (LHQ). Burston was appointed KBE in the Military Division in 1952. Burston was involved in thoroughbred racing both as a punter and owner. As Chairman of the Moonee Valley Racing Club oversaw the construction of the Burston Grandstand. Sir Samuel Roy Burston died at his home in South Yarra from a ruptured aortic aneurysm on the 21st August 1960.

Sources:
Photo; Burston in London 1915, from Grandson A. R. Sangster.
http://recordsearch.naa.gov.au/NameSearch/Interface/ItemDetail.aspx?Barcode=6231489
http://www.adb.online.anu.edu.au/biogs/A130354b.htm
MJA Feb 4th 1961; p. 184

CAIRNS Sir Hugh William Bell

KBE DM MD FRCS

1896 - 1952

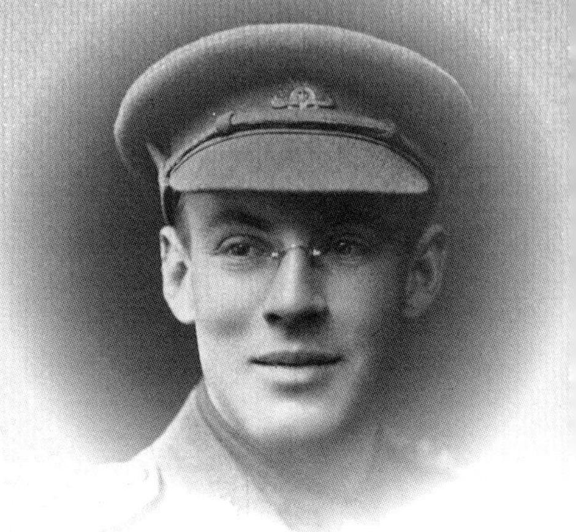

Hugh William Bell Cairns was born on the 26th June 1886 in Port Pirie, South Australia. He was the only son of William Cairns, a Scottish timber contractor, and Amy Florence, nee Bell. He was educated at Riverton High School and Adelaide Boys High School, where he was co-dux with John Besley Gillen, before his tertiary education at the University of Adelaide as an exhibition scholar. He reported that he spoke English and German.

Cairns joined the AIF on 11th May 1915 as a private soldier. He was nearly 19 years old and had already served in the 23rd ALH at Riverton for 11 months. He was 5ft 11ins and weighed 161lbs. He travelled with reinforcements for 3 AGH on HMAT *Mooltan* to the Middle East and joined his unit on Lemnos. He undertook medical orderly and nursing duties. He was promoted to Lance Corporal in September 1915 and, during this time, was admitted with influenza. He returned to Australia to complete his medical training on 13th March 1916 again performing nursing duties on the ship. He graduated from Adelaide University in 1917 as the Davies Thomas and Everard Scholar and South Australian Rhodes Scholar. He re-joined the army in August 1917 and on 9th November 1917 travelled on the *Port Sydney* to England and subsequently France where he served with 2 AGH, 3 AGH, 47th British Division and 15 Fd Amb.

He did not return to Australia following his service in France as he took up his Rhodes scholarship at Balliol College, Oxford in 1919. He rowed bow in the University Boat Race and was President of the Balliol Boat Club. He continued his training in pathology and then surgery at The London Hospital; he obtained the FRCS in 1921 and in this year married Barbara Forster the youngest daughter of AL Smith the Master of Balliol. His initial surgical interests were related to genito-urinary problems and he lectured on these topics at the RCS where he was the Hunterian Professor of anatomy. A growing interest in neurosurgery saw him take leave to study with Cushing in Boston in 1926-7. He returned to establish a neurological surgery unit at The London Hospital and with others established the new school of British neurosurgery. Cairns had an international reputation when TE Lawrence was fatally injured in a motor bike accident in 1935 and he was summoned to treat him. His enthusiasm for neurosurgery was instrumental in encouraging Lord Nuffield to endow the new Nuffield chair in Surgery in Oxford in 1937 to which Cairns moved from London. He rejoined the Army in WW2 rising to the rank of Brigadier; he was advisor to the Ministry of Health on head injuries, and stressed the advantages of early air evacuation of the injured, Cairns established mobile neurosurgical units early in WW2. Nearly 20,000 patients were treated by these units in which Cairns and Florey (Adelaide Rhodes Scholar successor) were amongst the first to use penicillin in neurological injury. Widespread use of penicillin was born. A young RAMC surgeon, Dick Jepson, was in one of these units and later he moved to Adelaide and became the Professor of Surgery at the University of Adelaide and the Adelaide Hospital, 1958-1968. Early in the WW2 Cairns persuaded the army to make crash helmets for dispatch riders compulsory; this, now routine protection for bike riders, is one of Cairns many lasting legacies. He was appointed KBE in 1946 and the next year, when the Sims Commonwealth Professor appointed by the RCS, was awarded an honorary MD (Adelaide). Hugh William Cairns died of cancer in the Radcliffe Infirmary on 18th July 1952 leaving a widow, two sons and two daughters.

Sources:

Williams E. T. 'Cairns, Sir Hugh William Bell (1896–1952)', Australian Dictionary of Biography, National Centre of Biography, Australian National University, http://adb.anu.edu.au/biography/cairns-sir-hugh-william-bell-5464/text9283, accessed 14th December 2013

Photo: SLSA, GRG26_5_4_02328.

Notes from Dr Mary Jepson

† CARR Howard Bevan

Medical Student

1896 - 1917

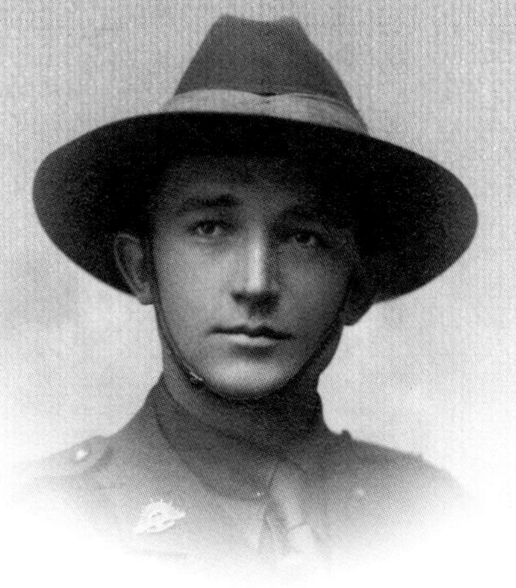

Howard Bevan Carr was born on the 28th July 1896 at Stirling West, Mt Lofty, eldest son of Dr. Hampden Carr and Emmie Bevan, nee Cooper. He was educated at St Peter's College and was believed to have been accepted to study medicine at the University of Adelaide.

Carr enlisted in the AIF at Oaklands Camp Adelaide on the 26th November 1914, just before he started studying at the University of Adelaide. He had 2 years of previous senior cadet training and served 1 year in the "C" Coy 78th Infantry. He was 18 years old, 6ft, and 174lbs, of dark complexion, dark brown hair and brown eyes. His father Dr Hampden Carr of "Roma", 30 Unley Rd, Unley was named as his next of kin. He was provisionally appointed Sergeant in the AAMC Base Depot and was posted in March 1915 entraining to Melbourne to the 1 ASH, 2nd reinforcement in Lemnos in June. He went to the 1 ACCS as a Private. He served in the Lowland CCS and Hospital ships throughout 1916 and in December transferred to Trinity College, Cambridge for Officer training with promotion to 2nd lieutenant in April 1917, then proceeded to France on the 24th April 1917 and taken on strength of the 50 Bn. He was promoted to lieutenant in July.

Howard Bevan Carr was killed in action on the 26th September 1917 near Zonnebecke in Belgium. He was 21 years old. His name is on the Ypres Menin Gate Memorial. His father was issued with his 1914-15 Star, British War Medal and the Victory medal. The Memorial Scroll and King's Message was delivered to his family in August 1921 and the Memorial Plaque in January 1923. His name is also in the St Peter's College Memorial Hall and on the plaque in the cloisters at the entrance to the large quadrangle at St Peter's. His brother Kevin Hampden Carr (1899-1977) was born in Moonta on the 21st January 1899. He served in the Flying Corps in England in WW1 and the RAAF in WW2.

Sources:
http://recordsearch.naa.gov.au/scripts/Imagine.asp?B=3207728
Photo: SLSA, GRG26_5_4_0_24 as a 2/Lieutenant taken in France.
NLA
The Adelaide Advertiser 24th October 1917
The Adelaide Advertiser 16 December 1914

Field Ambulance Work [Abdominal wounds] at ANZAC

By C.Mackie Begg, MD, FRCS, MRCP Ed.

It may be of interest to your readers to have a short note on the special difficulties and dangers which beset field ambulance work...at ANZAC...About fourteen days later, however, on making inquiries at the hospital ships, we found that the results in abdominal wounds were extremely bad...we determined to erect an operating tent on the beach and try treatment ashore unless the conditions for evacuation were very favourable. From this time til June 16th we operated on almost all cases of penetrating abdominal wound, and kept the patients on shore from twenty-four hours to four days afterwards....We found in about 60 per cent of the cases operated on that the condition was almost hopeless, whether the wound was caused by bullet, shrapnel, or shell fragment... Most of these cases died in a short time, but a few of them we sent off to the ship some days later in a surprisingly good condition. About 25 per cent of cases gave good hope of a favourable result...The conclusions we draw from our experience of abdominal wounds are:

Early operation if conditions are favourable and the operator is experienced in abdominal surgery. By early operation is meant any time up to six hours.

Rest at the place of operation for three or four days afterwards.

BMJ, 4th December 1915, p. 806

CATCHLOVE Sydney George Leyland

MS MB FRACS

1884 - 1968

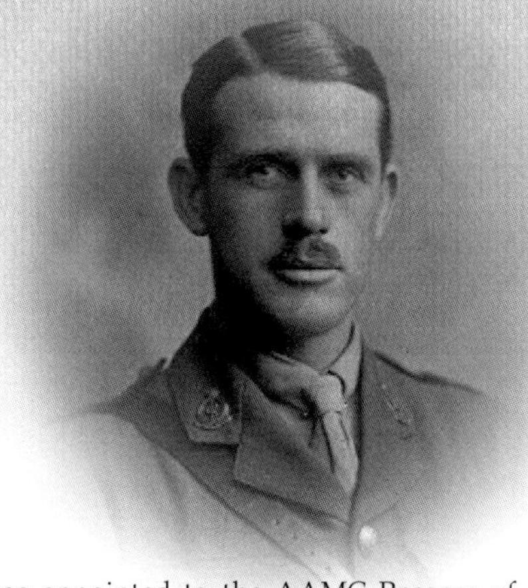

Sydney George Leyland Catchlove was born in Liverpool, England on 31st May 1884, the son of George Catchlove and Margaret, nee Leyland, both from Cheshire, England. They came to Adelaide and lived at Gover Street, North Adelaide. Catchlove attended Prince Alfred College and played football for the school. He went to the University of Adelaide achieving his MB BS in 1907. He also represented the Adelaide University at football. Following his graduation he was appointed as a Resident Medical Officer at the Adelaide Hospital. He married Una Heywood Cox and a notice in the Adelaide Register recorded that they had a daughter in Sydney in May 1913.

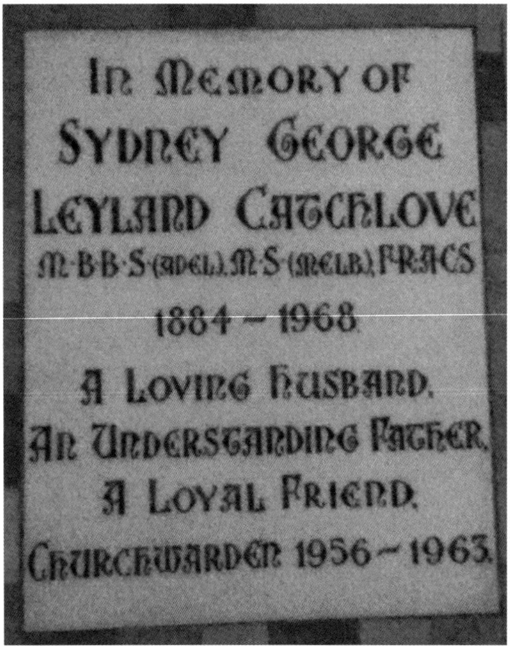

Catchlove was appointed to the AAMC Reserve of Officers on 1st July 1914, prior to WW1 as a Captain in the 2 MD in New South Wales. He was appointed to the AIF on the 8 July 1915, but this appointment was terminated on the 7 January 1916. It was recorded that he should not have been placed in the AIF. In England he was deployed in Australian Auxiliary Hospitals. He also served for some months on the staff of the Australian Head Quarters in London. He returned to Australia in November 1915 as the medical officer on the transport ship *Runic.* On return to Australia it was recommended that he transfer to the AAMC CMF in the 3 MD in Victoria. He was promoted to temporary major in August 1916 and appointed to 5 AGH. In June 1918 he became CO of 5 AGH and appointed lieutenant colonel. He was placed on the Reserve of Officers in 1921. He was issued with the British War Medal and although he requested the 1914-15 Star and Victory Medal, was told that he was not entitled to them as he did not serve in the AIF.

In 1938 Catchlove resided in Ellwood, Victoria and lived from 1947 in Collins Street, Melbourne, Victoria and was a surgeon at Prince Henry's Hospital until 1955. Sydney Leyland Catchlove died in Melbourne, Victoria on the 7th August 1968.

Sources:

http://recordsearch.naa.gov.au/NameSearch/Interface/ItemDetail.aspx?Barcode=3219530
NLA
The Adelaide Advertiser 17 Jan 1908
The Register Adelaide 28 May 1913
http://www.wikitree.com/wiki/Catchlove-21
Photo: Family and PAC Collection

CAVENAGH-MAINWARING
Wentworth Rowland
MB BS FRCS

1869 - 1933

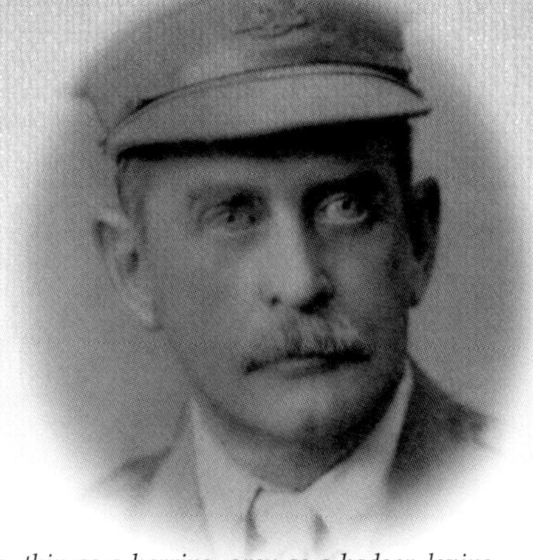

Wentworth Rowland Cavenagh-Mainwaring was born in Marryatville, South Australia, the son of the South Australian cabinet minister Wentworth Cavenagh and Ellen, nee Mainwaring. When Ellen inherited the estate of Whitmore Hall, Staffordshire in 1891, after the death of her brother, Cavenagh-Mainwaring's father added his wife's family name to his and was then known as Cavenagh-Mainwaring. Whitmore Hall remains in the family today. Cavenagh-Mainwaring was educated at St Peter's College and studied medicine at the University of Adelaide graduating in 1892. He proceeded overseas to gain surgical experience at The London Hospital and take the FRCS. He returned to Adelaide to be appointed Honorary Assistant Surgeon at the Adelaide Hospital in 1900. He taught anatomy at the University of Adelaide during the long absences of Prof Watson and was the first to fill the post of lecturer in pathology; for eight years he was the lecturer in surgery. His ability and knowledge was recognized by his colleagues who sought his advice and assistance. He served as the Honorary Medical Secretary of the SA branch of the BMA and of the Medical Defence Association.

Cavenagh-Mainwaring at the age of 45 years, on the 20th August 1914, and with no previous military experience, enlisted in the AIF. He was commissioned as captain in the AAMC and 3rd Australian Light Horse He was 5'10" tall and weighed 12st 2lbs. He served in a number of units in the Middle East. He served at Gallipoli from 9th May until September 1915 when he was evacuated to Malta with enteritis. He returned to the Gallipoli Peninsular later in October to re-join the 3 LH. John Corbin describes Cavenagh-Mainwaring at Gallipoli *"I could tell you many amusing stories of the soldiers and details of Cavenagh-Mainwaring, thin as a herring, grey as a badger, loving his work, doing it fearlessly and conscientiously, and loved by his men".* His heroic disregard of his own life and health won the love and admiration of the 3rd Light Horse. He was promoted Major in November 1916. Whilst in the Anzac Mtd Div in the Middle East under Major General Harry Chauvel, he was decorated with the White Eagle of Serbia (Third Class) and later with the White Eagle of Serbia (Fifth Class) with crossed swords. He was Mentioned in Despatches during action in the Clearing Stations in the First and Second Battles of Gaza in March and April 1917. He did a return trip to Australia in February 1918 as MO Transport Ship. He finally returned to Australia in 1919 with his appointment terminated on the 5th September 1919. He was issued with the 1914-15 Star, the British War Medal and the Victory Medal with Oak Leaves.

He was promoted to an Honorary Surgeon at the Adelaide Hospital in 1919 and continued there until his death. Wentworth Rowland Cavenagh-Mainwaring died from a bleeding peptic ulcer in 1933. He is described as entering life with great intellectual gifts, of a marvellous memory and a capacity for thinking clearly and of making sound judgements; he was a most loveable friend, cheerful, kind and gentle. His straight eye made games and shooting easy for him. He never married.

Sources:

Smeaton B., (1933) MJA 361 Obituary "Wentworth Rowland Mainwaring"

Photo: Christine Cavenagh-Mainwaring.

Likeman R., "Gallipoli Doctors" Slouch Hat Publications 2010

South Australian Chronicle 17th December 1892

Corbin J., 'Experiences with the AAMC at Gallipoli', MJA 5 Feb 1916, p. 111-114

CAW Alexander Ruan

MB BS

1879 - 1924

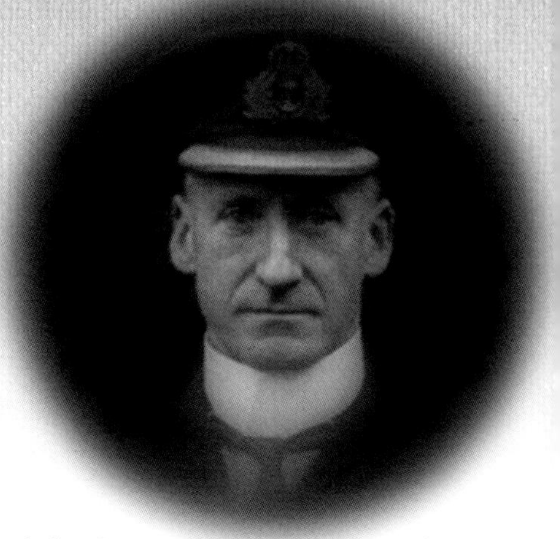

Alexander Ruan Caw was born on the 24th April 1879, the eldest son of W B Caw Huyton, Lancashire, England. He came to South Australia with his parents, a brother (Alfred Beech) and sister (Mary Olive). His father was a librarian at the Adelaide Circulating Library from 1884-1908. He was educated at St Peter's College and excelled academically and at the annual school sports in bicycle riding in 1897. He studied medicine at the University of Adelaide, and graduated MB BS in 1902. Caw was in the SA Junior Lacrosse Team to play NSW in 1901. He was in a medical practice with Dr McMillan in Naracoorte from 1906-1910. He returned to England in 1908 for further studies which included ship hygiene. Caw continued his position in Naracoorte on his return to Australia and, in March 1910, moved to Burra with new wife, Kathleen, to relieve Dr J L Sangster Jnr. who was moving to Glenelg. After the untimely death of his wife, aged 25 years, and son in childbirth at Kooringa, Burra in 1911, he passed his GP position to Dr David Steele from Adelaide. At his farewell he had said that he *always had a leaning towards the Navy, having for many years being in the Naval Reserves.*

Caw applied for a Staff Surgeon appointment for 3 years on the 1st August 1912. He served in *HMAS Australia*, and was on her delivery voyage from the UK and sailed on her from the 21st June 1913 until the 30th September 1919, with a promotion to Fleet Surgeon Commander on 1st August 1917. The AN&MEF was formed following a request by the British government on the 6th August 1914. *HMAS Australia* became the flagship of the AN&MEF that captured the German colonies in the southern Pacific. The force was assembled under the guidance of Colonel J G Legge, and was separate from the AIF forming under Major General W T Bridges. HMAS *Australia* led a force which captured Rabaul on 13th September 1914 before proceeding to Samoa. With no German forces left in the South Pacific, HMAS *Australia* was deployed to the United Kingdom. En route she sank the German auxiliary ship *Eleanore Woermann. HMAS Australia* became flagship of the 2nd Battle-cruiser Squadron of the Royal Navy's Grand Fleet on 8th February 1915. HMAS *Australia's* service with the Grand Fleet consisted of a series of frequent patrols and exercises. Caw was issued with the 1914-15 star, the British War Medal and the Victory Medal.

Caw married Lily Hewart daughter of South African surgeon Sir John Hewart in 1918. He resigned from his position in the Navy and his resignation was accepted. He was posted to HMAS *Penguin* for 3 months with his transfer to the Retired List on the 21st December 1919. He went to Johannesburg and entered medical practice as a Specialist ENT Surgeon in 1920. His decision to move to South Africa may have been influenced by his wife and father-in-law or by his year with Surgeon Lieutenant R W Hornabrook who was in HMAS *Australia* from August 1914 to August 1915, also of Adelaide, and who had served with the RAMC in the Boer War. Alexander Ruan Caw died on the 11th March 1924 six weeks after the death of his mother on 25th January 1924. He was survived by his wife Lily and two children.

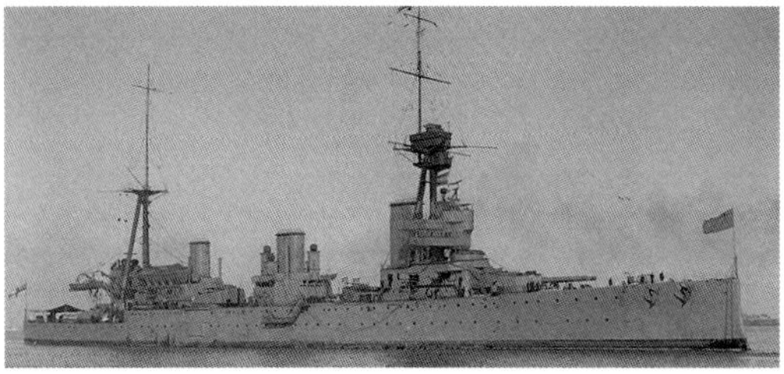

Sources:
NLA
Photo AWM EN0003,
HMAS *Australia*. The Burra History Group
St Marys Anglican Church, Burra http://catalogue.slv.vic.gov.au
The Register, Adelaide on the 26th March 1924,

CHAMPION de CRESPIGNY
Sir Constantine Trent
DSO VD MD FRCP FRACP

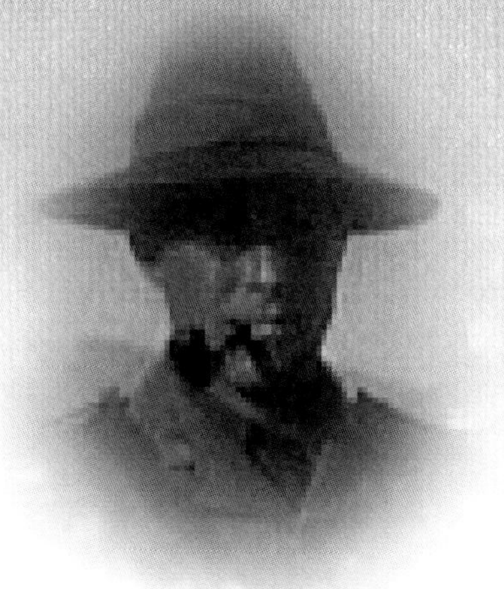

1882 - 1952

Constantine Trent Champion de Crespigny was born on 5 March 1882 at Queenscliff, Victoria, second son of Philip Champion de Crespigny and his first wife Annie Frances, née Chauncy. Champion de Crespigny was educated at Brighton Grammar School and Trinity College, University of Melbourne (MB 1903; BS 1904; MD 1906). He was a resident MO in Melbourne hospitals, from 1904 to 1907 then Glenthompson and married his first wife Beatrice in 1906. He was appointed to the Adelaide Hospital in 1909 and specialised in pathology. He ultimately became Honorary Director of the hospital's pathology services in 1912 and a lecturer in pathology in the University of Adelaide's medical school. He began a specialist physician practice at Gonville Chambers, 12 North Terrace and took residence at 132 Strangways Terrace, North Adelaide with his wife Beatrice.

Champion de Crespigny was commissioned in the AAMC in 1907. He was described as 36 years old and married. He joined the AIF in May 1915 as a lieutenant-colonel and was posted to 3 AGH which was based on the island of Lemnos during the Gallipoli campaign. He was promoted to temporary colonel on the 5th March 1917 and posted to command 1 AGH at Rouen, France. After becoming sick in August 1917 he returned to Australia from England in November 1917. He was appointed colonel on 18th September 1917 and returned to England and in 1918 become consulting physician at A.I.F. headquarters in London. He completed his MRCP in 1919 and returned to Adelaide. He was Mentioned in Despatches July 1916 during the period of General Sir Charles Munro's command of the Mediterranean Expeditionary Force. He was awarded the DSO in June 1917 for distinguished and gallant services. He was issued with the 1914-15 Star, the British War Medal and the Victory Medal with Oak Leaves.

Champion de Crespigny became an honorary physician at the Adelaide and the Adelaide Children's hospitals following WW1. He became FRCP in 1929 and was one of the senior Australian physicians involved in founding the Royal Australasian College of Physicians, of which he was president in 1942 to 1944. Champion de Crespigny was president of the South Australian branch of the British Medical Association in 1925-26. He was awarded the VD in 1927. He presided over the medical section of the Australasian Medical Congress in Sydney in 1929. He was knighted in 1941 and became known as Sir Trent. Four years later he visited the United States of America where he inquired into medical postgraduate education, especially as it affected medical officers returned from WW2. He had four children, two sons and two daughters with his first wife, Beatrice, who died in 1943. He remarried in 1945 to Mary Jolley and they had a daughter Charlotte. Sir Constantine Trent Champion De Crespigny died at his home in Stirling South Australia on 27 October 1952, survived by his second wife and his five children.

Remember

FEVER FOLLOWS FLIES;
FLIES FOLLOW FILTH
FILTH FOSTERS FEVER

J. R. Kaye, Lieut.Col.
Div. san. Officer WR Div. TF

BMJ, 19th September 1914, p. 517

Sources:
Charlotte de Crespigny, personal papers and photo.
Hackett Earle, Champion de Crespigny, Sir Constantine Trent (1882–1952), http://and.anu.edu.au/biography/champion
National Archives Australia
http://recordsearch.naa.gov.au/NameSearch/Interface/ItemDetail.aspx?Barcode=3230201

CHAPPLE Frederick

MB BS BSc

1871 - 1948

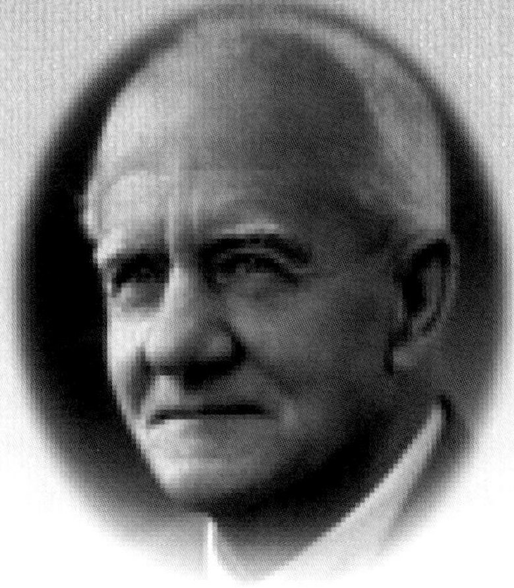

Frederick Chapple was born in England on 2nd February 1871. He came to Australia with his parents when his father was appointed Head Master of Prince Alfred College in Adelaide. Chapple was educated there and was awarded several scholarships; the Colton Scholarship in 1887, the Robb Scholarship in 1888, the Old Scholars Scholarship in 1888 and in 1889 he was awarded a University Scholarship to attend the Adelaide University where he completed his BSc. He continued on to study medicine and was one of the students who had to complete his degree at Melbourne University because of the Adelaide Hospital Row. He became the Superintendent of Rockhampton Hospital in Queensland on completion of his medical degree until 1905. He returned to Adelaide to become the Superintendent of the Adelaide Hospital and then took up a general practice at Nairne and Clarendon.

At the outbreak of WW1 he applied for military service overseas but was refused on account of his age of 43 years. He served throughout the war at the Hospital at Keswick Barracks. After the war he went into a general practice at Parkside where he remained until he had a serious accident in 1945 from which he never completely recovered. Frederick Chapple died on 22nd January 1948.

Sources:

Medical Journal of Australia, April 10, 1948, p. 483-484.
Photo: RAH Heritage Office

Need of the Army More Medical Men

Alfred Keogh
Director General Army Medical Services
War Office, Whitehall March 10th

Sir,–I should be glad if you would allow me to explain through your columns our position with regard to the employment of medical men for the army. It is briefly as follows:

1. The need of medical men, both for home and Foreign Service, is acute. We want every qualified man who is physically fit and willing to serve.
2. We are in special need of general practitioners, and would be glad to take on expert surgeons, ophthalmologists, radiographers, etc.
3. We would give suitable men immediate employment.
4. At present we are not, except in special cases, sending men of over 40 years of age overseas, but we should gladly take on older men for home service.
5. We do not wish to denude the country of civil practitioners, but every man who can arrange for his work to be done at home should come forward if we are to keep up an adequate supply of medical attendance to our armies in the field,

BMJ, 13th March 1915, p. 488

CHAPPLE Harold

MCh BSc FRCS FRCOG

1881 - 1945

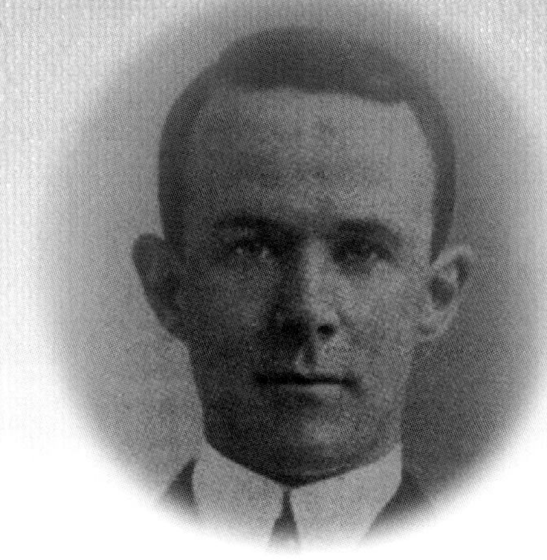

Harold Chapple was born in Adelaide on 13th February 1881. He was the seventh child and third son of Frederic Chapple and Elizabeth Sarah, nee Hunter and the younger brother of Phoebe Chapple. His father was Headmaster of Prince Alfred College and Chapple was educated there and then undertook a BSc at the University of Adelaide. He studied medicine at Cambridge, England and remained there for the rest of his life. He was prominent in tennis, rugby, swimming and acting. He began his clinical work at Guy's Hospital, London in 1905. He married Irene Briscoe Arbuthnot Lane, the daughter of Sir William Arbuthnot Lane, a noted surgeon at Guy's. Chapple then became an assistant in the obstetric department of the Charite-Krankenhaus, Berlin, and subsequently appointed obstetric registrar at Guy's.

Chapple joined the RAMC as a captain for the duration of WW1. After the war he returned to Guy's Hospital where he became a senior obstetrician and gynaecologist. He remained at Guy's Hospital all of his life. Harold Chapple died on 8th March 1945. He was survived by his wife Irene and two sons.

Sources:

Obituary, British Medical Journal, March 24 1945, page 425/6.
http://livesonline.rcseng.ac.uk/biogs/E003966b.htm

The Call to Arms [Australia]

On the twenty-ninth day of September His Excellency the Governor-General and Commander-in-Chief of the Commonwealth of Australia, by proclamation, called upon all male inhabitants of Australia who were then or thereafter became liable for service in the Citizen Forces, being then or thereafter of the age of twenty-one years and upwards, but under the age of thirty-five years, and unmarried or widowers without children, to enlist, and he further called upon every person referred to in the proclamation, unless exempted from service under any regulations made under the Defence Act. 1903-1915, and the War Precautions Act, 1914-1916, to render continuous military service within the limits of the Commonwealth and any territory forming part of the Commonwealth during the continuance of the present war....The attention of members of the medical profession may be directed to certain regulations dealing with certificates for exemption...

MJA, 7th October 1916, p. 297

The Empire has the right to demand of its citizens the service necessary to expedite victory. Individual interests cannot count; the honour and safety of the nation are at stake... The members of the medical profession have not shrunk from their duty under the voluntary scheme, and we feel convinced that they will now support the proposals of the Prime Minister and thus uphold the honour of Australia... Under these circumstances the Director-General has made provision for the future. He asks every member of the medical profession to enrol himself voluntarily at once. Those who do so will be given commissions in the Australian Army Medical Corps, and, in the event of a proclamation being issued calling up the classes to which they belong, they will be exempted from ordinary military duty. The object of this... is to enable the military authorities to make a wise decision, so that, while the necessary number of suitable men may be detailed for duty with the Army Medical Corps, the needs of the civil population may not be disturbed more than is unavoidable.

MJA, 14th October 1916, p. 321

CHAPPLE Phoebe

MM MB BS BSc

1879 - 1967

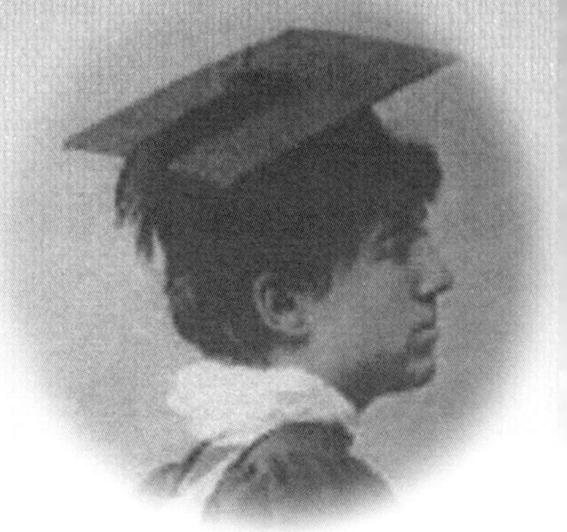

Phoebe Chapple was born on 31st March 1879 in Adelaide, the youngest daughter of Frederic Chapple and Elizabeth Sarah, nee Hunter. She was a confident and tall young woman and was educated at the Advanced School for Girls in Grote Street, Adelaide. Her father was Headmaster of Prince Alfred College and this family background enabled Phoebe to have an exceptional education. She was admitted to the University of Adelaide at the age of 16 and completed a Bachelor of Science in 1898 and her MB BS in 1904. She became a house surgeon at the Adelaide Hospital in 1905. She was appointed as the resident medical officer for the Sydney Medical Mission in 1906. However she soon returned to Adelaide where she had a practice at Prince Alfred College until 1914. Due to her interest in women's issues she became a committee member of the South Australian Refuge for Women in 1912 and in 1914 became Honorary Medical Superintendent of McBride's Maternity Hospital for unmarried mothers.

Chapple attempted to join the AAMC with the advent of World War One, but the Army refused to appoint women doctors for overseas duties. So she left Adelaide in February 1917 and joined the war effort from England. She still was not granted military status as a doctor and was attached to the Royal Army Medical Corps as surgeon at Cambridge Hospital in Aldershot. Later she was appointed to the Queen Mary's Army Auxiliary Corps and went to Abbeville, France in November 1917, and then in Rouen and Le Havre. She was accorded the honorary rank of Captain and was one of the first women to be sent to the front. She was inspecting the women's camps on the night of 29th May 1918 and sheltered from bombing in the trenches with 40 other women. They suffered a direct hit and nine of the women were killed and several others injured. She was awarded the Military Medal for her *'gallantry and devotion to duty during an enemy air raid. While the raid was in progress Doctor Chapple attended to the needs of the wounded regardless of her own safety'*. She was recommended for the Military Cross but this could not be awarded as it could only be awarded to commissioned military officers. She was originally recommended for an MBE but the Military Medal was decided upon as this could only be won in the field.

Chapple returned to Adelaide in 1919 and took up a practice on North Terrace. That year she decided to enter politics and stood for election in the Adelaide municipal elections. She was supported by the Women's Non-Party Association and was narrowly defeated. Phoebe continued her interest in women's health and in 1921 she became the honorary medical officer, night clinic (venereal diseases), for women patients at the Adelaide Hospital. She also continued her role as an honorary doctor at the McBride's Hospital, Medindie. She was Australian delegate to the Medical Women's International Association Conference in Edinburgh, Scotland in 1937. She also moved her practice from North Terrace, in 1937, to her home 'Tintagel" in Norwood where she continued until she was 85 years old. For many years she headed the Nursing Units in the Adelaide ANZAC Day March. She never married and died on 24th March 1967 and is still remembered by the bursary she left for St Ann's College, North Adelaide at the University of Adelaide.

Sources:

Gibberd Joyce, Chapple Phoebe 1879-1967, Australian Dictionary of Biography.
http://adb.anu.edu.au/biography/shapple-phoebe-5560
http://www.awm.gov.au/blog/2009/06/30drphoebe-chapple-the-first-woman-doctor-to-receive -the -military-medal/

CILENTO Sir Raphael West
MD LLB

1893 - 1985

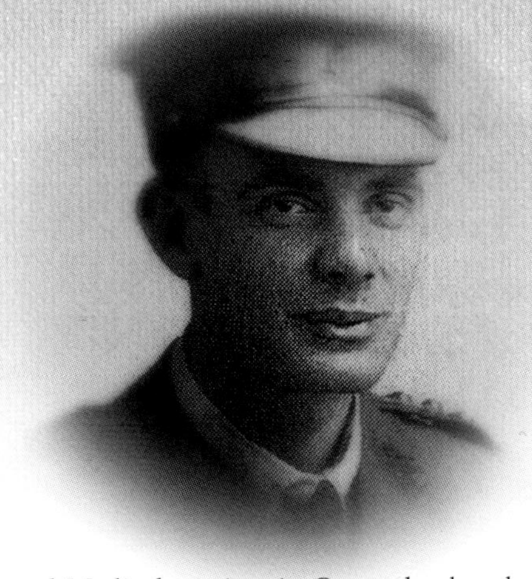

Raphael West (Ray) Cilento was born on 2nd December 1893 at Jamestown, South Australia, the second of five children of South Australian parents Raphael Ambrose Cilento, a stationmaster, and his wife Frances Ellen Elizabeth, nee West. His paternal grandfather was an Italian migrant who had a shipping business in Adelaide. Cilento attended Jamestown Public School and became a pupil-teacher in 1908. He taught at Port Pirie in 1910 to 1911. He completed his secondary education at Adelaide High School and then Prince Alfred College. He studied medicine at the University of Adelaide and graduated MB BS (1918) as Everard scholar and MD 1922.

Cilento joined the AIF in 1916 when still a medical student and was considered fit for home service. He was described as 5ft 8½ins tall weighed 128lbs with hazel eyes, brown hair, and medium complexion. He was promoted to corporal on 21st November 1916 and had uneventful service attached to the RMO of Murray Bridge War Service Camp until 1918. As soon as he graduated with his medical degree he was granted the rank of captain on 25th November 1918, and one month later on 18th December 1918 embarked on the *Melusia* in Sydney for Rabaul, New Guinea. He became familiar with tropical medicine and reported on medical conditions in New Guinea. He returned to Australia in September 1919 and his military appointment was terminated in South Australia on 18th October 1919.

Cilento married Dr Phyllis Dorothy McGlew on 18th March 1920. Later that year he obtained a post as a physician to the Sultanate of Perak, Federated Malay States, where he gained further expertise in tropical medicine. Cilento became a leading figure in the field of tropical medicine and was appointed director of the Australian Institute in Tropical Medicine in 1922. He was seconded to Rabaul in 1924 as director of public health for the Mandated Territory of New Guinea. He became Director of Tropical Hygiene and Chief Quarantine Officer in Brisbane, Queensland in 1928. He was appointed as the first State Director-General of Health and Medical services in Queensland and returned to Brisbane in September 1934. He was knighted for his service in 1935; he created a new public medical system, writing legislation for general medicine and for mental health. To assist this work, he studied law and was admitted to the Bar on 29 April 1939. Cilento came into conflict with the military over the awarding of his British War Medal, Victory medal and his returned soldiers badge in 1935. He applied for them to wear at the investiture of his knighthood in Sydney. Although he enlisted in 1916 as a medical student, he was not awarded the medals as he had embarked for Rabaul after 11th November 1918. Cilento attempted to re-join the Army with the advent of WW2 but was rejected by the Commonwealth Security Services because of rumours about his associations with the Italian government and with organisations such as the Dante Alighieri Society. Despite this he demonstrated his commitment to public service where his expertise in preventative medicine resulted in his appointment, in May 1945, with the United Nations Relief and Rehabilitation Administration. He was appointed a major general in the British Army, on the 25th August 1945, by General Montgomery. He worked first in the Balkans on malaria control and then in Germany, in July he was the first civilian doctor to enter Belsen concentration camp. Cilento was an active historical researcher; he was president of the Royal Historical Society of Queensland (1933-34, 1943-45, and 1953-68) and of the National Trust of Queensland (1966-71). Sir Raphael West Cilento died on 15th April 1985, at Oxley, Brisbane aged 92. He was survived by his wife, three sons and three daughters.

Sources:
Finnane M., 'Cilento, Sir Raphael West (Ray) (1893–1985)', Australian Dictionary of Biography, National Centre of Biography, Australian National University, http://adb.anu.edu.au/biography/cilento-sir-raphael-west-ray-12319/text22129, http://recordsearch.naa.gov.au/scripts/Imagine.asp?B=3249229
Photo from son Dr David Cilento, Brisbane.

CLARKE Cyril Lowther

MB BS

1884 - 1922

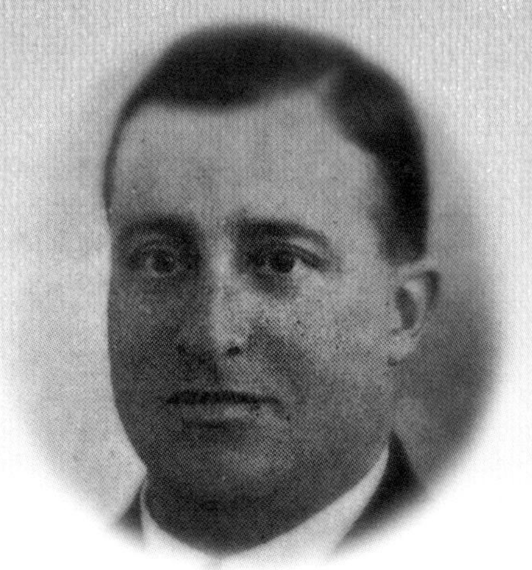

Cyril Lowther Clarke was born on the 6th August 1884 in York, England. He was the son of the Reverend Henry Lowther Clarke. His early school days were in Oxford, England and later at Bedford Grammar School. He moved to Australia at 18 years of age when his father was appointed the Archbishop of Melbourne in 1903. He attended Trinity College and the University of Melbourne, and graduated from medicine and surgery with honours in 1908. Later he practised in Kalgoorlie, WA. He settled in Peterborough, SA in April 1911 and was known as a sound practitioner, and a person of considerable ability and energy. He was appointed as the Medical Officer of Health for the Corporation of Peterborough. He married Constance Anderson eldest daughter of the Bishop of Riverina on 14th February 1912 at Hay, New South Wales. His father performed the ceremony.

Clarke joined the Australian AAMC as a captain in November 1911. He was employed at 4 MD. He enlisted in the AIF in early 1916. He was commissioned as a Major on 1st August 1916. He was 32 years old, 5 ft. 9 ½ ins. tall, He had a fresh complexion and brown eyes and brown hair. His wife was named as his next of kin care of his father Archbishop of Melbourne, Bishops Court, Melbourne, Victoria. He embarked from Melbourne on the *Karoola* on the 19th August 1916 and he was attached to 14 AGH in Egypt. Clarke was diagnosed with malaria during 1918 and had two relapses but he returned to duty by June 1919. He was transferred to Command the 5th LH FdAmb on the 13th January 1919. He was promoted to temporary lieutenant colonel on the 7th March 1919. Clarke had a glowing recommendation from Brigadier General Ryrie, and for a time served as ADMS with the Australian Mounted Division. He returned to Australia on the *Burma* on the 26th July 1919 with his appointment terminated on the 8th November 1919. He was issued with the British War Medal and the Victory Medal.

Clarke resumed his practice in Peterborough after his return to Australia. Also returning to the town was Dr Arthur Goode whose AIF appointment was terminated one month after Clarke. He was elected Chairman of Finance of the Municipal Council in 1920. In December 1921 he was elected Mayor of Peterborough and was considered a wise and capable administrator. He was also the President of the local branch of the Returned and Soldiers League. Cyril Lowther Clarke was killed in a vehicle accident on the 23rd September 1922, when returning from the races. There were four other young people in the car and a young boy of 13 years was also fatally injured. He was survived by his pregnant wife, Constance, and two sons aged 9 years and 21 months. Within weeks of his death Constance delivered a daughter.

Sources:

http://recordsearch.naa.gov.au/scripts/Imagine.asp?B=1968892

Photo: SLSA and Peterborough Council publication; 20th March 1922.

The Independent 23rd February 1912.

Military Medical Service at Home (45-55)

It seems that in some quarters misapprehension has arisen with regard to the appeal recently made in these columns for whole-time medical officers over 45 years of age....War is for young men, and there is no doubt that every available young man should be serving with the armies in the field.... Of medical men under 45 years of age only those should remain at home who are either physically unfit or unacceptable to the military authorities or absolutely indispensable in their civilian work. The indispensable men under 45 are comparatively very few. The majority of medical men of military age should be in khaki, and should only remain in the country long enough to be trained in their army duties.

BMJ, 1st July 1916, p. 19

CLAYTON Arthur Ross

DSO MB BS MRCS (Eng) LRCP (Lond)

1876 - 1963

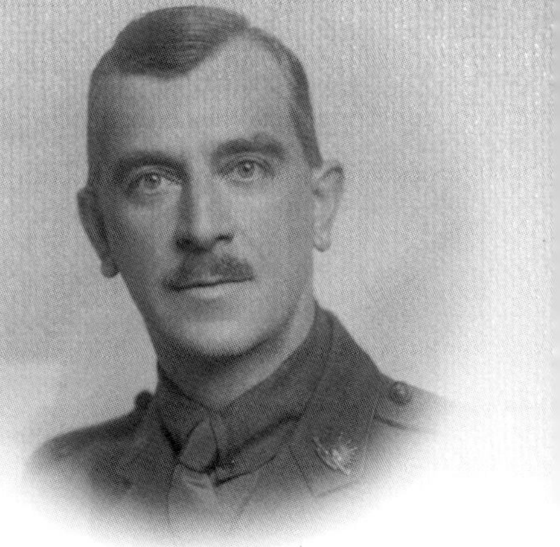

Arthur Ross Clayton was born on 14th May 1876 at Yankalilla, South Australia, son of John Woods Clayton and Elizabeth, nee Cornish. He was educated at St Peter's College and studied medicine at the University of Adelaide graduating in 1902. He became a resident surgeon at the Adelaide Hospital in 1903 and then undertook postgraduate study in England (MRCS England; LRCP London; 1905). After returning to South Australia In 1907, he went into general practice at Moonta. He subsequently was appointed surgeon to the Wallaroo and Moonta Mining and Smelting Company in 1908 and medical officer of health for Moonta in 1909. He joined the AAMC Reserve in 1912 and was the regimental medical officer to the 24th Light Horse.

Clayton enlisted the AIF on 10th September 1915 as a Captain at the age of 39 years. He was described as single, 5ft 8ins tall and weighed 164lbs. His mother Mrs Elizabeth Clayton of Medindie was named as his next of kin. He was posted to the 1 AGH in Egypt and then the 3 AGH at Heliopolis. He was promoted to major on 11th October 1915. He served in 7th and 6th FdAmb from March 1916 and then posted to 12 FdAmb on 10th November 1916 and placed in charge of the 5th Divisional Rest Station at Vignacourt. He went to the 1st Anzac Corps Rest Station at Bellevue Farm during operations at Bapaume in early 1917. During the battles of Bullecourt he served at the 5 Division's main dressing stations and from October to December was acting commander of his unit. Clayton assumed temporary command of 8 FdAmb on 22nd January 1918 and remained with the 5th Division on the Somme. He was promoted to the temporary rank of lieutenant colonel in May 1918 and remained in command of 8 FdAmb until the end of WW1. He was wounded in action in April 1918 but only suffered minor wounds. He was mentioned in Sir Douglas Haig's Despatches on 7th April 1918 and on 4th June 1918 he was awarded the DSO. His promotion to lieutenant colonel was substantiated in November 1918. He became the Commanding Officer of the AIF's remaining divisional field ambulances in Belgium in April 1919. He was issued with the 1914-15 Star, the British War Medal and the Victory Medal with Oak Leaves.

Clayton returned to Australia in August 1919 and was discharged in December 1919. After demobilisation he resumed his medical practice at Moonta and continued to serve in the Australian Military Forces Reserve as area medical officer at Moonta and Kadina before being placed on the unattached list in 1922. He married Nellie Mabel Mary Harbison on 12 September 1922 at St Mary's Anglican Church, Wallaroo He was among the community's most prominent citizens and was mayor of the Moonta Corporation in 1923-1926 and again in 1939 – 1940. He was a warden of the local Anglican Church and a Freemason. He and his wife had no children and Arthur Clayton remained at Moonta until his death on 2nd September 1963; his wife had predeceased him.

Sources:

http://adb.anu.edu.au/biography/clayton-arthur-ross-5675
Land William A, 'Clayton Arthur Ross' (1876-1963) Australian Dictionary of Biography
http://naa12.naa.gov.auB=3251481=10&T=R

The Use of Gas in Warfare

When gas was first used by the Germans it was assumed that the constituents relied on were bromine and chlorine...it has been clear that phosgene gas has played an important part...the accounts include references to "mustard gas"... The war has thus become quite different from all other wars, and, to a certain extent, it is being fought in the chemical laboratories.

MJA, 13th July 1918, p. 29

CLINDENING Frederick Talbot Driffield

MRCS (Eng) LRCP (Lond)

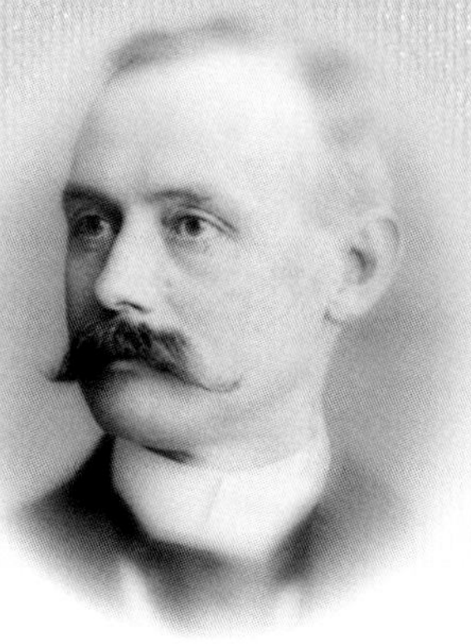

1859 - 1959

Frederick Talbot Driffield Clindening was born on 20th June 1859 in Port Elliot, South Australia. He was the second son of Dr William Talbot Clindening and Mary Rebow Jane, nee Driffield (1826-1925). He, with his parents and three siblings returned to England from 1861-1863. He was educated at the North Adelaide Grammar School and Prince Alfred College. He began BA at the University of Adelaide, but withdrew due to financial problems after passing first year. Clindening took up employment, from 1878 to 1879 with the South Australian Government in the Telegraph Survey and Surveyor-General Office as a draughtsman, surveyor and a warden of gold fields. He served in the militia from 1883 to 1887 in the Adelaide Rifles and Artillery. He married Clara Brooke, single, aged 39 at St Luke's Church Adelaide in September 1889 and in the same month he was cited in a divorce case by George Anderson, against his wife Jessie Maud Anderson. Clindening and his wife then moved to London where they lived at 20 Gordon Mansions, Francis Street, London WC1. He then studied medicine at St Bartholomew's Hospital, London, 1890-1895. After graduation he travelled and worked in many places including China, where he worked as a medical officer for the Kiukiang port, to Her Britannic Majesty's Consulate, and the Chinese Imperial Maritime Customs, in 1898.

Clindening enlisted in the RAMC in London in April 1915 and served for 23 months on the staff of the Netley Military Hospital and was in charge of the hospital trains running between Southampton and Scotland. He was promoted to captain in April 1916 and discharged on 3rd January 1920 in China. He and his wife, finally settled in England in the 1920s. It is recorded that he was on the reserve list in 1928.

Clindening remained with his family in England after the war and they never returned to Australia. They had six children. Frederick Talbot Driffield Clindening died on 23rd March 1959, aged 99 years, when he was living at 301 Clive Court, Maida Vale, London.

Sources:

South Australian Register 18 December 1885
South Australian Register 26 November 1886
South Australian Register 18 March 1878
South Australian Register 13 September 1889.
South Australian Register 24 September 1889
Chronicle Adelaide 15 August 1925
SLSA Clindening Family Collection
Military records LTCOL Neil C. Smith AM

CLOSE Walter John Westcott

MB BS FRCS(Ed) FRACS

1891 - 1979

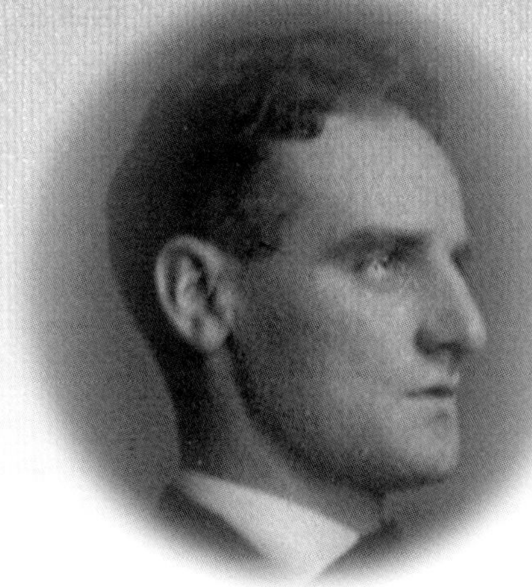

Walter John Westcott Close was born on the 7th May 1891 at Laura, SA, the son of John and Frances Close. He was educated at the Highgate State School and Prince Alfred College and studied medicine at the University of Adelaide where he graduated in 1913. At University he was proficient at tennis and was awarded a Blue for lacrosse.

Close enlisted in the AIF in February 1915 and had previous experience as the RMO of the 74th Boothby Infantry Regt in 1914. He was commissioned as a Captain on the 6th March 1915. He was 23 years old, single, 5ft 9ins, and weighed 11st 5lbs. His mother of "Exmoor", Prescott Terrace, Rose Park was named as his next of kin. He was posted to 4 LHFA, and sailed with the unit to the Middle East. Close was posted to 15 FdAmb when the 4 LHFA was disbanded and went to France in June 1916. He was at the Battle of Fromelles, and afterwards was posted as RMO of 58 Bn. He worked near and in the trenches and devoted his attention to the sanitary conditions of the soldiers. He paid special attention to providing hot baths for the soldiers within 400-500 yards of the front line and where possible clean clothes for the soldiers after bathing. This contributed to the reduction of medical illness amongst the soldiers in the trenches. He was promoted major in February 1917 and transferred to 14 FdAmb. He served with distinction as Adjutant of the unit at Vaulx and Warloy, and in September he was granted the Brevet Rank of Major, *'in recognition of* especially *meritorious work rendered on Active Service'*, at the conclusion of the Third Battle of Ypres in November 1917. Close was appointed DADMS of 5 Div. During the winter he fell ill, and in February 1918 was evacuated to England with pleurisy. He was Mentioned in Despatches for this period of service. He spent some time in 3rd LGH, and was repatriated to Australia in May 1918 with a recommendation that his appointment in the AIF be terminated on the 13th September 1918. Close was issued with the 1914-15 Star, the British War Medal and the Victory Medal with Oak Leaves.

He married Gladys Cilento, sister of Raphael West Cilento, on the 8th October 1918 at St Columba's Church, Hawthorn. Close followed a surgical career on his return to South Australia with successful post graduate studies in Great Britain and Europe. Initial appointments include honorary medical officer at Port Pirie Hospital followed by more senior appointments at the Adelaide Children's Hospital and the Adelaide Hospital. He consulted at 175 North Terrace with his private address as Kurrajong Cottage, Gilles St East, Adelaide. He was appointed as a tutor in Anatomy and Surgery at the Adelaide University Medical School in 1934. During WW2 he worked from September 1942 to November 1943 at the Isolation Hospital at Keswick. Walter John Westcott Close died at the age of 87 years on the 24th March 1979 and is buried in the Centennial Park Cemetery.

Sources:

http://recordsearch.naa.gov.au/scripts/Imagine.asp?B=3260356 ;
SA. Who's Who, 1936.
Likeman R., "From the Tropics to the Desert", Slouch Hat Publications, Port Melbourne, 2012.
Photo: PAC collection.
Letter to the University of Adelaide dated 8/12/16.
www.geni.com/people/WalterClose/6000000005250027135.

COCKBURN Patrick

MB BS

1888 - 1960

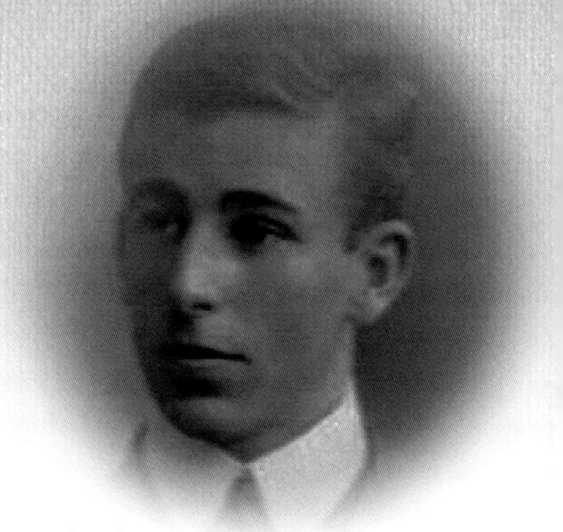

Patrick Cockburn was born on 2nd May 1888 in Wirrabara, South Australia the son of Tom Cockburn and Alice, neé Battern. His father was the brother of Sir John Cockburn KCMG, who at the age of 38 years, was the Premier of South Australia from 1888 to 1890. His father owned a large property "Lorraine" just outside of Wirrabara. He was educated at St Peter's College, Adelaide. His parents took him out of school to work on their property; however he insisted that he wanted to study medicine, so they reluctantly let him return to St Peter's College to matriculate and he then studied medicine at the University of Adelaide graduating in 1914. He became the resident medical officer at the Broken Hill and District Hospital from March 1915 and in December of that year was the Acting Surgeon Superintendent of Broken Hill and District Hospital. He returned to Adelaide in 1916 and was resident medical officer at the Adelaide Hospital until he enlisted. Prior to enlisting in the AIF he married Hester Lilias Berry.

Cockburn had previous experience in the AAMC Reserve in South Australia and had been posted as a Captain in the AAMC on 21st June 1916. Cockburn enlisted in the AIF on 23rd October 1916. He was 28 years old and his wife was named as his next of kin. Her address was care of Mrs Spencer Robinson, "Willunga", Dudley Ave Roseville, NSW. He is described as 5ft 9½ins, weighed 154lbs, of medium complexion with fair hair. He was allotted to General Reinforcements and embarked on the *Orontes* from Melbourne on 12th December 1916 and arrived in Plymouth, England on 20th February 1917, where he was posted to the Officer Corps School for Medical Officers. Soon after his arrival in England he was hospitalised with bronchitis. He proceeded to France on 19th June 1917 attached to 2 AGH. He was transferred on 29th July to the 3 Australian Division and 9 FdAmb. During this time Cockburn had several short term attachments between 9 FdAmb and 10 FdAmb. Cockburn was transferred for England on the *Jan Breydal* with a gunshot wound to his right elbow on 2nd January 1918. He re-joined the 10 FdAmb on 24th February 1918. He was admitted again to hospital in June 1918 with pyrexia and diagnosed later as influenza. He returned to 9 FdAmb in January 1919 and then posted back to England in March 1919 reporting to the DMS. He was subsequently transferred from 10 FdAmb to the regular forces of the British Army for retention against the time of his return from active service. He returned to Australia on the *Suffolk* in April 1919 and his appointment was terminated on 19th August 1919. He was issued with the British War Medal and the Victory Medal.

Cockburn became a general practitioner in Lambton, Newcastle in New South Wales after the war. He later separated from his wife, who remained with their son Alexander in New South Wales. He returned to live on the family property of "Lorraine" in South Australia. Patrick Cockburn died in February 1960 when he lived at Norwood, South Australia.

Sources:

Personal family interviews.

Photo: The Cockburn family

http://recordsearch.naa.gov.au/NameSearch/Interface/ItemDetail.aspx?Barcode=3264998

COLLINS William Kendall

MB BS

1896 - 1944

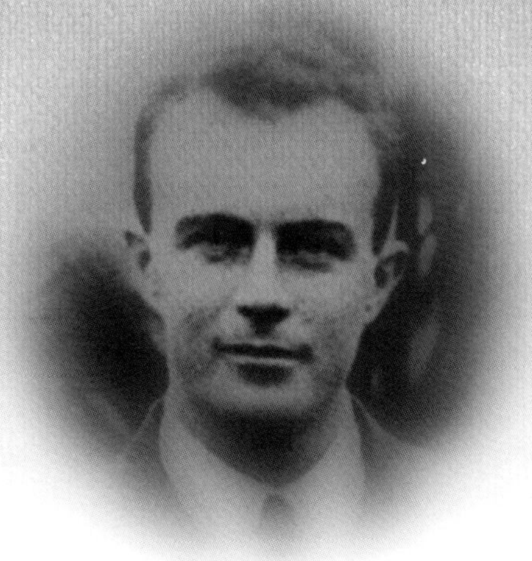

William Kendall Collins was born on 25th December 1896 in Williamstown, SA, son of William Thomas Collins and Ann Harris. He was educated at Gawler School and Prince Alfred College. He was awarded an Exhibition in 1910. He studied medicine at the University of Adelaide commencing in 1914 and graduating in 1918.

Collins enlisted on 17th June 1918 in Adelaide whilst he was still single and a medical student. He was living at Prince Alfred College and his father was named as his next of kin. He had served four years in the senior cadets and had transferred to the citizen forces. He claimed 120 days of prior service in the AIF and records of his service in 1916 are not available. He was 5ft 8ins tall, weighed 145 lbs. He was described as being of medium complexion with grey eyes and brown hair. He had a small scar above his right knee. He was not called up for duty and was discharged on 18th November 1918. He was appointed a Captain in the AIF on 9th December 1918 after graduating and the appointment was terminated on 2nd September 1920.

There is no record that he married but in 1934 he was recorded as working in Donnybrook, Western Australia. However, at some time he returned to South Australia and William Kendal Collins died in South Australia on 31st January 1944.

Sources:

Photo: Adelaide University Archives, Medical Graduates 1918, he is noted as C Collins
http://recordsearch.naa.gov.au/NameSearch/Interface/ItemDetail.aspx?Barcode=3016188
The Chronicle Adelaide 8 January 1910
The Adelaide Advertiser 23 November 1917
The West Australian Perth 17 July 1934
Ancestry.com
Biographical Index of South Australians 1836-1885

Volunteers for Medical Service with the Army

Several inquiries have been received at the offices of the British Medical Association from practitioners who are anxious to make themselves useful, but do not know where to apply: or who, having applied to the War Office have not yet received an answer... These applications have been coming in so freely as to tax to the uttermost the clerical staff of the War Office, so that those received from older men or from men who are only able to offer their services in certain conditions of time and place have either not yet received a reply or merely a formal one. We are asked to assure all such applicants that their offers have by no means been over-looked, and are, on the contrary, being carefully filed for future use. We are further asked to request all applicants who offer their services not to make merely general statements of their willingness to make themselves useful, but to give their age, qualifications and experience, and state what they are prepared to do; that is, whether they can only accept service locally or in this country, or are prepared, if ordered, to go abroad. Intending applicants must further understand that though their special qualifications may be of a surgical nature they must be prepared, until such special experience is required, to do ordinary general medical work. The War Office is anxious to have this made clear, because a small number of those applying whose work have recently been purely surgical, have stipulated that they should only be used in this way. Such a stipulation tends to make their offer less useful than it is doubtless intended to be. There is no fear that if and when the time comes their surgical abilities will be utilized to the full.

BMJ, 15th August 1914, p.343

CORBIN Cecil

MB BS

1871 - 1944

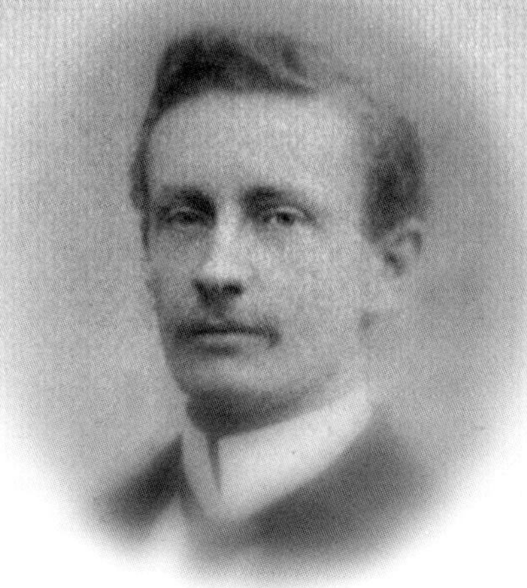

Cecil Corbin was born on 28th August 1871 at Riverton, South Australia. He was the son of Dr Thomas W. Corbin and Laura, nee Hardy and brother of John Corbin and their six other siblings. He was educated at St Peter's College and studied medicine at the University of Adelaide, graduating in 1894. Cecil was a member of St John Ambulance while he was practising in Woodside. He was the medical officer of Onkaparinga Board of Health. Corbin was one of four junior medical officers which included Drs E.E. Moule, J.A. Bonnin and H.R. Letcher, who complained of the competence of 'strike breaker' Drs Napier and Ramsey Smith after the 'Adelaide Hospital Row. They also criticised the manner in which the hospital was run. The Board considered that these house surgeons had *a distinct but covert spirit of antagonism to Drs Napier and Smith which destroyed all hope of harmonious co-operation.* Corbin was dismissed from the Hospital on charges of disobedience and insubordination but the other three were allowed to resign.

Corbin married Ethel Margaret Glen on 23rd October 1901 in Mount Gambier. He was appointed to look after the destitute poor in the Onkaparinga area in 1903. He was also a Scout Master. For a time he practised in Fremantle, Western Australia. Corbin left Adelaide in June 1914 on a health trip arriving in England a fortnight before World War I was declared. He was a captain attached to the 10 Bn in the South Australian militia prior to the war and had seven years of experience in the militia. He was one of the large number of Australian Medical men in London who volunteered for the RAMC whilst in England. After a week in training camp at Woolwich on 16th August 1914 they were ordered to the front. They sailed to Rouen France. An Australian Voluntary Hospital had been established with Colonel Evans in command. Corbin however, was sent to 11 General Hospital. Because the four British Hospitals were close to the front, and the British Forces were withdrawing, it was decided to move the hospitals all on one ship back to St. Nazaire. They stayed there for a month before moving to Boulogne. Casualties from Ypres took six hours to be evacuated to them. Some 2,700 casualties passed through 11 General Hospital in one month. They also treated many Germans who were apparently pleased to be in the hands of the British. Many Medical Officers were wounded and some were highly decorated. Corbin went on to say that the Australian Hospital was moved to Wimmereux 5 miles from Boulogne. It was the only hospital able to get the x-ray equipment to work and the Australians were highly praised for their ingenuity. Because of ill-health he left Boulogne before Xmas 1915 for England. He returned to Adelaide on the *Morea* with his wife and son. There was case of smallpox on board the ship and it was quarantined when reaching South Australian waters. Corbin, his wife and a son were landed on Torrens Island. He continued his interest in military matters and was an instructor at an Officer training unit and had been promoted to Major in 1916.

Corbin was practising in Hyde Park and on North Terrace, Adelaide in 1918. He was Chairman of the Royal British Nurses Association taking up the position very early after his return from overseas. He campaigned for more trained nurses. He also was a supporter of the South Adelaide Crèche which had been started by his mother and he was an office bearer in that organisation. All his family as a whole were great supporters of the Home for Incurables. He purchased 33 acres on the corner of Nottage Terrace and Main North Road in 1922. Cecil Corbin died on 24th August 1944 at Parkside, South Australia.

Sources:

Adelaide Advertiser 1889-1931 and 1931-1959

Personal interview The Mail 10th April 1915

South Australian Indexes of Birth Deaths and Marriages

"The Adelaide Hospital, Adelaide", South Australia

Adelaide, W.K. Thomas & Co., Grenfell Street, 1906

Estcourt Hughes J. "The "Hospital Row", a History of the Royal Adelaide Hospital, 1982 pages 189-205.

CORBIN John

FRACS MRCS (Eng) LRCP (Lond)

1878 - 1930

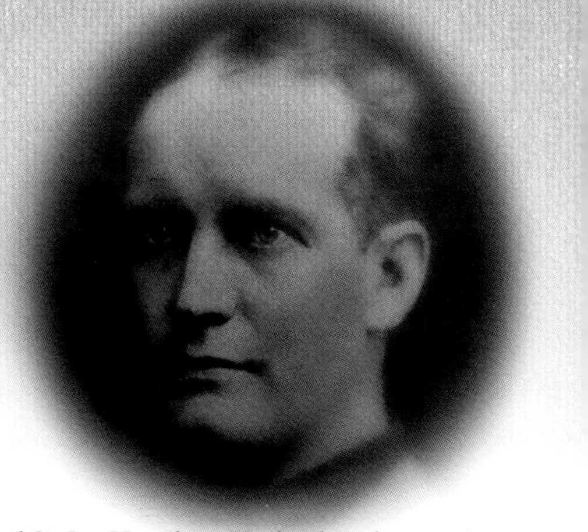

John Corbin was born in Adelaide on 1st June 1878, the third son of Dr Thomas W Corbin an Adelaide general practitioner. He was educated at the Queen's School and St Peter's College. After leaving school he spent some time working on the West Australian goldfields. Through the generosity of an uncle he sailed to England and entered St Bartholomew's Hospital Medical School. There he played Rugby and represented the Hospital XV although he had never played previously. He graduated MRCS (England) and LRCP (London). He returned to Adelaide in 1903 to join his father in practice in King William St where Muirden College is now situated. When his father retired in 1904 he and his brother, Cecil, who had returned from Fremantle, continued at the same practice. Prior to the outbreak of WW1, Corbin was a captain in the AAMC 1905-1908 and later, on the Reserve of Officers of the AAMC.

He joined in the AIF on 23rd October 1914 and was posted to 1 ASH at the rank of major. He was 6ft, and weighed 14st. His wife, Margaret Watt, nee Ogilvie of Brougham Place, North Adelaide was named as his next of kin. He departed Melbourne on the *Kyarra* and arrived in Egypt on 23rd January 1915 with 4 other Hospitals. He spent 2 weeks in 1 AGH with broncho-pneumonia until 28th February. The 1 ASH was divided leaving himself, TG Wilson and F Le Messurier at Maadi. In early March his group went to Mudros harbour and were joined by the rest of the 1 ASH on the 24th March 1915. Then on the 26th March he transferred to the 1 ACCS in the hope of getting closer to the front. This unit boarded on the 18th April and left Mudros on the evening of 24th April 1915. At 0530 the following morning he wrote, *I could see the cliffs and could recognise the difficulties,* of the landing. Corbin landed with the 1 ACCS. He records that *during the first 4 days 3,300 wounded passed through our hands.* Corbin gave a full account of his experience of the Gallipoli invasion in the Medical Journal of Australia in 1916. He was promoted Major on 27th July 1915 and in August was Mentioned in Despatches by General Sir Ian Hamilton. He developed a pyrexia, transferred to Egypt, and invalided to Australia, arriving 17th October 1915. After being declared fit again for active service Corbin re-enlisted on 17th March 1916 as lieutenant colonel in the 3 ACCS. He returned to France in October 1916 in Command of the 3 ACCS. He transferred to England for duty at AIF HQ in July 1917. He was struck off strength in August 1917 and returned to Australia. His appointment was terminated 4th October 1917. He was again Mentioned in Despatches by Sir Douglas Haig gazetted in May 1917. He was issued with the 1914-15 Star, British War Medal and Victory Medal with Oak Leaves. Corbin wrote extensive diaries of his military experiences.

Corbin was appointed an honorary assistant surgeon on his return to Australia, then honorary surgeon at the Adelaide Hospital in 1925. He was appointed surgical tutor and subsequently lecturer in Clinical Surgery at the University of Adelaide. Corbin also bought the practice and home of Dr M Jay at North Adelaide. He was surgeon at the Repatriation Hospital and *was always anxious to do all he could for the deserving soldiers.* He was prominent in the South Australian Branch of the BMA and President in 1928. He involved himself locally and interstate in study and reports to improve clinical care. He was also elected to positions with the Massage Association of SA and the Adelaide Medical Students Society. His hobbies and interest encompassed a flutter on the horses, golf, fishing and shooting. He was a great raconteur and even a repeated story was never dull. John Corbin died on 1st February 1930 aged 51 years at his home in North Adelaide and is buried in Mitcham Cemetery. He was survived by his wife Margaret, a son John, a medical student, and two daughters, Betty and Suzanne.

Sources:
Corbin J., MJA. Vol 1. No. 6 Feb 5th 1916
Newland HS, MJA. March 22nd 1930, p402.
http://recordsearch.naa.gov.au/scripts/Imagine.asp?B=3419959,

CORRY Samuel Lloyd

MB BS

1886 - 1983

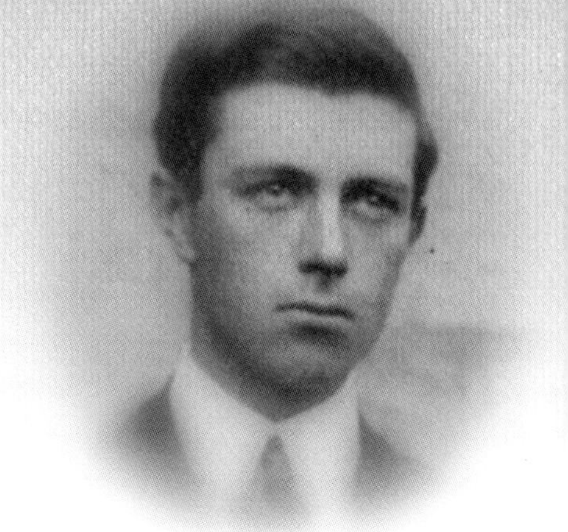

Samuel Lloyd Corry was born in Adelaide on 8th February 1886. He was the son of Samuel Corry and Annie Maria, nee Lloyd. His father, Samuel, died on 27th Oct 1896. He was educated at Prince Alfred College, and at the School of Mines in 1904 where he studied chemistry and building construction; he had been awarded a scholarship. He studied medicine at the same time, graduating MB BS in 1910.

His mother, of Brougham Place, North Adelaide told the Advertiser on 1st June 1915 that her eldest son had received a commission in the RAMC. He had been in Africa on his way to England when war was declared. He was offered a post at the Paddington Green Children's Hospital and completed this post before accepting his RAMC Commission in May 1915. Corry served in France with the Royal Engineers before returning to Australia after the death of his brother. His mother also reported that her younger son, Corry's brother, left with the AIF and was a motor cycle dispatch rider now with the Australian Forces at the Dardanelles. Thomas Edison Spurgeon Corry, a motor cycle mechanic with three years training at the School of Mines, joined the AIF on 18th August 1914 at the age of 19 years and 9 months. He was to die at sea, between Gallipoli and Malta having received a gunshot or shrapnel wound to the abdomen on 10th August 1915.

It is presumed that Corry married as the birth of a son, Gordon Edison Corry, in Uraidla is recorded in the Advertiser on 5th October 1917. It was reported, at the unveiling of the WW1 memorial obelisk in Uraidla, that he was involved in the purchase of the land for the Uraidla Memorial Park. He had been secretary of the fund raising committee and was reported as having personally raised most of the funds. He was overseas at the time the obelisk was unveiled as he took up a general practice in Hereford, England, where he remained for 35 years before retiring, at 70 years of age, in 1956. He took his first flight ever to New Zealand in 1979 where he spent the last 4 years of his life with his granddaughter, who had married a GP. Samuel Lloyd Corry died at the great age of 97, in Christchurch, NZ, on 21st May 1983. His son, Officer Cadet Gordon Edison Corry married Pamela Davies which was recorded in the Gloucester Echo 10th Jun 1940. He was commissioned in the British Army later that year. Gordon Corry was also to live to a great age dying in NZ at the age of 93 in 2011.

Sources:

The Adelaide Advertiser 1JUN15
BMJ 1983 11 298 "S L Corry
The Adelaide Register 27th March 1922

The following letter was sent to the University of Adelaide in late 1916 in response to a request about Corry's military service.

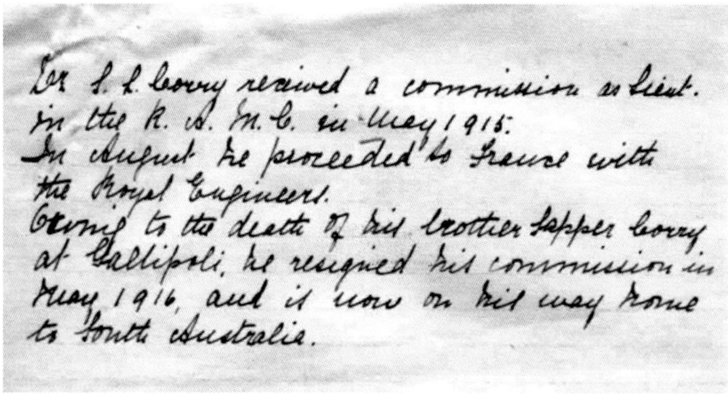

Dr S. L. Corry received a commission as Lieut. in the R. A. M. C. in May 1915.
In August he proceeded to France with the Royal Engineers.
Owing to the death of his brother Sapper Corry at Gallipoli, he resigned his commission in May 1916, and is now on his way home to South Australia.

COWAN Sir Darcy Rivers Warren

MB BS FRACP

1885 - 1958

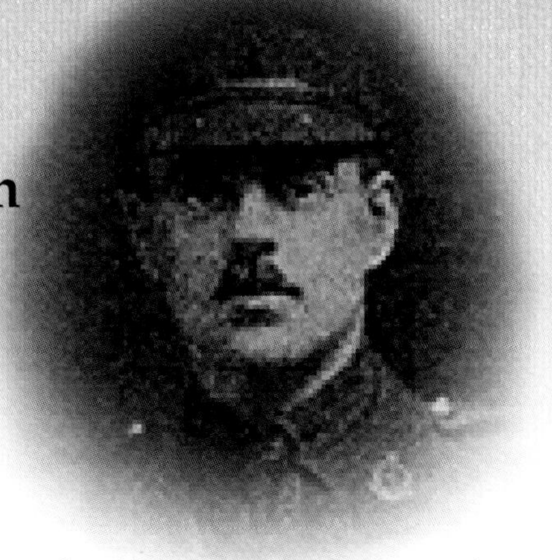

Darcy Rivers Warren Cowan was born on the 8th August 1885 at Norwood, Adelaide. He was one of eight children of James Cowan, a merchant from Ireland, and his wife Sarah Ann, nee Warren. His father was a prosperous flour miller and investor in Broken Hill; subsequently he was a Member of Parliament in South Australia. Cowan was educated at Prince Alfred College and studied medicine at the University of Adelaide where he won a triple Blue in lacrosse, football and tennis, and also played cricket. He married Effie Hewitt Cox on the 19th April 1910; they were to remain childless. Cowan was in England with his wife at the outbreak of WWI; on the 5th November 1914 he was appointed temporary lieutenant in the RAMC. Returning to South Australia, on the 22nd May 1916 he joined the AAMC Reserve as an honorary captain.

Cowan was an honorary physician to the Adelaide Hospital in 1924-35 where he furthered his interest in tuberculosis, and was especially concerned that the disease was infecting nurses and doctors occupationally exposed to it. He visited the United States of America to investigate methods of control of tuberculosis in 1937. As a result of his determination in the control and treatment of tuberculosis the Chest Clinic at the Adelaide Hospital was established. This included a ward for tuberculosis patients, of which Cowan was physician-in-charge from 1938 to 1950. He founded the South Australian Tuberculosis Association in 1943. Then in 1948 he helped to form the National Association for the Prevention of Tuberculosis in Australia and forged links with kindred societies in Britain and America. Cowan founded Northcote Home, which was a residence for children whose parents were in hospital with tuberculosis. He also founded Bedford Industries, which offered work opportunities for the rehabilitation of those afflicted with tuberculosis. This later became a factory at Panorama, SA, which provided those with different mental and physical disabilities with work opportunities. He was involved with the James Brown Memorial Trust which owned and managed Kalyra Sanatorium and Estcourt House, Grange from 1947 to 1957. Cowan was also President (1935-36) of the South Australian branch of the British Medical Association. He became a foundation fellow of the Royal Australasian College of Physicians in 1938. Cowan was knighted in 1955 for his work on tuberculosis. Despite a busy life he enjoyed gardening and was an office-holder in the South Australian Lawn Tennis Association; he had helped to organize the Davis Cup challenge rounds at Memorial Drive in 1952 and 1956. He belonged to the Adelaide Club from 1929 and was a life member of the BMA. Sir Darcy Rivers Warren Cowan died on 9 June 1958 at Calvary Hospital, North Adelaide, and was buried at Payneham cemetery. He was survived by his wife Effie. He was commemorated by the Australian Laennec Society with the establishment of the Sir Darcy Cowan prize for research into respiratory disease.

Sources:
Med J Aust, 1959, 1, 612-14.
Photo the PAC collection.
Woodruff P., 'Cowan, Sir Darcy Rivers Warren (1885–1958)', Australian Dictionary of Biography, National Centre of Biography, Australian National University, http://adb.anu.edu.au/biography/cowan-sir-darcy-rivers-warren-9845/text17415.

CUDMORE Sir Arthur Murray

CMG MB BS FRCS FRACS LRCP

1870 - 1951

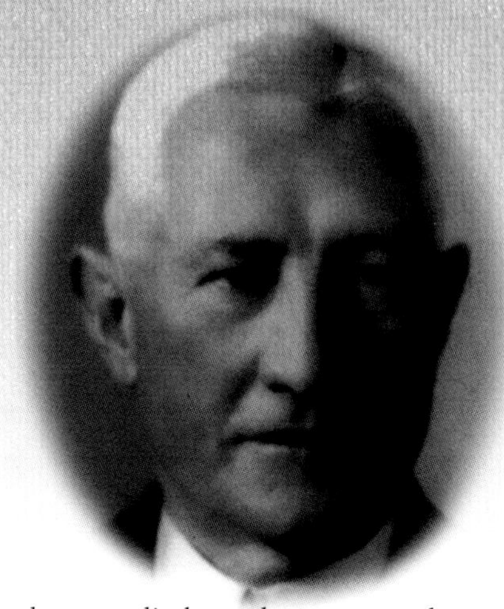

Arthur Murray Cudmore was born at 'Paringa,' second son of James Cudmore, on his family's sheep station on the River Murray near Renmark. His love of the country was a life long interest as was an interest in duck shooting. A left eye dominance required a curved stock for his Evans shotgun so that the gun at his right shoulder was brought up under his left eye. He was educated at St Peter's College and the University of Adelaide where he graduated MB BS in 1894. He then travelled to London where he took the MRCS-LRCP in 1896 and trained in surgery at The London Hospital and at St Mark's Hospital for diseases of the rectum. He obtained the FRCS in 1899 before returning to Adelaide where he was appointed Honorary Assistant Surgeon in 1901 and Honorary Surgeon from 1905-1925 when his 20 year appointment expired. He was lecturer in Clinical Surgery at the University of Adelaide from 1908-1919. He married Kathleen Cavenagh-Mainwaring in 1901 and they had two daughters.

Cudmore, aged 44 years, 5ft 10ins and weighing 11st 6lbs, joined the reinforcements for 3 AGH in April 1915. He embarked for the Middle East on the RMS *Mooltan* on 15th May 1915. He served at Gallipoli and on Lemnos before contracting paratyphoid in December 1915. He was admitted with the diagnosis of paratyphoid, emphysema and myocardial insufficiency. He returned to South Australia where he was discharged permanently unfit for service. Notwithstanding this he was consulting surgeon to 4 MD at Keswick and, mid 1918, returned overseas in the rank of lieutenant colonel and served in Great Britain and France before returning to Adelaide and was discharged in mid-1919.

Cudmore returned to surgical practice where he was remembered for his quiet voice, courtesy, and his simple sometimes delightfully repetitive teaching and his safe gentle surgery. He was a significant contributor to founding of the Dental School at the University of Adelaide and was Dean of the Dental Faculty and President of the Dental Board of SA. His hobbies included golf and motoring. He helped found the Royal Automobile Association of SA and was President in 1935. He was President of the Royal Adelaide Golf Club from 1925-1927. He appointed CMG in 1935 and knighted in 1945. Sir Arthur Murray Cudmore died on 27th February 1951 and his wife passed away on the 8th March 1951.

Sources:

McEachern AC 'Arthur Murray Cudmore 'The Founders of the Royal Australasian College of Surgeons p51, Smeaton Bronte 'Arthur Murray Cudmore' MJA 12May 1951 p 706.

Photo; Guy and Christine Cavenagh-Mainwaring.

http://recordsearch.naa.gov.au/scripts/Imagine.asp?B=3474108.

The Regimental Medical Officer

A medical man on taking a commission must be prepared to become a specialist in a subject which is entirely new to him, having a wide scope, and as remote from the nature of his ordinary routine of work as the subjects of public health, medical jurisprudence, etc., are from that of a newly qualified medical practitioner...When his regiment is not in action the regimental medical officer must be prepared, apart from routine instruction of his stretcher bearers and the usual supervision of general sanitation, to advise, *in anticipation,* on the course of procedure to be adopted in any matter which directly or indirectly affects the health of the whole unit or its individuals...When he has established his position in a unit, and when he has gained the confidence of experience, his energies may be directed towards enlightening the company officers on their own obligation in this direction.

BMJ, 14th October 1916, p. 527

DAVIES Harold Whitridge

ED MB BS FRACP

1894 - 1946

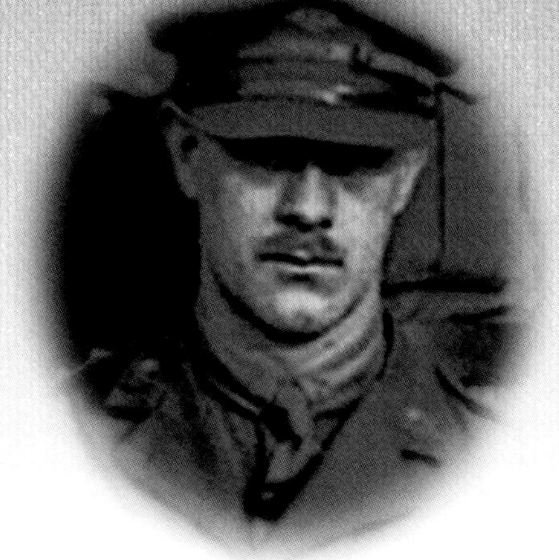

Harold (Pete) Whitridge Davies was born on 27th June 1894 in Adelaide. He was the eldest son of Dr Edward Harold Davies, and Ina Jane, nee Deland (daughter of a Gawler businessman). His father was a musician and Professor of Music and Director of the Elder Conservatorium of the University of Adelaide. Davies went to Prince Alfred College where he joined the Army Cadet Corps. He studied medicine at the University of Adelaide, graduating in 1917 and whilst at the University continued his military career in the Citizen Military Forces as a lieutenant in the 78th Infantry Bn. He started medical practice as the Acting House Physician in the Isolation Block and assistant in the Venereal Night Clinic at the Adelaide Hospital.

Davies was appointed as a captain in the AAMC on 6 July 1917. He was described as 5ft 11ins in height, of medium complexion and fair hair with grey eyes. He was attached as general reinforcements and embarked in Sydney for England in August 1917. He went on to France and was posted to 1 AGH in Rouen in November 1917. He was posted to 9 FdAmb in January 1918, and in April 1917 he was posted as MO to 33 Bn. He subsequently became sick with what was described as 'debility' and sent on leave to England in July 1918. He was posted to 3 Pioneer Bn in France as the medical officer in September 1918. Davies returned to London in early 1919 and was given leave to attend a Medical Research course. He then was given 3 months leave without pay from June 1919 to study the effects of dust inhalation at Ashhurst Military Hospital in Oxford in the laboratory of Dr J.S. Haldane. It was reported that he had taken an 'exceptionally keen' interest in the subject of his research and he rendered 'valuable service' throughout his stay at Ashhurst. He returned to Australia in July 1920 and his appointment was terminated on 12th August 1920. He was issued with the British War Medal and the Victory Medal. Davies' younger brother George, a teacher at Prince Alfred College, enlisted in the AIF 27th Battalion in May 1915. He was killed in action in France on the 29th June 1916 whilst in 8 FdAmb. He was awarded the Military Medal.

Davies continued with his research interest after the war and went to Edinburgh with Professor JC Meakins with whom he had worked at Oxford. He was appointed a Rockefeller Foundation Fellow for one year in 1923 at the Rockefeller Institute of Medical Research in New York. Davies returned to Australia in 1930 as the Professor of Physiology at the University of Sydney. He encouraged others to undertake significant research. To this end he supported staff members to be awarded Rockefeller fellowships and made two expeditions to Central Australia to study the adaptation of aboriginal people to water deprivation in hot and arid conditions. Due to the depression of the 1930s and work pressure of teaching Davies was not able to advance research in his department as he envisaged. However, he was an honorary consultant at three teaching hospitals and a Foundation Fellow of the Royal Australasian College of Physicians in 1938. Throughout this post war period Davies was a member of the Army Reserve. He was promoted to major in 1935 and lieutenant colonel in 1938 commanding 9 FdAmb in NSW. At the outbreak of WW2 he was mobilized and continued to command 9 Fd Amb. Due to health problems he relinquished his appointment in January 1942 after 7 months of service. He was awarded the Efficiency Decoration. Harold Whitridge Davies never married and left Sydney University in May 1946. He died one month later after falling down stairs in the Imperial Service Club in Sydney.

Sources:

Photo; AWM.EO1625

Family History from Dr Walford Thyer

http://recordsearch.naa.gov.au/scripts/Imagine.asp?B=1902307Text?

Bishop P.O., 'Davies, Harold Whitridge (1894–1946)', Australian Dictionary of Biography, National Centre of Biography, Australian National University, http://adb.anu.edu.au/biography/davies-harold-whitridge-9913/text17553,

DAWSON Dean

MB BS

1881 - 1939

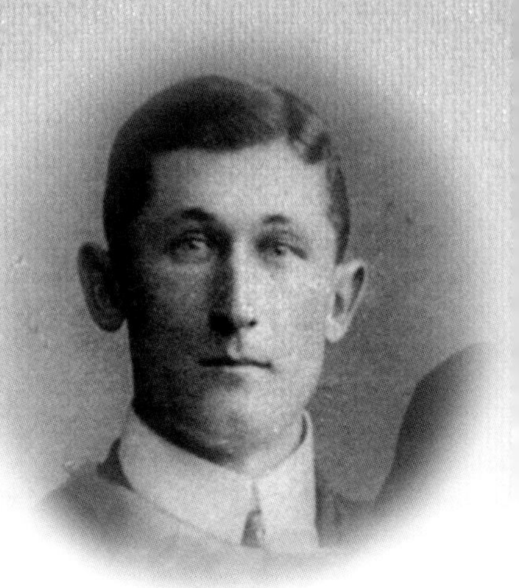

Dean Dawson was born at Gumeracha, SA on 13th March 1881. He was the third son and fifth child of Henry Dawson, a farmer, and Mary, nee Lillecrapp. He was educated at Prince Alfred College and studied medicine at the University of Adelaide graduating in 1905. He was an athletic man, playing football, cricket and lacrosse. In 1901 Dean joined the Norwood Football Club and was a renowned and successful player for the club. He was a house surgeon at the Adelaide hospital in 1906. He married Eulalie Burnard, also a medical graduate, and younger sister of Renfrey Gershom Burnard. She died in childbirth in 1907. After the death of his wife he took up a practice in Laura where he met and married his second wife Lorna Muriel Deeley. They were married on 4th August 1909. He moved to a practice in Port Pirie in July 1911, where his first two children were born.

Dawson enlisted in the AIF on 15th July 1915 for one years' service. He had previously had 12 months service as a captain in the AAMC Reserve at the Port Pirie Training Area. He was described as 5ft 9ins tall weighing 11st 6lbs, and was able to ride. He was initially posted to the 2 AGH in Egypt and was taken on strength on the 9th September 1915. He then proceeded to 1 AGH at the Heliopolis Red Cross Hospital in Cairo on 30th September 1915. He was posted for duty to 1 FdAmb in France on 1st August 1916. He returned to Australia on the *Kanowna* from Southampton for completion of his 12 months service on 23rd September 1916. His appointment was terminated on 20th November 1916, with the following warning; *"This Officer should be informed that the termination of his appointment in AIF does not relieve him from duty when required."* His appointment in the AAMC Reserve was also terminated. Dawson had some concerns with the return of his personal effects from the AIF and engaged in several letters with the military to recover his belongings. He was issued the 1914-15 Star, the British War Medal and the Victory Medal.

Dawson went back to Port Pirie for two more years on his return from the war. During this time he was involved in an inquest of a Mrs Fletcher, who died as a result of domestic violence, from Port Pirie on 21st November 1916 and was reported in the *Adelaide Advertiser* the following day. *"Dr Dean Dawson said the woman had a deep cut extending from the back of the neck and continuing towards the left ear. Her condition was serious from loss of blood and shock. Immediate attendance on the spot might have given her a chance".* He moved back to Adelaide with his family in 1919, and set up a practice at Clarence Park and North Terrace, Adelaide. He then moved with his wife to Mount Lofty where, after a year's illness, he died on 18th March 1939 aged 58 years. He was buried at Mitcham Cemetery. He was survived by his wife Lorna and their four children, two sons and two daughters. His wife lived until the 9th December 1971.

Sources:

The Adelaide Advertiser Monday 20th March 1939, p15.
http:nla.gov.au/nla.news-article74405379
The Adelaide Advertiser 22nd November 1916.
National Archives
http://recordsearch.naa.gov.au/scripts/Imagine.asp?B=3493117
Photo: Adelaide University Archives; 1905 Graduates
Person Family Records

† DEANE Edward Wilkinson

MD (Melb)

1872 - 1916

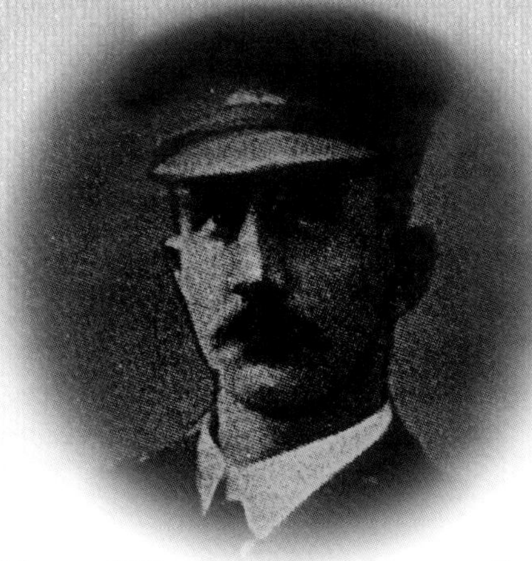

Edward Wilkinson Deane was born in Lancaster, England on 11th March 1872. He came to South Australia at the age of two years and attended Prince Alfred College, Adelaide. He moved to Victoria and he attended Geelong College and studied medicine at Melbourne University graduating in 1895 with MD ChB. He became a senior resident surgeon at the Melbourne Hospital and subsequently a senior resident at the Alfred Hospital. He started a private practice at Kaniva and later Maryborough in Victoria in 1898. He married Ada Maude Wilcox of Auburn, SA in 1897 and they lived at Park Road, Maryborough.

Deane enlisted in the AIF on 10th May 1915. He was described as 43 years old and a British subject. He was 5ft 10ins tall and weighed 150lbs. His next of kin was his wife. He was posted to 1 AGH at Heliopolis. He was admitted to 1 AGH with a bladder infection on 29th February 1916 and was deemed temporarily unfit for duty and to be returned to Australia. He was transferred to 3 AGH at Abbassia and his wife was informed that he was dangerously ill. He died of gastritis and acute cystitis on 4th April 1916. His leather trunk containing all his belongs was despatched back to Australia in November 1916. His wife received his medals, the 1914-15 star, the British War Medal and the Victory Medal in 1922. She also received a memorial plaque and a pamphlet "Where the Australians Rest". Edward Wilkinson Deane was buried in the Cairo British Cemetery in Egypt.

Sources:
National Archives
http://recordsearch.naa.gov.au/scripts/Imagine.asp?B=3495308
http://trove.nla.gov.au/ndp/del/article/74507247?searchTerm=EdwardWilkinsonDeane&searchLimits=

After visiting the Wardroom I returned to No. 1 theatre and found that the stretcher party had returned from the upper bridge… It had been a difficult place to get at however with the aid of a Neil-Robertson folding stretcher it had been achieved with no great loss of time. This stretcher by the way was found to be most useful and well adapted to a ship of this class with steep stairways and narrow passages and hatchways. The wounded man was Hoy AB RN he was working the range finder on the fore bridge when it was struck by a shell which did not explode. His left leg had been shot away at its junction with the body and was a horrible sight. He had lost a tremendous amount of blood and was almost dead on arrival below. I sent for Surg. Todd and got the patients clothes cut away rapidly and had him placed on the operating table.

…Cease fire sounded at 11.15 am after we had been working two solid hours in a very confined atmosphere and a temperature of 110°. The strain had been tremendous and SBS Mullins who had done wonderfully well with me started off to faint but a drink of brandy saved him and I was very glad of a similar drink at the time. Our clothes we [sic] saturated in blood and perspiration and altogether it had been a terrific two hours of high tension… The wardroom now contained eleven (11) cases and most of them were restless and groaning in agony. The initial dose of morphia, in no case less than gr ½ had been of slight value and I have good reason to suppose that the solution in the ampules supplied had deteriorated. Fresh doses of morphia were administered and iced water soda water and brandy to various cases as thought fit…

…During the action the space below seemed like a mad inferno. The tube was full of men belonging to the ammunition and fire parties and at the best of times there is little room here so the constant supply of wounded men was considerably hindered… At one time we keeled over, and the operating table with Hoy upon it took charge. It seemed as though we had been hit but it was only a sudden alteration of course as we soon discovered.

Excerpt from the record by
LEONARD DARBY, M.B., Ch.B. S.M.0. Surgeon, R.A.N
On the medical experience of the Action with SMS Emden of Cocos Isle Nov. 9th 1914

DOLLING Charles Edward

MB BS

1886 - 1936

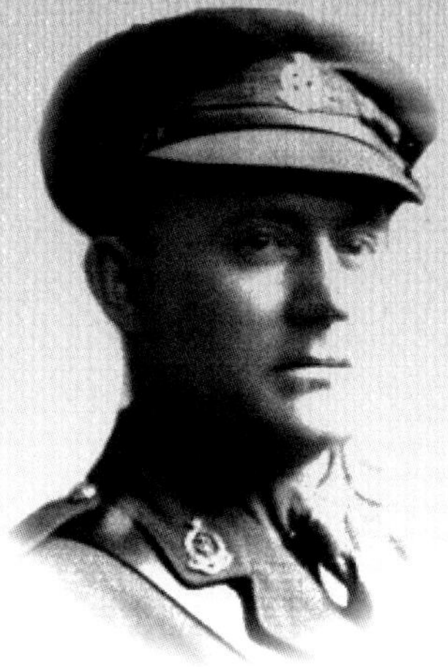

Charles (Charlie) Edward Dolling was born on the 4th September 1886 in Wokurna, SA. His parents were Johann Gustav Dolling and Minna Marie, nee Spoehr. He was educated at the Way College, Prince Alfred College in Adelaide and studied medicine at the University of Adelaide graduating in 1911. He began his medical career at the Adelaide Hospital. He moved to country practices in Minlaton and then Streaky Bay, SA in 1912. He took a position at Guy's Hospital, London, England in December 1914.

Dolling joined the RAMC as a captain on 6th July 1915. He served in Egypt and France and lost all of his instruments when undergoing a hasty retreat on the Western Front.

Dolling continued medical practice in England and Wales after the war until his return to South Australia in 1921 when set up a medical practice on Port Road, Hindmarsh, which continued until 1934. He married Dorothy Eleanor Ethel Victoria Georgina Barber Scott on 13th February 1923, at St Pauls Anglican Church in Adelaide. She was the only daughter of Edgar Scott and Alice Jane, nee Clarke; she was born in Dunedin New Zealand. Dorothy Dolling was a notable person in her own right and, though unusual for a woman of her time, taught mathematics and physics at the University of Leeds in England before coming to Adelaide. She also worked as a journalist and community worker in Adelaide. She was the treasurer of the South Australian Country Women's Association and was well known for her community work. Dolling travelled with his wife to Europe to study dermatology in Vienna and London in 1934. On return from England he set up a practice as a skin specialist on North Terrace, Adelaide. Dolling was a first class cricketer for South Australia with a batting average of 71. He was an Australian Cricket selector and he took part in the selection of the Australian Cricket XI for the Test matches in England in 1934. Charles Edward Dolling died following a stroke in his surgery in 11th June 1936 at 50 years of age. Dorothy Dolling continued to be a leading figure in community service in Adelaide after his death. She was on the committee to establish the Pioneer Women's Memorial garden adjacent to Torrens Parade Ground in Adelaide. She developed an interest in aviation and became the State President of the Royal Flying Doctor Service. In 1944 she was awarded an OBE and died 27 June 1967.

Sources:
Dolling Alison M., Dolling, Dorothy Eleanor Ethel Victoria Georgina Barber, (1897 -1967), Australian Dictionary of Biography
http://www.cricketarchive.com/SouthAustralia/Players/15/15951/15951.html
http://www.london-gazette.co.uk/issues/31530/supplements/10976

DORSCH Carl Emil

MB ChB (Edin)

1897 - 1938

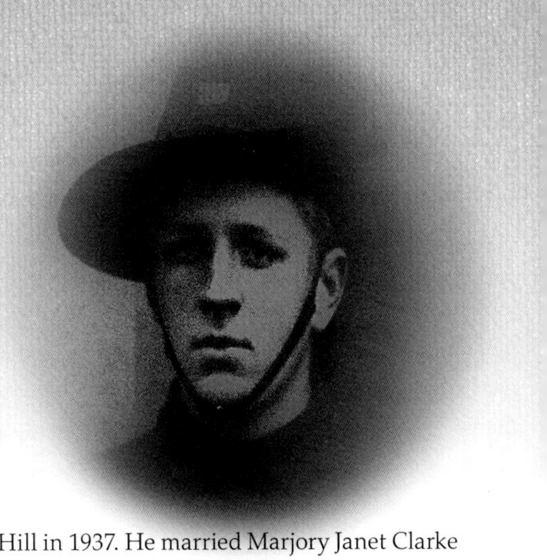

Carl Emil Dorsch was born in Adelaide, South Australia on 13th May 1897. His parents were Reverend Caspar Dorsch and his second wife Agnes, nee Heyne, of Clifton Street, Prospect. They had eight children and his father had five children from his previous marriage. Dorsch's father later suffered health problems leaving his mother to be responsible for this large family. His mother, Agnes, was an academically brilliant woman with a Bachelor of Arts (with Honours). The children were assisted in their study as their mother enabled them to gain scholarships to support their education. Dorsch, like his brothers, was educated at Prince Alfred College and studied medicine at the University of Adelaide. The girls were educated at Tormore House at North Adelaide.

Dorsch enlisted in the AIF on 17th June 1918 when he was a second year medical student. He had served in the Senior Cadets for four years and had then transferred to the Citizen Military Force. He was 5ft 8ins tall and weighed 170lbs, of fair complexion with blue eyes and fair hair. He was allocated to the AAMC Reinforcements at Mitcham Camp as a private. He embarked in Adelaide on *SS Gaika* on 6th August 1918 for the United Kingdom disembarking in London on 13th October 1918. He developed influenza and was admitted to hospital on 28th October 1918 and was discharged to the AAMC Training Depot on 5th November. He was posted to the 3 AAH at Dartford on 2nd December 1918. He was again in hospital from the 16th to 24th February 1919 and he was sent to London and was discharged in London on 11th September 1919. It is stated in his discharge documentation that he received the British War Medal but elsewhere it is indicated he was not entitled to any service medals.

Dorsch completed his medical studies at Edinburgh University after discharge. He was awarded a medical degree ad eundem gradum in Adelaide. He was practising in Loxton in 1931 and was practising in Broken Hill in 1937. He married Marjory Janet Clarke on 3rd October 1936. Carl Emil Dorsch died on 31st July 1938 in Loxton. Members of the Dorsch family between them won five Tennyson Medals for English Literature.

Sources:

National Archives of Australia.
The Chronicle of 17th December 1931, 4th August 1938
Adelaide News 27th December 1929
The Adelaide Advertiser 23November 1917, 5th January 1937
Biographical Indexes of South Australia.

Waterloo

One hundred years have passed away since the battle of Waterloo was fought on June 18th 1815, and Napoleon's power finally crushed by the British army under Wellington, aided by that of Prussia under Bluecher. After the lapse of a century we see the same combatants, differently grouped as allies, again locked in a life and death struggle… During the present war a dozen battles have been fought beside each of which Waterloo seems but a skirmish. The battle of Waterloo was lost and won in one long summer day, or, if we include the preliminary battle of Quatre Bras, in three days. The numbers engaged were about 70,000 on each side, the British and allied casualties about 27,000, the French about the same. These numbers are small compared to the first battle of Ypres, fought through October and November of last year, which lasted some six weeks, and in which the casualties on both sides together are said to have amounted to about half a million. Yet Waterloo settled the destinies of Europe for about half a century; can the present titanic struggle do more?

BMJ, 19 June 1915, p. 1050

DOWLING Donald Augustus

OBE MB BS DPH

1896 - 1979

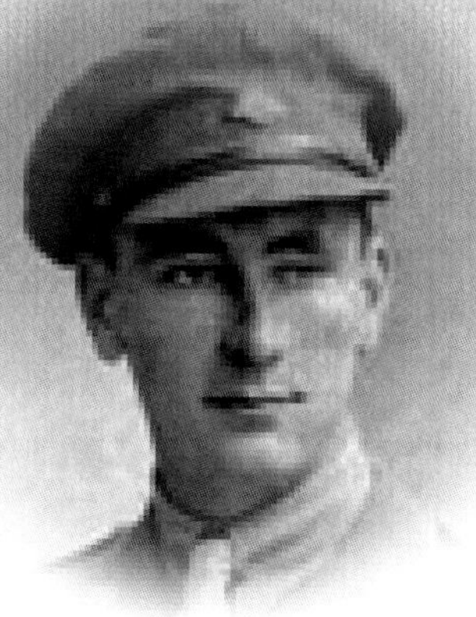

Donald Augustus Dowling was born on the 7th July 1896 at Farina, South Australia. He was the son of James Patrick Dowling of Manoora, SA. He was educated at Port Pirie and gained a bursary to Adelaide High School where he was a fine athlete in football, cricket and rowing. He began medicine at University of Adelaide in 1914 and rowed in the university eight.

Dowling enlisted in the AIF, on 14th September 1914, at Morphettville, as a 19 year old medical student. He had 2 years experience in the 50th AAMC and was a private soldier. His father gave permission for him to join and was named his next of kin. He was described as 5ft 10ins, 160lbs, of fair complexion with blue eyes and fair hair. He had four vaccination marks on his left arm. Dowling was posted to B section of 4 FdAmb. His unit proceeded, on the 12th April 1915, to join the MEF for the landing at Gallipoli. Whilst there he was hospitalised twice first with a dental problem and then in July with gastroenteritis but returned to duty and served with them until the end of the Gallipoli Campaign. He was promoted Lance Corporal in 1916 and transferred to a brief course as a Cadet with the 6th Officers Bn at Balliol College, Oxford. He was commissioned in November 1916 as a 2nd lieutenant and proceeded to France with the 27th Infantry Bn and served with them throughout 1917 and 1918. He was wounded in September 1917 in Belgium and from Rouen transferred to the 3rd London General Hospital with a gunshot wound to the neck. After 2 months care in November he returned to France and later served as the Brigade Gas Officer with the 7th Inf. Bde. Dowling returned to Australia in September 1918 with his appointment terminated in the 4 MD on the 22nd January 1919. He was issued with the 1914-15 Star, the British War medal and the Victory Medal.

Dowling resumed his medical studies at the University of Adelaide in 1919 graduating in 1923. He also gained sports blues in lacrosse and rowing and held executive positions in University sporting clubs and the Adelaide Medical Student Society. He then became a resident at the Adelaide Hospital. He entered private practice and returned to London in 1927 for further study. He joined the Commonwealth Department of Health as a medical officer at Port Adelaide in 1928 followed with a Diploma of Public Health and Tropical Disease from the Sydney University in 1933. He then continued as a Medical Officer on quarantine duties across Australia until 1946 followed by three years as Chief Medical Officer at Australia House, London. This led to a period of senior positions as the Australian Delegate to World Health Assemblies until 1951 when he returned to Australia. He was appointed as Commonwealth Medical Officer for Queensland until his retirement in 1960. Dowling's interest in sport and public life was sustained in Brisbane; he was a delegate to the Australian Olympic Federation, and the manager of the Australian Swimming Team to South Africa in 1959. He served on several industry and war appeal tribunals, and was a President of the AMA, Queensland Branch. He was appointed OBE in 1952. He was made a Fellow of the Australian Medical Association in 1978. Donald Augustus Dowling died in Brisbane aged 83 years on the 8th March 1979.

Sources:
http://recordsearch.naa.gov.au/scripts/Imagine.asp?B=3519026
AWM: P08858-013
MJA: December 1st1979.p598-589

DOWNEY Michael Henry

DSO MB BS (Melb) LRCP LRCS (Edin)

1877 - 1933

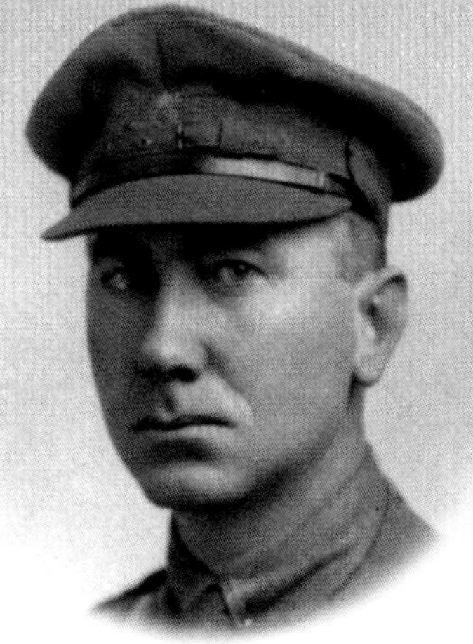

Michael Henry Downey was born on 20th October 1877 in Toolleen, Victoria. He was the son of farmer William Downey and his wife Ann, nee Lynch. He went to Echuca Grammar School and later began medicine at the University of Melbourne in 1896. During his school years he joined the Victorian Rangers, which was a citizen military organisation. He joined the University Officers Corps at the University of Melbourne in 1898. Before completion of his MB BS he moved to the University of Edinburgh where he completed his LRCP, LRCS in 1901. He served in the Boer War in 1902 at Cape Colony and at the western Transvaal as surgeon to the RAMC. Downey then returned to the University of Melbourne and completed his MB BS in 1904. He showed an interest in mental diseases and studied with Sir Thomas Clouston whilst in Edinburgh. He continued this interest in Melbourne with William Beatie and, on the 15th June 1905, was appointed assistant resident medical officer at Parkside Mental Asylum in Adelaide, South Australia. He lectured in psychiatry at the University of Adelaide in 1912, and in 1914, on the retirement of Dr C L Cleland, he became the Superintendent of the Parkside Mental Asylum. Downey continued his military service in the Reserve in South Australia and, in 1909, was commissioned as a captain in the AAMC. He was promoted to major in 1912 and lieutenant colonel in 1915.

Downey joined the AIF on the 10th February 1916 and posted in command of the 11 FdAmb. After initial training in England 11 FdAmb was sent to France in November 1916 to take over the rest station at Steenwerck. Downey was admitted to hospital with bronchitis on 10th February 1917 and returned to duty later that month. During the battle of Messines on 7th June 1917 he was awarded the DSO for his ability as a leader in the evacuation of the 3000 wounded from the Advance Dressing Station at Kandahar Farm. He was posted as ADMS to the 5th Division as temporary Colonel in October 1917, and confirmed as Colonel on 26th April 1918. He was Mentioned in Despatches three times including a special mention in General Haig's despatches for distinguished and gallant services and devotion to duty in the field on the 8 November 1918. He returned to Australia in June 1919. Downey was issued with the 1914-15 Star, the British War Medal and Victory Medal with Oak Leaves.

Downey continued his career in the Reserve and commanded the 6th Cavalry Field ambulance from 1920 until he retired from the Army in 1926. After the war he went back to his work at Parkside Mental Hospital and continued to give lectures and examinations in psychiatry at the University of Adelaide. It was said that he had an *'orderly brain'*, was slow to make decisions but once made never altered his mind and was rarely wrong. Michael Henry Downey died at the early age of 56 years from a heart attack at Calvary Hospital North Adelaide on 17 April 1933. There are two buildings at Glenside Hospital named in his honour; Downey House and Downey Grove. He was survived by his wife Eva Agnes, nee O'Brien and their son Don.

Sources:
http://anzacsonline.net au/2012/03downey-michael-henry-dso. Parkside Historical Society,
Fielding, Jean P. 'Downey, Michael Henry (1877–1933)',
Photo: AWM H19198
http://adb.anu.edu.au/biography/downey-michael-henry-6009/text10267 .
http://recordsearch.naa.gov.au/scripts/Imagine.asp?B=3520095

DREW Charles Francis

MC MB BS

1888 - 1960

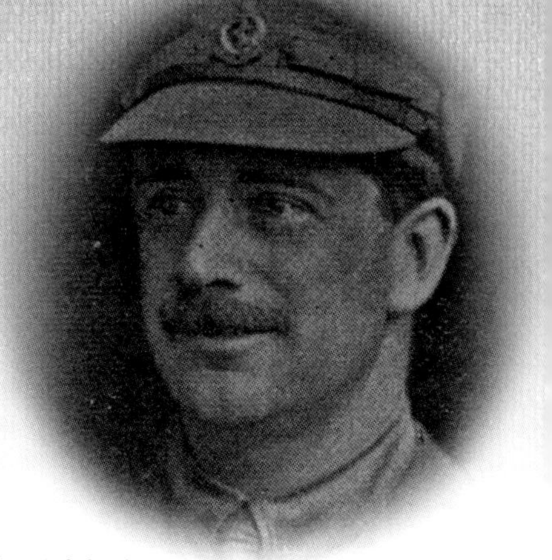

Charles Francis Drew was born on the 24th April 1888 at Kooringa, Burra. He was the son of Thomas and Catherine, nee Symons, one of 11 children all born at Burra. He was educated at Prince Alfred College and studied medicine at the University of Adelaide, graduating in 1911. He excelled in sporting achievements as an undergraduate. He was the first "triple blue" in Adelaide, played League football with North Adelaide and represented South Australia in cricket as a right hand bat. After graduation he joined in a practice with Henry Arthur Powell in Kadina for 18 months, with the intention to go to England for further study.

Drew decided to go directly to England after the declaration of war and joined the RAMC in 1915. His war service was distinguished. He served in Advanced Dressing Stations in France for the whole of the war, except for a spell of six months spent in a Base Hospital. When in the line he served with the Guards divisions. He attained the rank of major and was Mentioned in Despatches in 1917. He was awarded the Military Cross in 1918 and finally was attached to the Army of Occupation, based at Cologne.

Drew returned to Adelaide in 1920 and married Mary Isobel Gall, on the 27th April 1921, daughter of T B Gall, solicitor, at All Saints Church, St Peters. He acquired the practice of Dr Gregerson at Hindmarsh in 1921 and worked as a GP in that area for the rest of his working life. He was held in high regard by his professional colleagues especially for his medical ethics. He was a councillor of the South Australian branch of the BMA from 1939-1943 and declined the nomination as President as he could not spare the time away from his practice. He did find time however for leisure with tennis and golf. He was living in John Street, Hindmarsh in the 1930s. During WW2 he conducted the practice of two of his associates in Hindmarsh who had gone on active service; this was a strain on his health which he accepted uncomplainingly. Charles Francis Drew died in Adelaide on the 19th February 1960, aged 71 years. He was survived by his wife and two sons, the younger of whom was also a member of the medical profession.

Sources:

MJA: April 30th 1960 p 709,
Photo; PAC Collection.
The Adelaide Advertiser 14 Dec 1911
The Adelaide Advertiser 14 Aug 1936

Bacilli and Bullets

What I wish to urge is a true knowledge of your foes, not simply of the bullets, but of the much more important enemy – the bacilli. In the wars of the world they have been as Saul and David – the one slaying thousands, the other tens of thousands… It is bitter enough to lose thousands of the best of our young men in a hideous war, but it adds terribly to the tragedy to think that more than one-half of the losses may be due to preventable disease. Typhus fever, malaria, cholera, enteric and dysentery have won more victories that powder and shot.

An address to the Officers and Men in the Camps at Churn
By Sir William Osler – Regius Professor of Medicine, Oxford
BMJ, 3 October 1914, p. 569

DUGUID Charles

OBE MA MB ChB FRACS

1884 - 1986

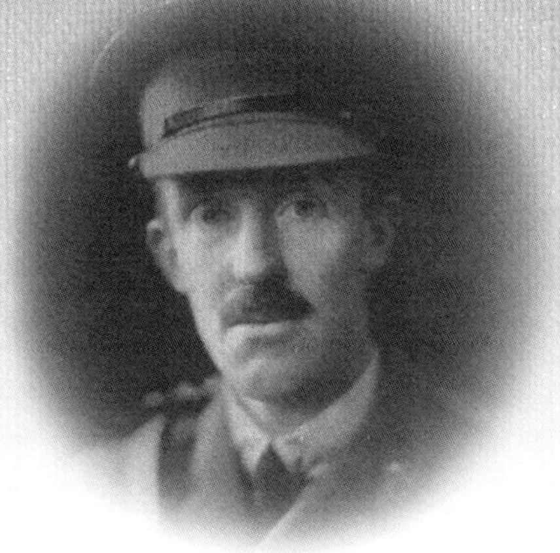

Charles Duguid was born on the 6th April 1884 in Saltcoats, County Ayr, Scotland the eldest child of Charles Duguid a school teacher and Jane, nee Kinnier. He attended Glasgow High School and University of Glasgow graduating with MA (1905) MB, Ch.B (1909). He served in the Territorial Force from 1904 to 1906 whilst at University. He left Scotland for Australia as a ships medical officer in 1911. During the journey he met and became engaged to Irene Isabella Young who was travelling back to Australia. He immigrated to Australia the following year working his passage as a ships surgeon. He married Irene on 23 October 1912 in Melbourne and took up a practice in Minyip, Wimmera before moving to Adelaide in 1914.

Duguid enlisted in the AIF aged 32 years as a Captain in the AAMC on 12th February 1917. His service was relatively short but he was sent to the Middle East moving between 2 AH at El-Arish, 3 LHTH at Moascar and 14 AFGH at Abbas Sin. He was returned to Australia on 17th July 1917 for a posting to 4 MD in Adelaide and his appointment terminated on 5th December 1917. Nevertheless he wrote about his experiences in two publications; *From the Suez Canal to Gaza with the Australian Light Horse* (1917?), and *The Desert Trail* (1919).

Duguid set up a general practice in Magill on his return to Adelaide, and also worked as a surgeon at the Memorial Hospital, Adelaide. He was active in local branches of the RSL, Legacy and Toc H. He returned to the United Kingdom for further study in 1927. His wife died suddenly at sea whilst returning to Australia with their son. He returned to Australia and in 1930 married Phyllis Evelyn Lade. He was elected as a fellow of the Royal Australasian College of Surgeons in 1930. Duguid became interested in the plight of aboriginal health and in 1934 he went to Darwin to see for himself. When he arrived in Alice Springs by train he was asked to perform emergency surgery. He missed his connection to Darwin and stayed in Alice Springs for 3 weeks. During this time he was appalled by the treatment of the Aborigines and so began his lifelong work in the protection of Aborigines. Duguid became the first lay moderator of the Presbyterian Church in South Australia and the President of the Aborigines Protection League in 1935. He went on to investigate conditions for Aborigines in the Musgrave Ranges in South Australia. Duguid was again appalled and with RM Williams journeyed to Ernabella and met the Pitjantjatjara people resulting in a Christian mission to serve as a *"buffer between the Aborigines and the encroaching white man"*. He provided medical care with the view that the responsibility be passed to the local people as soon as possible. Duguid strongly and publically criticised the British proposal to test guided weapons from a base at Woomera and resigned from the Aborigines Protection Board when it approved the proposal. Duguid was president of the District and Bush Nursing Society in South Australia from 1944 -1960. He was awarded the OBE in 1971. He received a letter from the Ernabella people requesting that on his death his body be buried at the mission, *"so that the Aboriginals will always remember that he was one of us and that he faithfully helped us"*, in 1972. He supported the Pitjantjatjara people in their claim for land rights in 1980 which was granted in 1981. Charles Duguid died on 5th December 1986 in Kent Town and was buried in the Ernabella Mission cemetery. He was survived by his second wife, their son and daughter and his son from his first marriage.

Sources:

Photo; SLSA

http://recordsearch.naa.gov.au/scripts/Imagine.asp?B=3525322

Edwards WH., 'Duguid, Charles (1884–1986)', Australian Dictionary of Biography, National Centre of Biography, Australian National University, http://adb.anu.edu.au/biography/duguid-charles-12440/text22369.

DUNSTAN Harold Frank

MB BS BSc

1890 - 1953

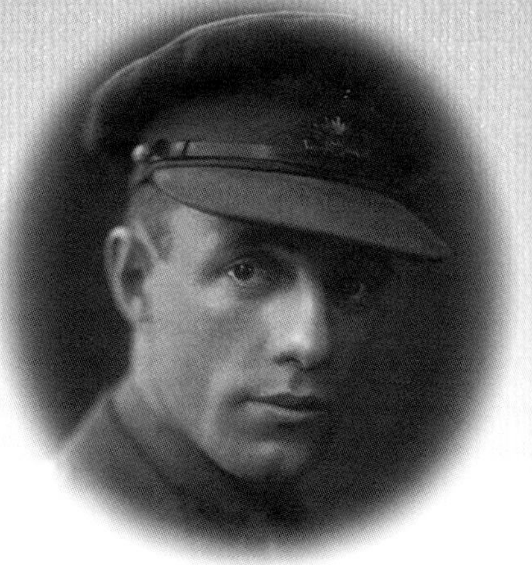

Harold Frank Dunstan (Kollosche) was born at Semaphore, South Australia on the 3rd March 1890, the eldest son of John Kollosche and Bayliss, nee Dunstan of Croydon Park, South Australia. His father was formerly a school master at Clare. Dunstan studied medicine at the University of Adelaide. It was during his university years that he changed his name from Kollosche to Dunstan, his mother's maiden name. He graduated in 1914.

Dunstan enlisted in the AIF at Adelaide on 1st March 1916 at the age of 26 years. He had 3 months experience in the AAMC Reserve from the 1st December 1915. He was 5ft 10ins, and weighed 150lbs. He was appointed as a captain in 11 FdAmb. He embarked, after three months training, on the 31st May 1916. His unit was sent to France in December and moved into the front line near Armentieres where they spent a very bleak winter. Dunstan was evacuated to hospital for over five weeks with bronchitis In January 1917. On return to duty his unit was sent to Belgian Flanders where Dunstan took part in the Battle of Messines in June and distinguished himself. He was recommended for a Military Cross but this was downgraded to a Mention in Despatches. He was attached to the 3rd Brigade after the battle, an artillery unit, for four days as Acting Regimental Medical Officer. He was involved in the Battle of Broodeseinde Ridge on the 4th October 1917. The 11 FdAmb was earmarked to take part in the Battle of Passchendaele on the 12th October and Dunstan moved to the forward area to make medical arrangements for the coming battle. While in the forward area, he received a gunshot wound to his abdomen on the 11th October. The bullet penetrating to his right thigh and he was evacuated to 3rd London General Hospital in England. Dunstan was invalided to Australia in January 1918 aboard the *Dunluce Castle,* transhipped to the *Karoola* at Cape Town in February. He disembarked at Melbourne on the 10th March and proceeded by rail to Adelaide where he was discharged from the AIF on the 5th October 1918. He was issued with the British War Medal and Victory Medal with Oak Leaves.

Dunstan worked in general practice in Renmark from 1919-1928 and then moved to Prospect where he remained until 1948 when he was admitted to the Repatriation Hospital. After a long illness Harold Frank Dunstan died on the 8th August 1953. He was survived by his wife and three sons; John of Melbourne, Dr Richard Dunstan of Grange and Dean Dunstan of Crafers. Another son, Thomas E, Dunstan was killed serving with the 2nd AIF in the Pacific.

Sources:

Photo....http://recordsearch.naa.gov.au/scripts/Imagine.asp?B=3529495.

RSL, Renmark.

Kollosche Family personal interview.

DUNSTONE Leonard John

JP MB ChB

1880 - 1962

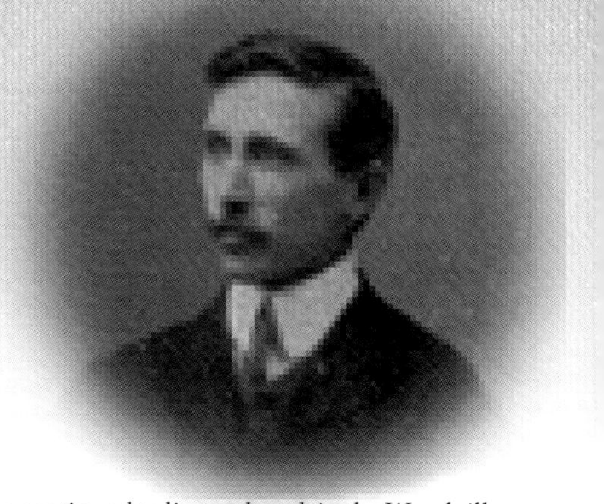

Leonard John Dunstone was born on the 3rd December 1880 in Port Augusta, son of John Dunstone, an accountant. They later moved to Largs Bay. He was educated at Prince Alfred College and studied medicine at the University of Glasgow, Scotland. He graduated MB ChB in 1907. Dunstone returned to Australia, and took up a medical practice in Lameroo, South Australia. He married Stella Marion Salter at the Lockleys Baptist Church in August 1912. She was the only daughter of Mr MH Salter of Lockleys, South Australia.

At the start of WW1 and on the 1st February 1915 he was appointed as the District Naval Medical Officer at Port Adelaide. Dunstone also joined the AAMC Reserve, 4 MD, as an honorary captain on the 22nd May 1916. He continued with the Navy and was promoted to surgeon lieutenant commander in 1924 and surgeon commander RANR in 1930. He was subsequently transferred to the retired list in 1935 but re-engaged under the National Security Regulations for 2 years from November 1943.

Dunstone continued to live and work in the Woodville and Port Adelaide areas of South Australia after the war. He lived on Woodville Road, Woodville. Dunstone was fined for exceeding the speed limit of 15 MPH in St Vincent Street, Port Adelaide on the 17th January 1919. He was a Divisional Surgeon for St John Ambulance, an Honorable Surgeon for Woodville Volunteer Fire Brigade for 15 years and president of the South Australia Operatic Society. Leonard John Dunstone died on 5th August 1961 in Malvern. He was survived by his wife and son.

Sources:

http://www.universitystory.gla.ac.uk/browse-graduates/?start=820&max=20&o=&l=d

Trove

http://trove.nla.gov.au/ndp/del/article/5336013?searchTerm=LeonardJohnDunstone&searchLimits=l-title=34

http://archive.org/stream/armylistoctvol31917grea#page/120/mode/2up/search/dunstone

Who's Who South Australia 1936

Interview of son of John Dunstone

Experiences with the AAMC at Gallipoli by John Corbin

I exchanged into the Clearing Hospital with Captain Mattei...I obtained a senior position in the unit, and some opportunity of obtaining surgical work.Owing to the weather, I believe, our starting was postponed until the 24th of April, when we left Mudros at 11am...Everyone was on deck, and as the grey of the coming dawn became less dense, we turned in towards the Gallipoli Peninsula and slowly crept in towards the land...Concentration on your own job and total disregard of the other fellow was the only way the whole thing got pieced together and was carried through. Fortunately, we had work to do from the moment of landing, and no room for fear...During those first four days 3,300wounded passed through our hands. We gave up recording them, as our only book was filled up on the first day, and simply counted them. During this time all urgent operations were done, including necessary amputations, tying of arteries, several belly cases, depressed, compound fractures of skull, bladder cases and big compound fractures of the thigh. All these necessitated anaesthetics, which were administered in nearly every instance by non-commissioned officers or by privates... The men of the [1st Australian] Casualty Clearing Station behaved in the most exemplary manner. The beach... was described by men in the fighting here as the most "unhealthy" spot in the whole position. I can vouch for the unpleasantness of life upon it...in 18 weeks there were only five days in which no shrapnel was fired on it.

MJA, 5 February 1916, p. 111-114

EAST Edwin Charles

FRCS(Ed) MRCS (Eng) LRCP (Lond)

1881 - 1961

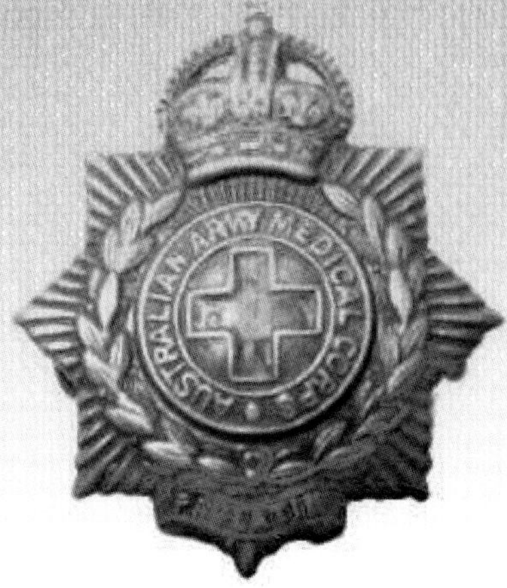

Edwin Charles East was born on the 24th June 1881 in King's Norton, Worcestershire, fourth of the five sons of a builder, Edward James East, and his wife Elizabeth, nee Main. East started work as a dispenser, and then progressed to medical school. After obtaining his licence, he worked in the Queen's Hospital in Birmingham until he was able to sit for the FRCS Edinburgh examination in 1913. Having passed the examination he looked for a wider horizon, and migrated to Australia. He and his wife Beatrice were fined 1/- (20 cents) and costs of 16/-($1.60) by the Gawler SM for failing to enrol in accordance with the Commonwealth Electoral Act. He was in a practice in North Adelaide, South Australia in 1914.

East was commissioned in May 1915 and allotted to 1 AGH Reinforcements. He was 34 years old, married with his wife, care of JH Bennett, Daly St, Gawler, named as his next of kin. He was 5ft 8ins, and weighed 146lbs. He sailed from Melbourne for Egypt in June 1915. In December he was posted to 2 ASH at West Mudros, but his time with this unit was brief. Back in Egypt in January 1916 he was transferred to 1 ACCS, which left for France in March. The unit opened at Estaires in support of I ANZAC Corps. It played no part in the management of casualties after the Battle of Fromelles, and spent the year largely in expansion and consolidation. East was recalled to England in October, and posted for several months to 3 AAH at Dartford. He returned to Australia at his own request in February 1917 with his appointment terminated on the 28th April 1917. He settled in Fremantle, Western Australia. He was issued with the 1914-15 Star, the British War Medal and the Victory Medal.

East took over the practice of Dr Landon in Perth Western Australia. He was appointed as an HMO at the Fremantle Hospital from 1917-1941, initially as a General Practitioner who acted as a surgeon and physician. He was always available for Residents to leave the Hospital premises and later a member of the Board. In 1922 East volunteered for the RANR and was appointed a surgeon lieutenant. He served until 1926, when he was placed on the Retired List. He purchased Woodside Hospital, 18 Dalgety St, East Fremantle for £3,000 in December 1926. It was built as a home in 1896 by the Hon William Dalgety Moore MLC (1835-1910), and converted to a private hospital in 1924. It continued to operate as such until 1945, and is now Heritage Listed. East also built Haslam House (since demolished) in Queen St, Perth which became the site of Brands Department Store. He was prominent in the social and sporting life of the community as a senior member of the management committees of the Fremantle Public Hospital Board, the Royal Fremantle Club, the Fremantle Association, the Fremantle Club and the Fremantle Tennis Club. Edwin Charles East died in Fremantle in 1961. He was survived by his 3 children, June, Vaughn and John.

Sources:
http://recordsearch.naa.gov.au/scripts/Imagine.asp?B=3532647
Likeman R., From the Tropics to the Desert, Slouch Hat Publications, Port Melbourne, 2012
Stubbe J.H., Being a History of Fremantle Hospitals and Doctors with Appendix - The Fremantle Hospital 1897-1967, University of Western Australia Press, 1969.

† ELLIS John Chute

MRCS (Eng) LRCP (Lond)

1886 - 1917

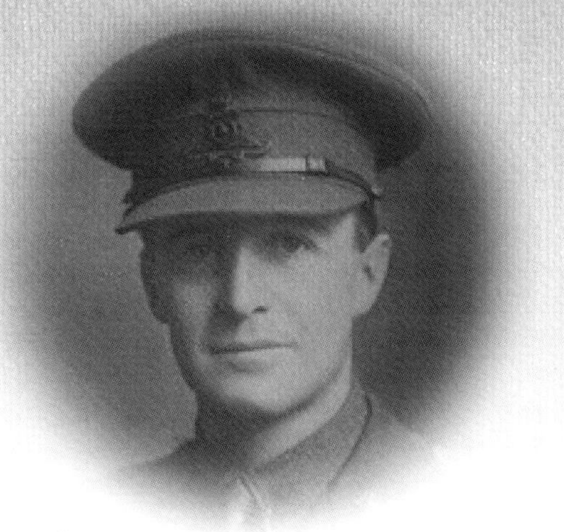

John Chute Ellis, was born in Mount Gambier the third and youngest son of. T. C. Ellis, of Benara, one of the early members of the old South Australian Provincial Council who was born near Adelaide on the old Port Gawler and Hummocks Station in 1848. Ellis spent his boyhood at Mount Gambier, and began his education at the Rev. Hartley Williams's Grammar school; and finished it at Christ College, Christchurch, New Zealand. He studied medicine at the Dunedin University followed by four years in London.

He and his two brothers were joint owners of Eremeran and Burrabogie stations in the Murrumbidgee District of New South Wales, his place of residence being Burrabogie. He returned to Mt Gambier in September 1915 to see his father and be farewelled by the town and his friends before returning to England to join in the 106th Brigade Royal Field Artillery as a combatant. He had already received an appointment through The London Hospital. John Ellis died of war wounds in Belgium on the 6th June 1917 and is interred in Lijssenthoek Military Cemetery, Belgium.

Sources:

National Centre of Biography, Australian National University,' Ellis, John Chute (1886–1917)', Obituaries Australia, http://oa.anu.edu.au/obituary/ellis-john-chute-350/text351

Photo: http://nla.gov.au/nla.cs-pa-http%253A%252F%252Fcas.awm.gov.au%252Fphotograph%252FP07904.001

Extracts from the Diary of Major John Corbin No 1 Stationary Hospital

December 5th [1914]–Left Melbourne 6pm SS *Kyarra*

January 1st–Everything dirty-dirty food, dirty linen, dirty servants...orders come out and are contradicted, continually verbally.

January 14th–Entered into Alexandria

January 16th–Still no news as regards destination

Saturday 24th April–Left Mudros Harbour at 11am. Steamed out with Piper's Band playing cheerily at my suggestion through the remaining ships and round to a rendezvous on the North side of Island...We are to be fed at 3.30am, start landing at 5am.

Monday 26th April – Worked continuously to 8am...Had a bathe under fire and come out refreshed and invigorated to work on until 8.50, then on to 12.30 hard at it.

Saturday 1st May – 304 Wounded – It is extraordinary how phlegmatic one becomes, the risk of being hit becomes such a usual thing that you cease to regard it a possibility.

Wednesday 5th May–145 Wounded Fleet Surgeon McMillan still sends us bread. You cannot imagine the comfort this is instead of biscuits. Our food is plentiful but plain. It is amazing what one can eat and enjoy when hungry. I devoured a slab of stale crust with Marmalade at 1230 am.

Friday 14th May – Up and a swim, which certainly bucks one up greatly...General Birdwood got a scratch on the top of his scalp this evening. I shaved and dressed it. If it had been two inches lower and a full bullet it would have been nasty.

Wednesday 16th June- While dressing a patient a man stopped on the beach to look over the canvas screen alongside me. He gave a grunt as a shell burst, and fell down. I looked over and found his chest blown in by the casing and quite dead.

Wednesday 23rd June – Went for a walk on my lonesome to read a letter from "Mum-O", which came this morning, with papers and a pair of socks, also photograph on "M" in evening dress, very ripping it is. While on the hillside I saw the beach being bombarded and especially in the neighbourhood of the Hospital.

Source: Anne Stott (Corbin family)

FLECKER Hugo

MB BS FRCS(Ed) FFR FRCRA LRCP

1884 - 1957

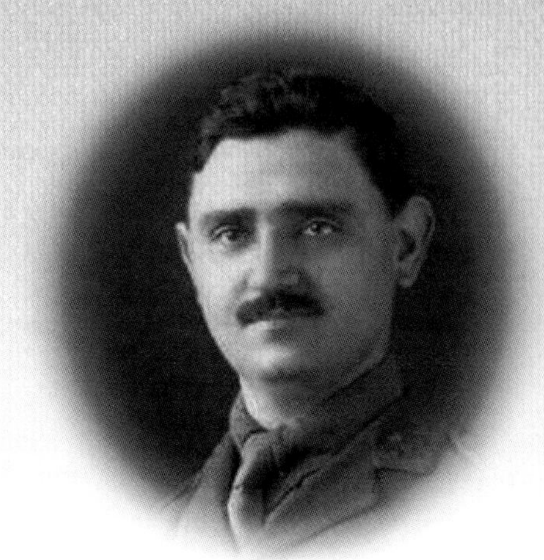

Hugo Flecker was born on 7th December 1884 at Prahran, Melbourne, Victoria third son of George Flecker and Emma, nee Ziffer. They moved to Adelaide where his father managed the South Australian Hotel. Flecker was educated at Prince Alfred College and initially began medicine at the University of Adelaide in 1904 but transferred to Sydney University where he graduated MB in 1908. He then went to England and gained his LRCP and became a fellow of the Royal College of Surgeons, Edinburgh in 1912. Flecker returned to Sydney and undertook several positions including as a demonstrator in anatomy at Sydney University. He was an honorary physician at the Mater Misericordia Hospital and in general practice in Neutral Bay.

Flecker joined the AAMC militia prior to WW1 as Captain and enlisted in the AIF on 20th August 1914, the first week of the war. He was attached for duty with 27 Bn. He was 30 years old, and described as a British born subject, 5ft 6ins tall, weighed 11st 6lbs. He was recorded as single and his mother Mrs Emma Flecker is recorded as his next of kin. However he had a girlfriend Miss Thelma Arnold, later to be his wife, in Lindfield, NSW, who was also to be notified of any changes in his circumstances. He embarked on the *Ayrshire* on 20th Dec 1914 and served initially with 7 LH in Egypt. He was then transferred to 1 AGH on 16th April 1915 and proceeded to Marseilles, France and then transferred to 37 Bn in August 1916. He was posted to the 6 FdAmb in October 1916. He was promoted to major on 1st January 1916. He became ill with dermatitis in January 1917 and his mother was informed that he was in the 14th General Hospital. He returned to duty in Australia in April 1917. He was issued with the 1914-15 Star, the British War Medal and the Victory Medal.

Almost immediately on his return to Australia Flecker married Thelma Arnold on 21st April 1917. He remained in the Reserve of Officers and commenced a practice in Temora, NSW. He set up a practice in Collins St, Melbourne in 1921 as a radiologist and was an honorary radiologist at the Austin Hospital for Incurables. He was also responsible for the change of name of the hospital to the Austin Hospital for Chronic Diseases. Flecker and his family moved to Cairns in Queensland in 1932 where he continued as a radiologist/radiotherapist. He gained his diploma of Radiology in 1937 and became fellow of the Faculty of Radiology (England) in 1939. He was amongst the first Australian radiologists to employ deep X-ray therapies. Flecker was a keen naturalist renowned for his research on the effect of scorpions, snakes and marine venom on humans. His life work is commemorated in the names of a number of rare species including the world's most poisonous creature the 'box jellyfish', *Chironex fleckeri*. Flecker continued with his military service and served during WW2 enlisting on 10th February 1942 at the age of 57 years. He was posted to 116 AGH and served throughout the Second World War in Queensland and Horn Island in the Torres Strait. He was admitted to 116 AGH with Dengue Fever in 1942. He was transferred to the Reserve of Officers in August 1942. Flecker's son, Patrick Oscar Flecker, also a doctor, enlisted during WW2. Flecker was a prominent Freemason and a member of Legacy. Hugo Flecker died on the 25th June 1957 in Cairns and was survived by his wife Thelma and his son and daughter. He was posthumously award the JP Thomson medal of the RGSA in the year of his death. The Flecker Botanic Gardens, Cairns, were named in his honour in 1971.

Sources:

http://recordsearch.naa.gov/NAAMedia/ShowImage.asp?B=4913001&S=18&T=R

http://farnothrqueenslandsgottalent.blogspot.dom.au/2012/06/flecker-dr-hugo.html

Pearn John H., 'Flecker, Hugo (1884–1957)', Australian Dictionary of Biography, National Centre of Biography, Australian National University.

Obituary, Medical Journal of Australia November 30 1057 p 808/9.

Ryan J, Sutton K, Baigent M, 'Australian Radiology A History' McGraw Hill Books Australia Pty Ltd, 1996

FLEMING Thomas Gordon

MC MB BS

1888 - 1946

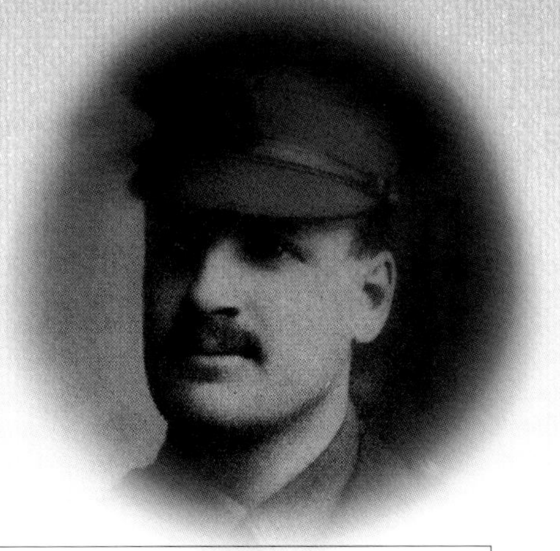

Thomas Gordon Fleming was born at Parkside, South Australia in 16th April 1888. He was the youngest son of a solicitor Thomas Wilson Fleming SM and Fanny Ellen, nee Everett. He was educated at Prince Alfred College and studied medicine at the University of Adelaide and graduated MB BS in 1909. He worked one year at the Adelaide Hospital and then took up a practice for the next two years at Hawker, South Australia.

Fleming travelled to England in 1913 for postgraduate studies and enlisted as a lieutenant in the RAMC on the day that war was declared, before completing his studies. He went to France in February 1915, was promoted to captain and appointed to the divisional staff of the Army Director of Medical Services. He was Mentioned in Despatches twice and awarded a Military Cross for bravery during the Somme offensive. He was later promoted to major. After the war, due to war injuries and a serious illness, he was unable to complete his postgraduate studies and returned to Australia.

Fleming took up a medical practice in Goodwood, South Australia. He continued to have problems with his health for the rest of his life. He appeared not to have married. Thomas Gordon Fleming died on 12th January 1946.

Sources:

http://discoverhttp://discovery.nationalarchives.gov.uk/SearchUI/Details?uri=C1074870y.nationalarchives.gov.uk/SearchUI/Details?uri=D3497490

Photo: Adelaide University Archives; Medical Students 1906

The Advertiser 13th January 1946

http://histfam.familysearch.org/getperson.php?personID=I152688&tree=SouthAustralia

Experiences with the AAMC at Gallipoli by John Corbin

It is sufficient to describe the trip on the *Kyarra,* which carried five hospital units from Australia, as one of great discomfort, lasting six weeks before we arrived at Alexandria...With regards to the sickness prevalent, a great deal of it was due, in my opinion, to the fact that measles occurred on nearly every transport carrying troops from Australia to Egypt, and in practically every camp, coupled with the fact that influenza was also prevalent in the same manner... the No. 1 Australian Stationary Hospital disembarked on the 23rd of January...we were sent to Maadi, an English suburb of Cairo... half this hospital was detached on the 27th of January, under Major Powell, for duty at Ismalia. Colonel Bryant detailed Major Newland and Captain Verco to accompany the half unit, and there was much sadness in the hearts of Wilson, Le Messurier and myself who were left behind to attend to the measles, coughs, colds and venereal cases at Maadi.

...We arrived at the harbour of Mudros on the 6th of March, a huge land-locked harbour, surrounded by bare, undulating country, with occasional high stony hills...the scene ashore was like a piece from a comic opera. The small quay was crammed with soldiers of every description: British territorials, Navy men, French territorials, with officers in the most splendid uniform, ditto their naval men. Heaps of Zouaves, in their fanciful uniform, Senegalese, big black men of fine physique, in elaborate uniform, chattering Greek peasants in a variety of national garbs and, through them all, the husky Australian, swearing, grumbling and rough to look at, but doing more work than any equal number of other troops...

MJA, 5 February 1916, p. 111-114

FLOOD John Wellesley

MB ChB BA BAO (Dublin)

1883 - 1929

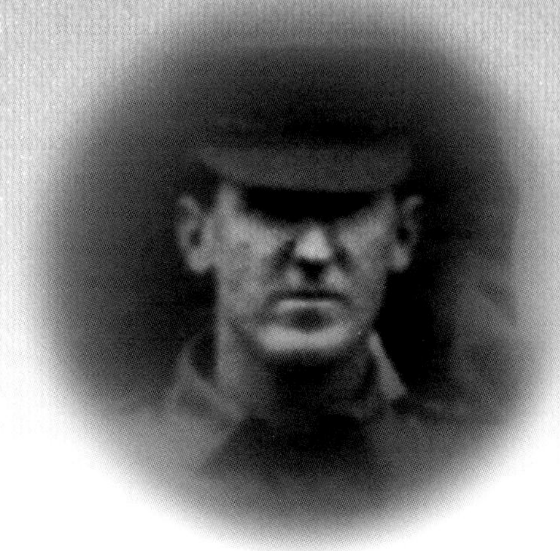

John Wellesley Flood was born at Yorketown, South Australia. He was the second son of Dr John W Flood and his wife Annie, nee Cammell. He was educated at St Peter's College and studied medicine at Trinity College, Dublin. Whilst overseas, aged 23 years, he married Rose Elise Coombs in a Registry Office, London on the 17th July 1907. Flood returned to Australia after graduation and set up practice first at Blyth, SA and then at Brinkworth.

Flood served in the Citizens Force in 4 MD, where he was on the Reserve of Officers. He enlisted in the AN & MEF in November 1914 and served in New Guinea. He travelled to Madang with a group of seven doctors under the command of Cecil Strangman. He was sent to Herbertshöhe (present day Kokopo) on arrival, where there was a large Native Hospital to run. Flood remained there until March 1915, when he was moved to Rabaul. Malaria control and the securing of clean drinking water were the primary objectives. Flood was made temporary major in March 1916, and in April 1917 he went on furlough to Australia, returning in August on the *Matunga* with Lieutenant Colonel Strangman and several other officers of the administration in New Guinea. The ship failed to arrive in Rabaul on time, and after a general search was posted missing, presumed lost. It was seized by a German auxiliary cruiser, the *Wolf*, which had lain in wait for her after intercepting her wireless transmissions. The Officers, passengers and crew were taken on-board as prisoners of war and, in unusual circumstances, they were released among 467 prisoners from other captured ships, in Denmark in February 1918. The *Matunga* was eventually sunk by the *Wolf* after her cargo and coal were removed. The Officers and some American prisoners from the *SS Matunga* were given special privileges whilst POW's and were referred as the Wolf's "top deck Prisoners". After release from Denmark, Flood, his wife Rose and other prisoners went to London for rehabilitation. He was given a commission as major in the AIF and was posted to the 2 AAH in Southall England. He was posted to 2 ACCS in October 1918, which was at that time in the Armentières-Bethune area in support of General Birdwood's Fifth Army.

Flood was among the first to be repatriated as a former prisoner of war after the Armistice, and he left England for Australia in January 1919. After his arrival he was re-appointed to the AIF as PMO, and once again set sail for Rabaul from Sydney. This time he arrived safely, and took up his new position at the end of May. He was promoted lieutenant colonel in June 1919. Flood held this appointment until May 1921. Flood took up an appointment as GMO at Kokopo in East New Britain, and practised there until 1928. He then set up in private practice. He died of heart problems on 23rd March 1929 and is buried in the C of E portion of the Rabaul Cemetery leaving substantial debts. The Rabaul Times records that *"he took a lively interest in athletics and sports generally, being a cricketer of no mean ability; an excellent tennis player and a swimmer above the average. He was a keen judge of horses and an enthusiastic race goer. His loss seems irreparable professionally. There can be few that can surpass him in his knowledge of all tropical complaints, particularly malaria."* His wife Rose returned to England after his death; they had no children.

Sources:

http://recordsearch.naa.gov.au/scripts/Imagine.asp?B=4039255
Likeman R., 2010 'From the Tropics to the Desert', Slouch Hat Publications, Port Melbourne.
Guilliatt R., Hohnen P., "The Wolf", 2009.
Photo: AWM A02241 Flood at Rabaul, 1915.
Rabaul Times March 1929.

FOOKS Edward Verdon Russell

MRCS (Eng) LRCP (Lond)

1871 - 1922

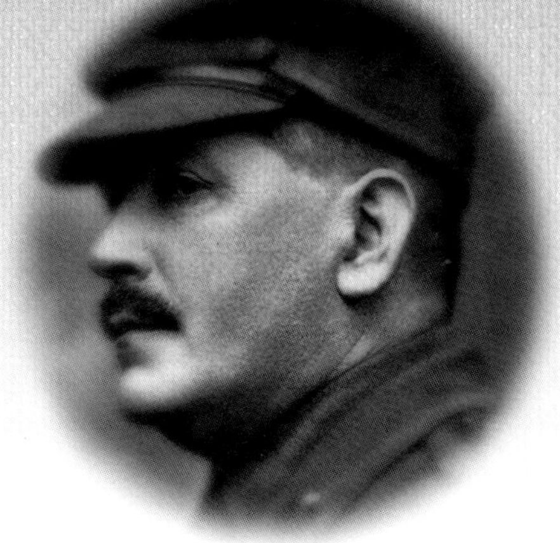

Edwin Verdon Russell Fooks was born on the 24th November 1871 at Otahuhu, Auckland, New Zealand. He was the son of William Pemberton Fooks of Auckland and grandson of William Haycroft Fooks QC, an English barrister. He was educated at Mercers School in England and studied medicine at Charing Cross Hospital graduating in 1894. He married Hilda Jane Maud Bains of York, England in 1901. Fooks had visited Australia previously, so in 1902, he and Hilda decided to settle in SA. They lived first at Lyndoch and subsequently at Gawler, where, in 1902, he was a public vaccinator and in 1903, appointed to attend to the destitute persons and aborigines in Barossa Valley (East and West wards). Due to his wife's health issues they moved to Adelaide in 1910. At the time he was President of the Gawler Bowling Club and in 1913 he became President of the Adelaide Bowling Club.

Fooks joined the British Forces as a lieutenant in the RAMC and was commissioned in January 1915. He served on a hospital ship and in France with 22 FdAmb, 7 Div from January – August 1915. He was permitted to resign his commission owing to the death of his child and was discharged in August 1915. Fooks returned to Australia and enlisted in the AIF on 22nd May 1916 in 4 MD Adelaide. He was 44 years old and his wife of 20 Clifton St, Goodwood and of 87 Wakefield St, Adelaide was named as his next of kin. He was 5ft 9ins tall, and weighed 14st. He could ride and noted previous hospital experience at St Saviours Infirmary, London. After embarkation from Adelaide on the 27th June 1916 Fooks was allotted to 2 AGH for one month and then 6 months with the 14 FdAmb. He went to the 3 ACCS in France from March 1917 until August 1917 when he was hospitalised with a fractured third left rib as well as prolonged enteritis. This was deemed to be a previous disposition aggravated by active service. He returned to Australia on the 14th March 1918 to the 7 AGH, Keswick and declared as *Medically Unfit for further Service* and his appointment was terminated on the 28th March 1918. After his incapacitation his wife and son of 87 Wakefield St, Adelaide, were respectively granted pensions of £1/1/3 and 10/- from the 29th March 1918. Fooks was issued with the 1914-15 Star, the British War Medal and the Victory Medal

He took over the practice of Dr William Thornborough Hayward on The Parade, Norwood for 2 years. He continued to suffer ill health so undertook several locum positions in country South Australia to build up his constitution. He became the medical officer for BHP in Whyalla SA. Edwin Verdon Russell Fooks died in Whyalla on the 5th October 1922 from heart failure aged 51 years. He was survived by his wife Hilda, son Walter and daughter Mary.

Sources:
http://recordsearch.naa.gov.au/scripts/Imagine.asp?B=3912717
NLA
The Register Adelaide 10 Aug 1906
Daily Herald Adelaide 5 Oct 1922

FRY Henry Kenneth

DSO MD BSc (Hons) BSc (Oxon) FRACP DPH (Oxon) Dip Anth (Oxon)

1886 - 1959

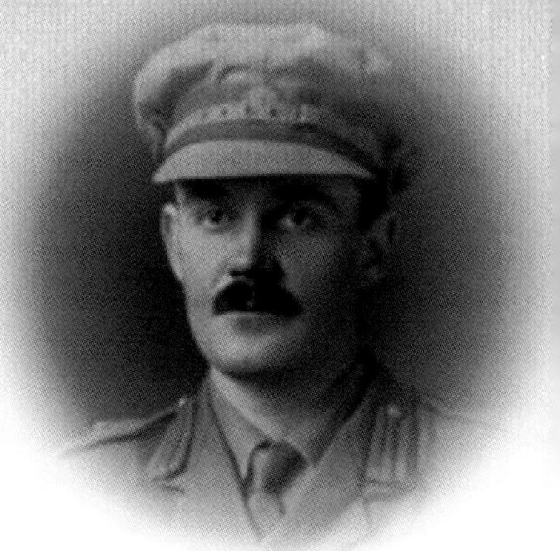

Henry Kenneth Fry was the fourth child of Henry Thomas Fry, a warehouseman, and his wife Margaret Hannah, nee Phillips. He was educated at Prince Alfred College and University of Adelaide where he excelled academically and at athletics, lacrosse and rowing. He graduated BSc (Hons) in physiology in 1905 and MB BS as Everard Scholar in 1908. His house surgeon year was at the Adelaide Hospital. He was Rhodes Scholar in 1909, and at Balliol, took another BSc and diplomas in Public Health and Anthropology. He returned to Australia and took up the post of Chief Medical Inspector of Aborigines in Darwin.

Fry enlisted in the AIF as a captain in August 1914. He indicated 3 years previous experience as a private soldier in King Edward's Horse and as surgeon captain in 79 Infantry Bn. He was single at the time of enlistment and his brother, NS Fry of Henley Beach, was named as next of kin. He was 5ft 8ins" and weighed 144lbs. He sailed for the Middle East with 3 FdAmb in October 1914 on the *Medic*. He landed at Gallipoli, with his bearers at Ari Burnu, on 25th April 1915. Surviving a storm of shots, he established his ADS in the vicinity of the Sphinx. He was later to establish ADS at Shrapnel and Victoria Gullies. As temporary major he was the Divisional Sanitary Officer from 3rd September 1915. He returned to Egypt in November with scurvy before returning to Gallipoli. Substantively promoted to major he was appointed DADMS for 2 Div. He served in this capacity throughout the battles of the Somme where he was decorated with the DSO for his achievements at Pozieres and Sausage Valley where he *was constantly under shellfire superintending and arranging the evacuation of the wounded....throughout the campaign similar thoroughness of work has been his characteristic.* He was promoted lieutenant colonel and given command of 13 FdAmb in October 1917. He married Dorothy Editha Deeley, during leave home, in the Church of the Epiphany, Crafers on 21st October 1918. He returned to France in December as honorary colonel, ADMS 5 Div. He had been Mentioned in Despatches 3 times.

He returned to Australia and established a general practice in Eastwood; the practice had a laboratory, surgery and X-Ray facility. He was to develop three distinct strands to his remarkable career. Firstly as a physician with an interest in therapeutics and psychiatry, secondly as an anthropologist and thirdly as a public health medical officer. He was initially honorary assistant physician at the Adelaide Hospital, later honorary physician; he lectured medical students in 'materia medica' and therapeutics (he wrote a small textbook on the subject).He promoted the use of the new antibiotic sulphonamides in the treatment of pneumonia and patients were admitted preferentially under his care. He was awarded MD (Adel) and was a foundation fellow of the RACP. He was physician to the Parkside Mental Hospital. He was a member and later President (1939) of the Royal Society of South Australia, established with others, the Board for Anthropological Research, and participated in numerous medical, anthropological and ethnological research expeditions to central Australia. He was the Medical Officer of Health for the City of Adelaide for over 20 years. He promoted the concept of mass chest X-rays and formulated plans for implementation in Adelaide and later SA. He tried to enlist again in WW2 but his employer, the City of Adelaide, refused to release him. Fry was a man of high ideals and filled several offices giving him opportunities of community service. He was a quiet, devoted and sincere worker and a sound and efficient administrator. Henry Kenneth Fry died on 22nd July 1959 and was survived by his wife, son and daughter.

Sources:
National Archives
http://recordsearch.naa.gov.au/NameSearch/Interface/ItemDetail.aspx?Barcode=4001291
Jones Philip 'Fry, Henry Kenneth' (1886–1959), Australian Dictionary of Biography, Vol. 14 (MUP) 1996
http://adb.anu.edu.au/biography/fry-henry-kenneth-10256

GARDNER John Forrest
MB BS

1890 - 1929

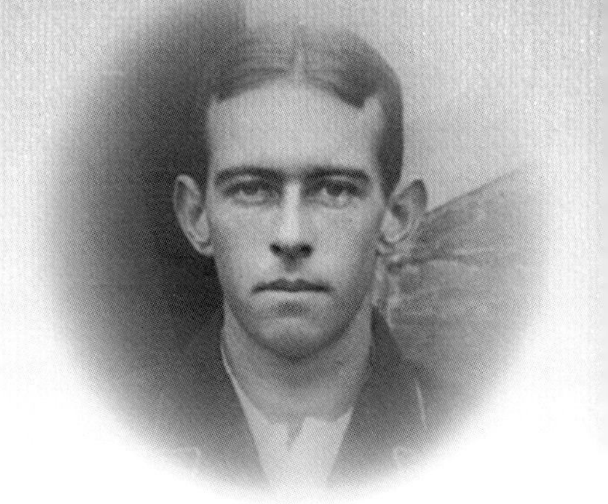

John Forrest Gardener was born on the 30th July 1890 in Adelaide. He was the younger son of Gavin J and Mary Josephine Gardner. He was educated at St Peter's College and studied medicine at the University of Adelaide graduating in December 1914. He lived with his parents at Trinity Street, College Park, South Australia.

Gardner enlisted in the AIF on 4th April 1916 at 25 years of age. His father, whose address was given as the Stock Exchange, Adelaide, was named as his next of kin. He had 2½ years experience in the Commonwealth Cadet Corp and 3 months in the AAMC. He was 5ft 11ins tall, weighed 142lbs, of fair complexion, grey eyes and dark hair. He was posted, as a captain, to the AAMC Transport Staff. Gardner undertook two Transport Trips from Melbourne to Suez and returning with invalided soldiers, between the 28th January 1916 and the 22nd July 1916. His appointment was terminated on the 23rd July 1916. He was issued with the British War Medal and the Victory Medal.

Gardner moved to Richmond, Victoria after the war. He married Hilda Josephine Florey from Mitcham, SA on 17th February 1917. She was the older sister of Howard Florey, whom he had met at the Adelaide University. Hilda Josephine Florey was born in 1890 at Malvern, South Australia. After leaving Miss Thornber's School for Girls, she entered the University of Adelaide in 1908, and graduated MB BS in 1912 and was an outstanding student. She held resident appointments at the Adelaide Hospital, the Adelaide Children's Hospital, and the Women's Hospital, Melbourne between 1913 and 1917. John Forrest Gardener died in Richmond Victoria at the beginning of August 1929 from tetanus. He was survived by his wife and his daughter, Joan, who became a distinguished microbiologist with a special interest in antibiotics, sterilisation and infection control. Gardner also had a son who died of septicaemia at the age of seven.

Sources:
Photo: Adelaide University Archives; 1912 Intervarsity Tennis team.
http://recordsearch.naa.gov.au/scripts/Imagine.asp?B=4028102
http://www.racp.edu.au/page/library/college-roll/college-roll-detail&id=395
The Adelaide Mail 27th December 1919.

Dearth of Doctors

The departure of so many senior men and the filling up of their places on hospital and university staffs, and still more the drain on the recently qualified members of our profession, have produced such an effect that it is well-nigh impossible to obtain qualified house-surgeons. The Adelaide Hospital is partly manned by fifth year students, whilst the Children's Hospital has to be content with third year men as resident clinical assistants; vacations have been dispensed with, and examinations have been held earlier so that students may become qualified in four and a half years instead of five, the understanding being that those who are eligible immediately enter on active military service. Meanwhile, too, the authorities are refusing to enrol medical students in any capacity, it being considered more important for them to complete their course and take a degree.

BMJ, 6 November 1915, p. 691

GAULT Arthur Kyle

MB BS

1894 - 1955

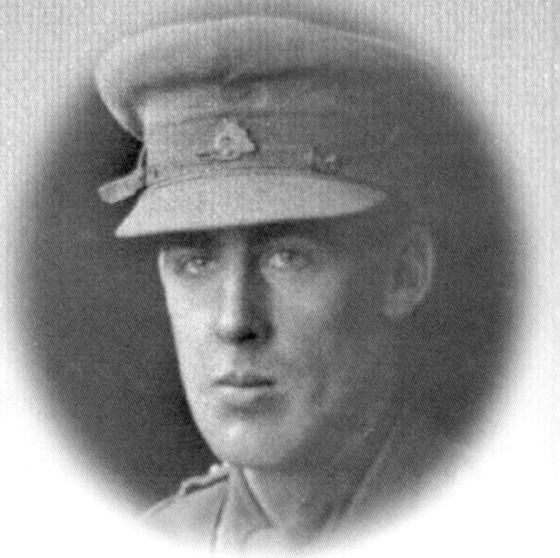

Arthur Kyle Gault was born on July 10th 1894 at Mitcham South Australia. He was the son of Dr Arthur Henry Gault (1864-1917) and Mary, nee Steele. Gault's father arrived in Mitcham in 1888, aged 24, and carried out his practice from a house called "Ardmeen" on Unley Road which had five acres of gardens, a tennis court, milking cow, chickens and horse stables. It is now better known as "Lenzerheide", a popular restaurant. Gault was educated at Prince Alfred College and studied medicine at the University of Adelaide where he enjoyed lacrosse and tennis

Gault enlisted in the AIF at Morphettville on the 19th August 1914 as a 4th year Medical Student. He had previous experience of 2 years in the AMC reserve. He was 20 years of age, 5ft10ins, weighed 155lbs, of dark complexion, blue eyes and brown hair. Gault was attached to "B " Section 3 FdAmb. He went with the unit to Gallipoli where he suffered a gunshot wound to the lower jaw on 1st June 1915 at Gaba Tepe. He was admitted to 1 AGH at Heliopolis and was repatriated to Australia on 28th July 1915 weighing only 62 lbs. According to family records his return to Australia was expedited by Professor Archibald Watson. It was deemed by the Military Medical Board on the 30th November 1915 that he was permanently unfit for Military Service. He was refused a military pension and he resumed his medical studies at the University of Adelaide. However after his graduation in July 1917, Gault enlisted again as a captain in the AAMC having completed 1 year and 107 days in the AIF of which 310 days were in overseas service. He now was deemed fit for re-enlistment. He embarked for Liverpool from Sydney 8th August 1917. He served as an MO in 2 Com Depot in Weymouth and was taken off strength in October when he requested and was granted leave to return to Australia because of the sudden death of his father. He returned to the 4 MD after Transport Duty with his appointment terminated on the 13th August 1918. Gault was issued with the 1914-15 Star, the British War Medal and the Victory Medal.

Gault took over his father's practice and in 1921 he married Ruth Hawker of Bungaree Station, Clare. His marriage to Ruth ended in divorce and he later married Evelyn. He retired suddenly in 1950. He left his assistant Dr Ken Crafter in charge after his retirement. The practice grew to include 5 doctors, and became known as the Sturt Clinic. Eventually the practice moved into a new building next door. It was renamed "The Crafter Medical Centre" in honour of Dr Crafter. Arthur Kyle Gault died on 7th April 1955 of a ruptured aneurysm and was cremated at West Terrace Cemetery and laid to rest with his parents in Mitcham Cemetery. He was survived by his former wife Ruth Marjorie Hawker and three children Richard, Yolanda and Avril. On the corner of Belair and Angus Roads, Memorial Gardens, Hawthorn stands a *"DR. A. KYLE GAULT MEMORIAL FOUNTAIN DONATED BY CITIZENS OF MITCHAM 1957."*

Sources:

http://recordsearch.naa.gov.au/scripts/Imagine.asp?B=4028450

Photo: AWM, 16073.

Ramsey AL., Gault Family History publication, Ch2.

GEORGE Mildred May

MB BS

1888 - 1933

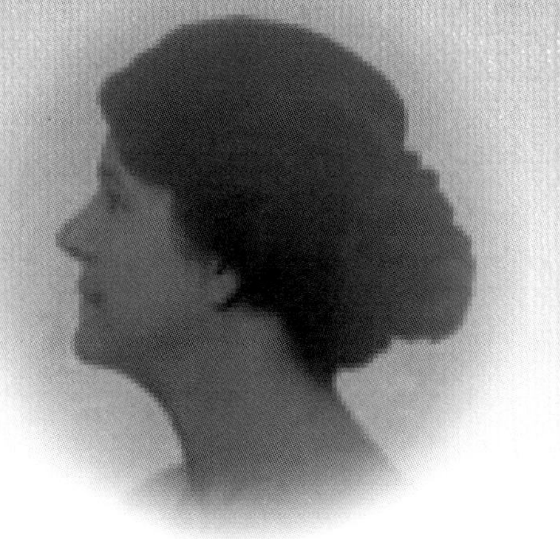

Mildred May George was born on 1st February 1888 the eldest daughter of W. J. George. She had one sister who was 14 years younger. She attended Sturt Street School where she was awarded an open bursary. She studied medicine at the University of Adelaide and graduated with MB BS in 1914. Her address is recorded as Riverton, South Australia. There is very little record of her life before WW1. During the period of the war she was appointed to the rank of captain and remained as a resident medical officer at the Adelaide Hospital. There is no indication of how she was appointed to this rank, but the University accepted her service and included her on their WW1 Roll of Honour.

George started a private medical practice in Perth after the war in 1918, and married the Reverend George Thomas Caton on 31st August 1921. She was honorary assistant gynaecologist at the Perth Hospital in 1922. She was the assistant honorary physician for the outdoor department of the Children's Hospital for some years. She was a champion for child and women's protection and was the honorary medical officer to the Children's Protection society and lobbied the government for funding for the establishment of clinics for child welfare. She was also a life member of the St John Ambulance Association and a member of the executive of the Australian Red Cross Association. Mildred May George died at sea whilst travelling to London on the *Ascanius* in an area south of Madagascar on 4th February 1933. Her death has never been explained; she just disappeared on the night of 4th/5th February. She was survived by her husband, her sister and nephew, they had no children.

Sources:
University of Adelaide archives.
http://trove.nla.gov.au/newspaper/result?q=Mildred+May+George
Foster, Peter C, family personal interview.

The Rum Ration

The following physiological effects have been observed by military and naval officers to follow from the issue of the rum ration.

1. Decadence of *moral*. Causation of grousing, friction, and disorder.
2. Drunkenness. Punishments. Degradations in rank.
3. Decadence of observation and judgement. Causation of errors and accidents.
4. Loss of endurance and diminution of physical vigour. Causation of fatigue, falling out, and slackness.
5. Loss of resistance to cold. Causation of chilliness, misery, and frostbite.
6. Loss of resistance to disease (particularly those occurring under conditions of wet and cold), namely, pneumonia, dysentery, typhoid fever.
7. Loss of efficiency in shooting (Half the rum ration causes a loss of 40 to 50 per cent. In rifle shooting. The navy rum ration causes loss of 30 per cent in gunnery shooting).

That all these evils, and increase of the difficulties our men have already to contend against on active service, are the direct and invariable result of issuing the rum ration is of course well known, and it is incomprehensible that Lord Kitchener's repeatedly expressed hatred of the alcoholic curse of armies should have been overborne, yet such is the case and the nation and the army must suffer in proportion.

BMJ, 30 January 1915, p. 204

GETHING William John

LRCP LRCS (Edin) LRCP LRCS (Glas)

1862 - 1915

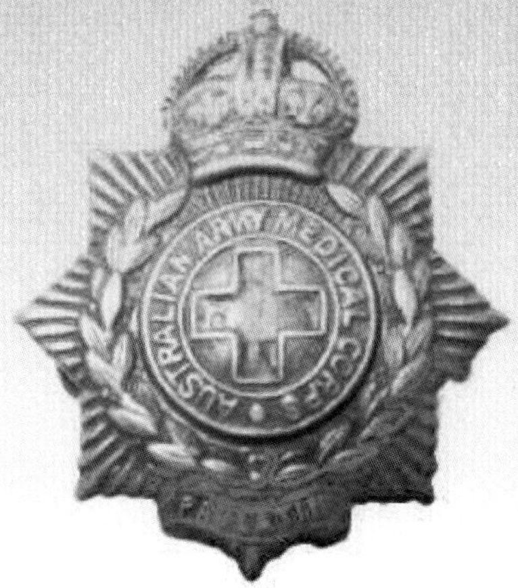

William John Gething was born at Port Adelaide SA on 8th September 1862. He was the eldest son of Dr Robert Gething and his wife Jane Tevanion, nee Toll, the daughter of chemist John Toll from Nairne, South Australia. Robert Gething had originated from Wales and qualified in medicine at Edinburgh University in 1847. Dr John Toll took over his practice later on his retirement. Gething was educated at Prince Alfred College. He left school at 17 years to begin legal training with George Downer at G&J Downer in Adelaide and was articled in 1880 for 5 years. When the Law Faculty at the University of Adelaide began in 1883 Gething enrolled in some subjects but was not required to complete his training. He was admitted to practice in 1885 and, at first practised at Port Adelaide and then set up practice as an agent for the Downers in Nairne. Gething, encouraged by his uncle Dr John Toll, studied medicine in Edinburgh and Glasgow from 1890 to 1894. He returned to Adelaide in 1895 and joined Dr John Toll's practice in Port Adelaide. He married Gertrude Rose in 1900 and they had a son and a daughter.

He joined the Volunteer Forces and the Port Adelaide Rifle Club as a student and became a Surgeon Lieutenant in the Medical Staff Corps of the South Australian Military Forces. He was promoted to captain in 1899. In January 1914 Gething became Chief Quarantine Officer and after the beginning of the war was appointed MO Permanent Troops Port Adelaide. William John Gething died after a short illness at 52 years of age on 22nd June 1915. He was survived by his wife and 2 children.

Australian Population WW1	4,870,000
Enlistments 416,809 = 8.5% of total population	
South Australian Population 1916	441,690
SA Enlistments 49,000 = 11% of total population	
Examined	34,959
Served overseas	27,770
Killed or discharged overseas	6,000
Casualties on the Western Front	
British and Empire	
Killed	1,000,000
Wounded	2,000,000
French	
Killed	1,250,000
Wounded	4,000,000
German and Austrian	
Killed	1,500,000
Wounded	3,500,000

Peter Last, *The Repat.* April 1994

Sources:

South Australian Register 18 March 1884, 29 March 1884, 19 February 1895
The Adelaide Advertiser 24 June 1915
http://histfam.familysearch.org/getperson.php?personID=I80795&tree=SouthAustralia

GILBERT Henry

MB BS FRCS FRACS LRCP (Lond)

1880 - 1947

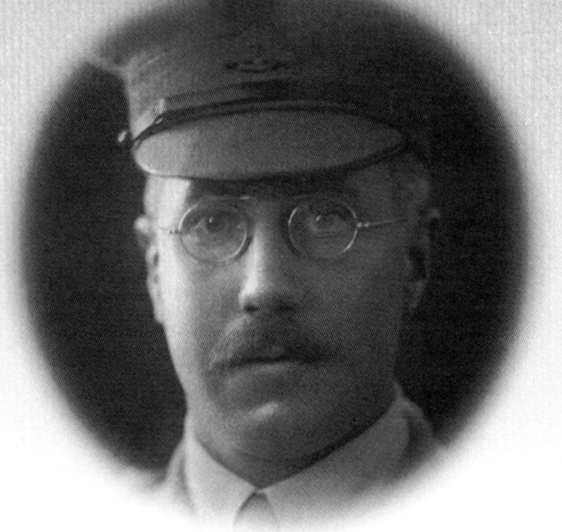

Henry Gilbert was born on 8th June 1880 at Pewsey Vale, Lyndoch in South Australia. He was the son of William Gilbert and the grandson of Joseph Gilbert, an eminent pastoralist in South Australia. He was educated at St Peter's College, and the Adelaide University and gained his MB BS at the University of Melbourne in 1901 due to the 'Adelaide Hospital Row'. After graduation he studied surgery in London and took the Fellowship of the Royal College of Surgeons in 1906. He became interested in the Opsonic Index and furthered this interest in Almroth Wright's laboratory at St Mary's Hospital, London. He went into general practice with Dr Humphrey Marten on his return to Adelaide in 1907. He was also a visiting surgeon to the Adelaide Children's Hospital.

Gilbert enlisted in the AAMC on 1st May 1915 at the age of 35 years and 10 months. He was unmarried and his father William was recorded as his next of kin. He was described as a British subject who could ride and was 5 ft 8ins tall, weighed 12st 10lbs. Gilbert embarked on HMAT *Geelong* for service as a medical officer on the transport ships. This appointment was terminated on 27th August 1915. He was re-appointed to the AIF on 28th April 1916 for duty with 1 AGH at Heliopolis. He was quickly re-appointed to transport ships in June of that year and returned to Australia from Egypt in July when his appointment was terminated on 27th July 1916. He was issued with the 1914-15 Star, the British War Medal and the Victory Medal. After the war Gilbert lodged a claim for a war gratuity based on his short service in Egypt, but this was refused.

Gilbert continued as an honorary staff member of the Adelaide Children's Hospital on return to Australia. He was a member and subsequently President of the Board of Management of the hospital. He was conferred Life Governorship of the Adelaide Children's Hospital in 1936. A wing of the Children's hospital was named the Gilbert Wing in his honour. He also served on the Council of the South Australian Branch of the British Medical Association and later became the President of the Medical Benevolent Association of South Australia. Gilbert had a long and active association with St Mark's College of Adelaide University. He retired prior to WW2 but returned to work to allow his younger colleagues to enlist. Gilbert was also a keen cricketer and slow bowler and formed a hospital cricket team in 1929. He married the granddaughter of Bishop Short, the first Anglican Bishop of Adelaide, and they had 2 sons who served in WW2. Henry Gilbert died suddenly in 27th October 1947 at the age of 67 years in his home on Le Fevre Terrace, North Adelaide and was survived by his widow, three sons and a daughter. He was described "as one of the State's most public spirited men"

Sources:

http://naa12.naa.gov.auB=5033756&S=6&T=R

The Medical Journal of Australia, January 23 1948, p 121/122.

Findlay M., 'Gilbert, Joseph (1800-1881)' Australian Dictionary of Biography, Vol 4 1972, http://adb.anu.edu.au/biography/gilbert-joseph-3610

Photo: SLSA GRG26_5_4_0_2289

The War: Some Immediate Duties

It is a clear duty of all members of the medical profession who remain at their ordinary civilian work to see that those medical men who have pledged themselves in advance to serve the country in any such emergency as has now arisen shall not suffer in their civilian practices, and that their patients shall be looked after. The country has to meet a situation such as it has never before been called upon to face for events moved less swiftly in the Napoleonic war and we must all stand by the men who are taking their places in the first fighting line.

BMJ, 8 August 1914, p. 307

GILLEN John Besley

MB BS DPM

1895 - 1937

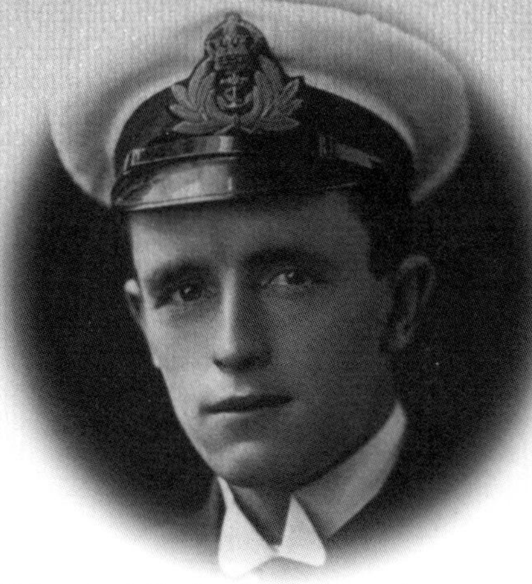

John Besley Gillen was born in Alice Springs on the 31st January 1895, the second son of Mr. F. J. Gillen, who was well known for his work with the Aborigines in Central Australia, and Amelia, nee Besley, daughter of a school teacher from Mount Gambier. Members of the Besley family were serving on the overland telegraph line. Gillen's father eventually became the Post Master of the Alice Springs Telegraph station and he was a Special Magistrate and Sub Protector of aborigines in the area. The family moved from Alice Springs to Moonta and eventually Port Pirie. Gillen had an early education at Moonta and Port Pirie and later boarded privately in Adelaide, and gained a Government bursary whilst a student with Hugh Cairns at the Adelaide High School. Gillen and Cairns were co dux of Adelaide High School in their final year. He studied medicine at the University of Adelaide and was the recipient of both the Elder Prize and the much-coveted Dr. Davies Thomas scholarship. He graduated in MB BS in 1917.

After graduating at the University of Adelaide, Gillen joined the Royal Australian Navy on the 20th November 1917 as a temporary surgeon lieutenant in the Permanent Naval Forces serving in HMAS *Cerberus* until March 1918 then the cruiser HMAS *Brisbane* and later in the Submarine Depot Ship HMAS *Platypus* from 1918 to 1920. HMAS *Brisbane's* complement was 31 officers and 454 sailors. The *Brisbane* was tasked to search for a German raider that was laying mines near the sea trade routes around Australia and New Zealand. The ship is known as the *Wolf* which in August 1917 captured the *Matunga* returning to Rabaul and retained Colonel Cecil Lucius Strangman and John Wellesley Flood as POW's. HMAS *Brisbane* returned to British waters until 17th April 1919, when she departed from Portsmouth for home. During the return trip, she caught up with the submarine depot ship HMAS *Platypus* and the six J class submarines transferred from the Royal Navy to the RAN after the war. J5 was experiencing problems, and HMAS *Brisbane* took the boat under tow; the two vessels reached Sydney on the 27th June 1919. All were sold before 1929. The cruiser was decommissioned on the 4th August 1922, and Gillen transferred to the Emergency List. He was issued with the British War Medal and the Victory Medal.

Gillen married Ellen McCann in 1920. After general practice in Morgan he joined Dr Tobin at Gawler, from whom he subsequently took over the practice. Gillen stayed in practice in Gawler until 1935. He became involved with the High School council at Gawler in 1929 and was a familiar figure on the local links and a keen tennis player. He had extensive involvement with the Gawler Jockey Club. He began a practice at Tusmore, a suburb of Adelaide, on leaving Gawler in 1935. Gillen was interested in psychiatry and went to England for further study. He gained his DPM in England and was to return to South Australia in November 1937. His success led to his wife, sister of the State Agent-General in London, making the trip overseas to join her husband expecting to share some time with him before coming home. John Besley Gillen died suddenly in London on September 6th 1937, as a result of a heart attack. Their children, Robert and Pamella, were attending school in Adelaide at the time. A letter on Sept 12th 1937 from Sir Hugh Cairns at Oxford to his widow said:–*Jack and I were class mates all through AHS and I know well what a sturdy and loyal man he was, it was a great pleasure to meet him here this year in London and learn of his great hopes and prospects for the future. It was characteristic of him to break away into new fields.*

Sources:
Wikipedia, Navy Lists WW1,
MJA October 2nd 1937 p 563;
Photos AWM: HMAS *Brisbane*, P01886 001.jpg
Photo and personal interviews with Dr R Gillen (son).
NAA: A6769, barcode 5225002

GODFREY Kirke Charles

JP MB BS

1888 - 1978

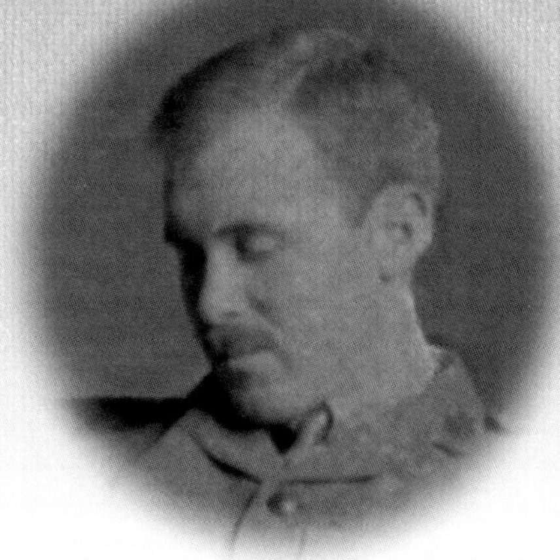

Kirke Charles Godfrey was born in Glenelg, South Australia on 8th March 1888. He was the son of Charles George Godfrey of Glenelg and his wife Mary Elizabeth, nee Kirkpatrick. Godfrey's father was the fourth member to join the Stock Exchange, his election had taken place on 27th January 1891. His father was also a fine opening bat and a notable cricketer in the eighties. He played in several international games. Godfrey attended St Peter's College in 1906 and studied medicine at the University of Adelaide graduating in May 1914.

Godfrey enlisted in the AIF and was commissioned on 1st May 1915 and allocated to 7 FdAmb. He was single, aged 27 years of Althorpe Place, Glenelg with his father of the same address named as his next of kin. He sailed the same month. On arrival in Egypt he was transferred to 2 AGH and sent to Mena Hospital. He did not go to Gallipoli with the rest of his unit. He was posted to 6 FdAmb in February 1916 and went to France with this unit in March 1916. During the Battle of Pozières in August, Godfrey was gassed, and evacuated to 4 LGH at Denmark Hill, London. As a result of this he became asthmatic, and was sent to No 2 Command Depot at Weymouth to await return to Australia for convalescence. He was taken off strength on the 12th November 1916 and sailed from Portland for Australia. Back in Australia he was passed as fit for Home Service only. He had served 624 days of which 579 were overseas. His appointment in the AIF was terminated on the 7th February 1917. Godfrey was issued with the 1914-15 Star, the British War Medal and the Victory Medal.

Godfrey married Beatrice Adelaide Gepp in the St Peter's College Chapel on 6th April 1918. She was the youngest daughter of the late Thomas Gepp, S.M., and Mrs. Gepp, of 'Hockky,' Kensington Gardens. He remained in South Australia in the near country of Mt Pleasant and Clare where he became a Justice of the Peace in January 1921. Godfrey eventually moved to Perth WA in the 1930s. Godfrey made a round trip to Singapore from Fremantle as ship's surgeon on board the *Centaur* in 1933. This ship's name became renowned in 1943 when as 2/3 AHS she was sunk off Point Danger, Queensland by a Japanese submarine. Godfrey's son Sgt David Kirke Godfrey, serving with 6 SQN RAAF as an air gunner, was shot down and killed over New Guinea in 1942. Godfrey became an anaesthetist, and joined the staff of Perth Public Hospital with his rooms in 222 St George's Tce and at 92 Thomas St, West Perth. He was elected to Honorary Membership of the Australian Society of Anaesthetists in 1961, recognising him as a pioneer specialist anaesthetist in Western Australia and a past president of the WA section of the society. Kirke Charles Godfrey died on the 13th November 1978.

Sources:
http://recordsearch.naa.gov.au/scripts/Imagine.asp?B=4818061
Photo, AWM.6060
The Daily Herald Adelaide 18 Dec 1914
The Mail Adelaide 24 November 1917
The Mirror Perth 15 July 1939
Ancestry.com

GOLDSMITH Frederick

MB BS

1867 - 1942

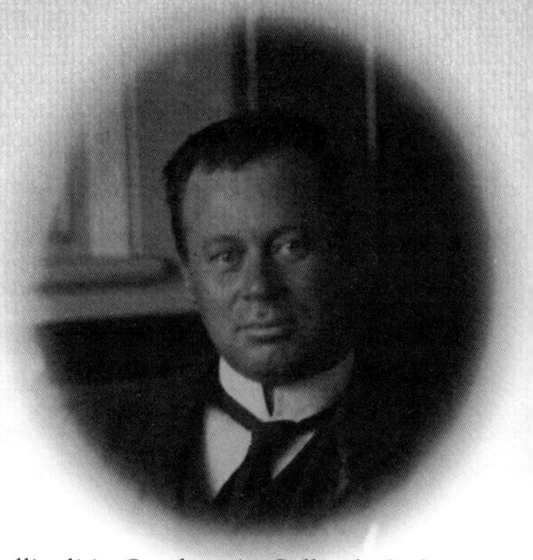

Frederick Goldsmith was born on the 12th July 1867 in Robe, South Australia. He was the son of Dr Francis Edmund Goldsmith and his wife Emma, nee Hallett. He was educated at St Peter's College. He was one of the first four graduates from the University of Adelaide medical school in 1889. He was resident physician and resident surgeon at the Adelaide Hospital in 1890. Afterwards he was in private practice at Balhannah, Port Wakefield and Hindmarsh. He served in the militia for 2 years, and transferred to the AAMC Reserve in 1903. He was the District Registrar for the Port of Darwin in 1904. He offered his services as a doctor with the Red Cross contingent from London to Montenegro during the Balkan Wars of 1912-13. He was awarded the Order of Prince Danilo for this service. He studied tropical diseases in the Northern Territory of Australia, New Guinea, where he became the Federal Medical Officer, and in India. He travelled to England several times. He married Edith Ellen, sister of a Mrs Ainslie a caterer of St Peter's College in 1912.

Goldsmith volunteered for the AIF on the 6th August 1914. He was a 47 year old surgeon, and his wife of Balhannah, was named as next of kin. He was 6ft tall, and weighed 13st10lbs. He was allocated to the tent sub-division of B Section, 3 FdAmb. He went ashore at Gallipoli on 28th April 1915 and was almost immediately sent up White's Valley to 12 Bn to relieve Captain Stewart. He established an advanced dressing station at the head of the valley which was maintained by the FdAmb for the rest of the campaign. Between June and September Goldsmith suffered from several episodes of febrile illness, and at the end of September he was evacuated to Alexandria and then to Cairo. He recovered sufficiently to rejoin the unit at Gallipoli in October. At Gallipoli Corbin described Goldsmith *'with a permanent cigarette in his funny little holder, quite unchanged by war's alarms'*. In March 1916 he was promoted major, and continued to serve with the unit in France until February 1917 when he was admitted to hospital in England with pneumonia. After convalescence he was attached to 2 AAH, and then transferred to the Sea Transport Section. He left England for Australia in October 1917. Undaunted, he then made two further return trips to England on transports, being finally discharged in January 1919 with his appointment with the AIF terminated on 28th March 1919. Goldsmith was issued with the 1914-15 Star, the British War Medal and the Victory Medal.

Goldsmith had a practice in Chatswood, NSW after his return to Australia, but moved back again to South Australia. He invested with others from Adelaide in the White Hope Junction Gold Mining Company in Western Australia which was not successful. He lived at Rose Park in 1922 and lived at 49 Kensington Road Norwood South Australia in 1937. Frederick Goldsmith died at his residence in Norwood on 4th March 1942. His wife Ellen died nearly three years later on 1st December 1944.

Sources:

Likeman R., Gallipoli Doctors, Slouch Hat Publications, Melbourne, 2010.
http://recordsearch.naa.gov.au/scripts/Imagine.asp?B=4818268,
Photo from the ACH Cup Book FG, taken May 1904
The Adelaide Register 12th October 1912
The Daily News Perth 2nd April 1942
The New Adelaide 9th August 1938.
Corbin J (1916) 'Experiences with the AAMC at Gallipoli.' MJA 1:6 p. 111-114

GOODE Arthur

MB BS

1871 - 1938

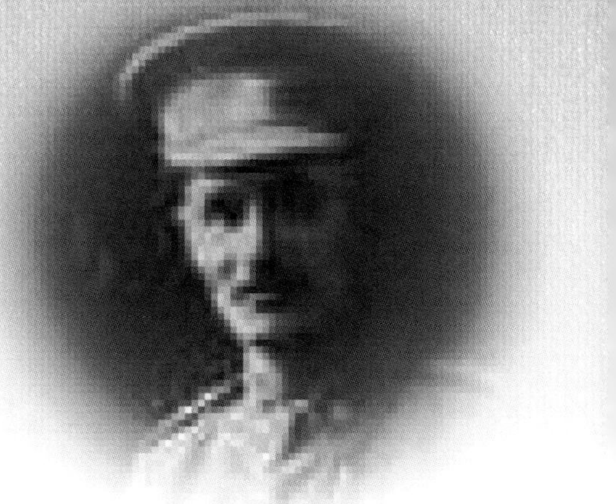

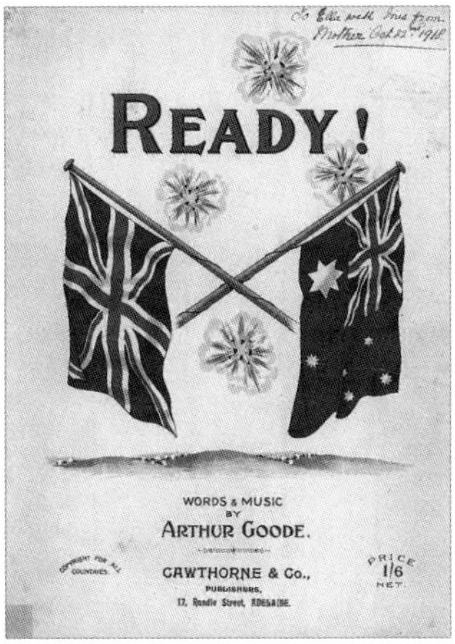

Arthur Goode was born on the 12th July 1871 at Canowie Station, south west of Terowie in South Australia. He was the one of thirteen children of Thomas Goode (1835-1926) and Margaret, nee Wilson. Thomas Goode had arrived in South Australia in February 1856 and was the Station manager for 35 years. Goode was educated at Glenelg Grammar School and Prince Alfred College. He studied medicine at the University of Adelaide and graduated in 1894. Goode was a fine runner, and a prominent player in the South Adelaide Football Club. After graduation Goode went to Broken Hill until 1896 and then Norseman, WA in 1897. Goode pleaded guilty to a crime in Norseman and was convicted and sentenced to 2 years imprisonment. However, he was not penalised in his medical registration. He came back to South Australia and moved to Peterborough and was in practice there until he enlisted for active service with the AIF in 1915.

Goode joined the AAMC on the 21st February 1916 at the age of 44 years. His next of kin was recorded as his father Thomas Goode of Westall St, Hyde Park, South Australia. He was 5ft 8ins tall weighed 12st and of dark complexion, brown eyes, dark hair and normal vision. He embarked from the 4 MD on the 20th April 1916 on the *Mooltan* as AAMC re-enforcements. He was attached to the 15th Training Bn on arrival then to 3 AGH, Brighton before moving to France on the 11th April 1917 to Abbeville and Rouen. He spent most of December 1917 in hospital and convalescence in France and England with respiratory problems, returned to duty to 1 AGH. Chronic bronchitis again caused intermittent service throughout 1918. He returned to Australia on the *Kashmir* as ships MO. His AIF appointment was terminated on the 10th June 1919. His records note *"Brought to the notice of Secretary of State for War for Valuable Services'*. He was issued with the British War Medal and the Victory Medal.

He resumed practice at Peterborough on returning to South Australia and purchased a house in Railway Terrace and took a prominent part in the effort which resulted in the erection of the fine Soldiers' Memorial Hospital in that town. Goode joined Dr Cyril Lowther Clarke, who had returned to Peterborough, from the war a month earlier. However, active service had seriously affected Goode's health, and he found it necessary to go to the milder climate of Queensland. He purchased a property at Cleveland in 1926 and established a small farm, however, in later years his chief recreations were gardening and music. He is reported to have opened the first Hospital in Mount Isa in 1926. Arthur Goode died on the 24th April 1938 in Rosemount Military Hospital, Brisbane. Goode did not marry, but was survived by five brothers and four sisters.

Sources:
Nla_mus-an6806487-s1-v with inscription "To Ella with love from Mother, Oct 22nd 1918"
NAA: B2455, Item barcode 4818471.
Family records and photo from David Newgreen and Michael Wilson Photo SLSA, B33019.
The Western Australian, Thursday December 9th 1897.
Chronicle Adelaide 26th May 1938.

GRANT Richard Longford Thorold

MB BS FRACP MRCP

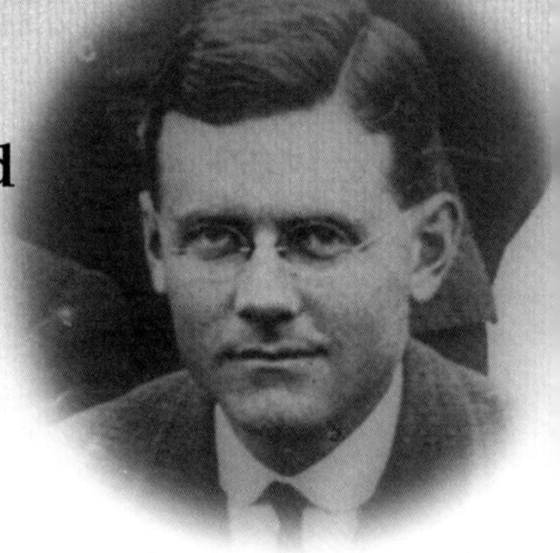

1894 - 1979

Richard Longford Thorold Grant was born on 22nd of April 1894 at North Adelaide. He was the son of William Thorold Grant and Emily, nee Jefferson. His parents were pastoralists and his father became known as a writer of rural affairs for *The Australasian* under the pen name "Benlbey". His parents later moved to Victoria. Grant was educated at Queen's School, North Adelaide. He had been in the Boy Scouts. His athletic abilities were cut short by renal tuberculosis necessitating a nephrectomy. He graduated from the University of Adelaide in 1918.

Grant enlisted on the 4th July 1918 when still a medical student. He had one year of school cadets and six years of citizen military forces experience. He was single and gave his address as 3 Brougham Place, North Adelaide. He was 5ft 7½ins tall, weighed 135lbs and of medium complexion, grey eyes and brown hair. His father was named as next of kin and his address given as 149 Kooyong Road, Toorak Victoria. He was not called up for service and discharged on 18th November 1918. He was appointed captain on 26th November 1918. The Principal Medical Officer recommended him for enlistment despite his blindness in his right eye. The appointment was terminated on 1st February 1919. He did not serve outside of Australia

Grant went to England after the war where he obtained his Membership of the Royal College of Physicians. He went on to be a founding Fellow of the Royal Australasian College of Physicians. He was appointed honorary assistant pathologist at the Adelaide Hospital in 1925 after the resignation of Dr Jose. He married Jane Nancy Lewis, daughter of Dr Brook Lewis, an ophthalmologist of Mount Lofty, on 23rd February 1927 at St Peters Cathedral. The wedding was reported in the social pages of the Adelaide Advertiser and considered to be a 'fashionable wedding'. They had two sons. He served again in WW2 and was a consultant physician to the RAAF with the rank of squadron leader. He was later promoted to wing commander. At the Annual Meeting of the BMA (SA Branch) in 1948 he was elected to Council. He had various senior positions following his return from the United Kingdom as Pathologist, Bacteriologist and later as Physician at the Adelaide Children's Hospital. He contracted a severe generalised dermatitis from chemicals in clothing which required long term treatment and instituted a long legal process eventually to the level of the Privy Council. During this time he was unable to work and his wife had to return to work. Grant eventually resumed his practice as a general physician with a particular interest in children's illnesses. Never very affluent he lived at Grange and also had honorary appointments at the Home for Incurables and Tennyson House. Despite his financial issues he maintained his membership of the Adelaide Club. Richard Longford Thorold Grant died on 29th March 1979. He was survived by his 2 sons.

Sources:

Trove Newspapers
http://trove.nla.gov.au/newspaper/result?q=Richard+Longford+Thorold+Grant
National Archives of Australia
http://recordsearch.naa.gov.au/NameSearch/Interface/ItemDetail.aspx?Barcode=4671236
Sims EB ,RACP College Roll, Obituary
http://www.racp.edu.au/page/library/college-roll/college-roll-detail&id=872
Photo: Adelaide University Archives; Medical Graduates 1918.

GREY William Charles

MB BS

1875 - 1930

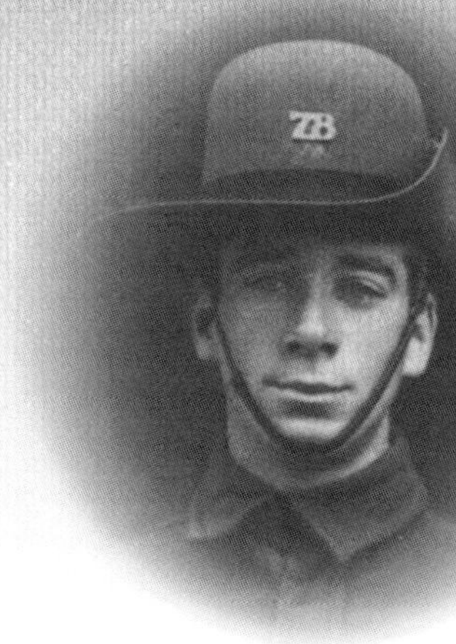

William Charles Grey was born 27th March 1875 at Balaklava, South Australia. He was son of Mr C S Grey. He was educated at Prince Alfred College. Grey went on to the University of Adelaide to study medicine from 1894-1898 but his university study was interrupted. It was reported at his death that he was a veteran of the South African War and this may have been the cause of the delay in his studies. There is no record in the National Archives of Australia of him enlisting in the Boer War. Nevertheless he continued his medical studies at the University of Adelaide and went on to complete them at Sydney in 1901, likely as a result of the Adelaide Hospital Row. Grey was in Western Australia in 1903 and appointed public vaccinator in Bulong, a now abandoned gold field town. He and his wife, Louise Fanny, had a son in 1905, in Boulder City Kalgoorlie, WA. However, in 1911 he was in Rookwood, Western Sydney, NSW where he had started a medical practice and living at "Bonarty" Victoria Ave Rookwood, Lidcombe NSW

Grey enlisted in the AIF on 24th November 1914 in 2 MD and left Australia on the *Kyarra* on 28th November 1914. He was 39 years old, 5ft 8ins tall, and weighed 15st 7lbs. He was appointed major with 2 AGH on enlistment. He was then seconded for duty as CO Mena Convalescent Depot. Grey was promoted to lieutenant colonel on 1st January 1916 and took command of the 3rd Auxiliary Hospital. He was in hospital at Ras et Tin in July 1916. His service commitment was completed in November 1916 and was returned to Australia on the *Wiltshire* with his appointment terminated on the 17th January 1917. He was issued with the 1914-15 Star, the British War Medal and the Victory Medal.

After Grey returned to Australia he resumed his medical practice in Rookwood, NSW. Later he moved to 57 Dudley Street, Lidcombe. William Charles Grey died on 12th March 1930 in Lidcombe.

Sources:
Photo: PAC Collection
National Archives
http://recordsearch.naa.gov.au/NameSearch/Interface/ItemDetail.aspx?Barcode=4711320
Trove
http://trove.nla.gov.au/ndp/del/article/4966754?searchTerm=WilliamCharlesGrey&searchLimits=

From our Special Correspondent [SA]

The War

By the mail which carries this letter some of the members of the Double General Hospital will leave us. It is to be equipped in England and will be under the command of Colonel Fiaschi D.S.O., of Sydney, a veteran of the Italo-Abyssinian and Boer wars. The Registrar and secretary is Dr de Crespigny, of Adelaide and Dr A.M. Cudmore FRCS, will be surgeon, both with the rank of Lieutenant Colonel. Amongst the juniors will be Drs Lance Hayward and E.A.H. Russell, and the Quartermaster is Captain Medlyn, Secretary to the Adelaide Hospital... Meanwhile our First General Hospital in Egypt is to be doubled, to contend with the casualties likely to come from the Dardanelles, and Drs C. Yeatman and Cunningham have been appointed to it; a special Convalescent Hospital has also been formed at Harefield Park.

BMJ, 3 July 1915, p. 31-32

GRIFFITHS Ernest William

MB BS

1881 - 1949

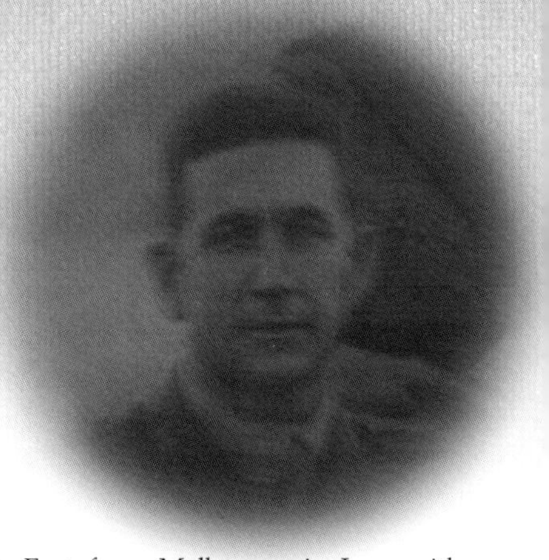

Ernest William Griffiths was born in Adelaide in December 1881, the son of William and Emily Griffiths. Griffiths studied medicine at the University of Adelaide and was one of the three to graduate in 1906 after the reopening of the medical school following the 'Adelaide Hospital Row'. He gained a first class pass. Griffiths first practised at Mannum, South Australia soon after the first telephone exchange was installed; his number was Mannum 7. He went to England in 1910 for further experience. He returned to Adelaide and went into general practice.

Griffiths enlisted in the AIF on the 14th May 1915 in 4 MD. He was 34 years old, single and his brother, G T Griffiths of Henley Beach Rd, Mile End, was nominated as his next of kin. He married Floris Clare Hay on the 2nd March 1916 and changed his next of kin to his wife of "Vespray" Prescott Terrace, Rose Park. He was 5ft 6ins, weighed 143lbs, of fair complexion and mid brown hair. Griffiths embarked for the Middle East from Melbourne in June with the reinforcements for 1 AGH. Soon after his arrival in Egypt he became ill from paratyphoid, and was sent back to Australia in December 1915 for three months rest. He returned to Egypt in September 1916. He expected to be posted to 3 AGH, however this unit had moved to England, so he was posted to 14 AGH instead. He was transferred to the RANBT in November 1916. He served at El Arish and Gaza, and when it was disbanded he returned to 14 AGH. He was promoted Major in June 1917 and posted to the Details Camp at Moascar. He returned to Australia in February 1918 and took up a position at Keswick Hospital. His appointment was terminated on the 5th April 1918. He was issued with the 1914-15 Star, the British War medal and the Victory Medal.

Griffiths returned to his medical practice in Adelaide after the war. He sued the Tramways Trust in Adelaide in 1924 over the resumption of a house and land which he owned. Griffiths claimed that the property was worth far more than the Trust's valuation. He had his car, a 1924 Dodge stolen from his residence at Henley Beach Rd, Mile End in 1925. Griffiths moved to Ryde, NSW in 1933 and was an Honorary Medical Officer at Ryde District Hospital. Here he started legal proceeding against a neighbour over a parcel of land rented for a market garden. Ernest William Griffiths died on 12th September 1949 at Gloucester House. He was survived by his wife Floris, 2 sons and 2 daughters and 6 grandchildren.

The Home-Coming

The medical profession in Australia comprises approximately three thousand members...During the period of the war about one half of the total number of medical practitioners offered their services for duty...the majority went overseas... the record of this service overseas is a wonderful one...These men are coming home now. After years of sacrifice they look for the opportunity to re-establish themselves and gradually to make up for the pecuniary loss associated with the prolonged period of war service.

MJA, 19 May 1919, p. 385

In April, 1917, Surgeon-General Fetherston recorded that no less than 994 medical men had gone abroad on active service since the beginning of the war.

MJA, 24 August 1918, p. 161

Sources:

http://rcordsearch.naa.gov.au/scripts/Imagine.asp?B=4703119
Photo extracted from a group of Australian Dr's on mules and camels in front of the sphinx; the possession of Dr R Brummitt of Adelaide.
The Register Adelaide 27 Nov 1906
The Register Adelaide 25 Mar 1915
The News Adelaide 23 Sep 1924
Adelaide Advertiser 06 April 1925
Sydney Morning Herald 14th September 1949.

GURNER Colin

MB BS FRCRA

1896 - 1962

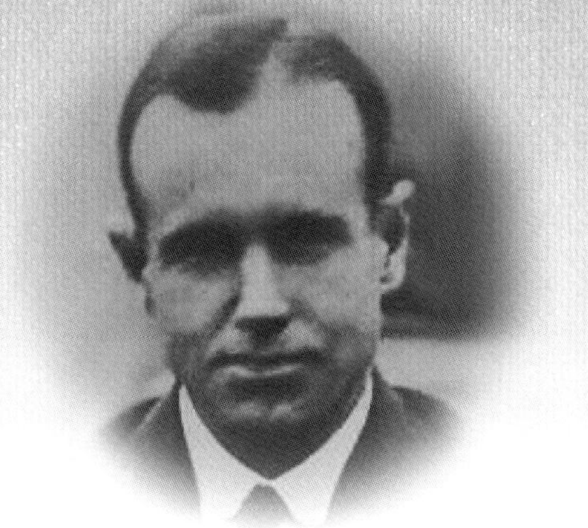

Colin Gurner was born on 25th May 1896 the second son of Walter and Hannah, nee Fry and brought up in Marryatville, SA. His great grandfather had migrated from England in 1849 eventually settling in Riverton, South Australia. He was educated at Prince Alfred College and studied medicine at the University of Adelaide where he graduated MB BS in 1918. He played football and tennis for the university eventually captaining both teams and being awarded a Blue for each.

During his medical course he had joined the Citizens Military Force and after his graduation was appointed captain in the AAMC on 26th November 1918. This appointment was terminated on 17th December 1919. His brother Leonard, a lieutenant in the infantry, was killed in action in July 1918.

Gurner entered general practice with Ernest and Lincoln Borthwick in the Payneham and Marryatville areas. He joined the radiology practice of Stanley Verco in 1930 and, with his wife and two sons, he left Adelaide to study radiology in Vienna, London and the United States in 1931. Not long after his return to South Australia and partnership with Dr Verco in Verco Buildings on North Terrace he was appointed honorary assistant radiologist and radiotherapist at the Adelaide Hospital and the Adelaide Children's Hospital. He became a member of the SA State Committee of the Australian and New Zealand Association of Radiologists in 1938 and remained a member until 1950. Gurner joined the AAMC in October 1939 and was posted to 2 AGH. Joining Leonard Charles Edward Lindon and Edmond Britten-Jones at Puckapunyal they found the circumstances offered at the Menzies Hotel in Melbourne more desirable than a shared tent and became known as the 'MX contingent (the Menzies Expeditionary Force)'. Gurner embarked for the Middle East in 1940 and set up at Kantara on the Suez Canal. He returned to Australia in March 1942 and Gurner was to take a number of military posts around Adelaide and did not go overseas again. The Gurner home became an unofficial 'officers mess' for officers billeted all over Adelaide. He returned to his work at Adelaide and Adelaide Children's Hospitals and the Verco, Gurner and Smeaton radiological practice much to the relief of Bronte Smeaton who had had the lion's share of the work as his partners were engaged in their military duties. After Smeaton's death the practice was joined firstly by Peter Verco, Stanley Verco's son and later Gurner's son, Colin. Gurner was a heavy smoker, and was showing signs of vascular degeneration. When his son joined the regular army in 1960 he retired from practice. Colin Gurner died on 15th February 1962. His wife, Jessie, died a few weeks later. He was survived by his children including Colin who later became Major General Gurner AO CBE ED QHP, DGMS.

Sources:

Ryan J, Sutton K, Baigent M., 'Australasian Radiology' McGraw Hill, Sydney, 1996.

http://recordsearch.naa.gov.au/NameSearch/Interface/ItemDetail.aspx?Barcode=4380383

http://recordsearch.naa.gov.au/NameSearch/Interface/ItemDetail.aspx?Barcode=4380385

GUYMER Arthur Howes

MB BS FRCS(Ed)

1893 - 1962

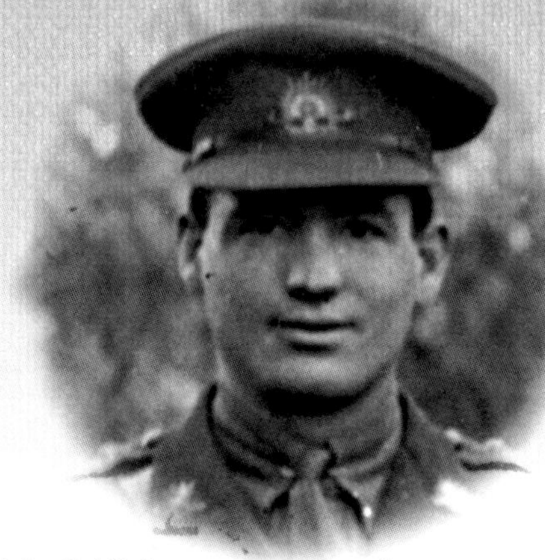

Arthur Howes Guymer was born at Kilkenny, SA on 6th March 1893, youngest son of George Huften and Mary Elizabeth Guymer, of 8 Wilpena Terrace, Kilkenny, and younger brother of Ernest Albert. He was educated at Prince Alfred College and studied medicine at University of Adelaide graduating in 1915. He was a junior house surgeon at the Adelaide Hospital for only a few weeks before enlistment.

He enlisted in the AIF on 1st October 1915 just 2 weeks after his older brother. He was single, 23 years old, 5ft 11ins, and weighed, 9st12lbs and his father was named as his next of kin. He had one year of previous AAMC reserve service and applied for a commission as a captain in the AAMC. He was posted for general duty to 43 Bn of the 11 Bde and attached on the 13th April 1916. This Bde was part of 3rd Div then assembling in Australia. They embarked from Adelaide on the *Afric* on the 9th June 1916 and did not go into action in France until late in 1916. He was transferred to Alexandria in October 1916 and then from 3 AGH to the RAMC base Depot at Mustapha and subsequently joined the BEF per *Minnetonka* finally posted to 43 Bn from 11 FdAmb. He suffered a severe gunshot wound to the left arm at Wimereux (Passchendaele), France on 18th October 1917 and transferred to the 3rd London General Hospital. After recovery he was posted for duty to 11 FdAmb in May 1918 and then to several field ambulance attachments in France. Whilst with 11 FdAmb in 1918 he was recommended for a Military Cross, but no award was made. At the cessation of hostilities he was granted leave from 7th March 1919 to 7th September 1919 with pay for medical experience at the Royal Berkshire Hospital at Reading. His appointment was terminated in England on the 11th October 1919. He issued with the British War Medal and the Victory Medal.

Guymer returned to Australia on the 30th March 1922 and by special dispensation of the Bishop he married Sylvia C Ninham, a singer and youngest daughter of Mr and Mrs F W Ninham of Croydon at St Margaret's Church, Woodville. At this time he had been appointed as the Health Office for the District of Morgan in South Australia. However Guymer then lived and had a general practice in Mosely St, Glenelg. The family moved to Ballarat from 1925-1935 where he worked with his brother. On return to Glenelg the family were prominent in the social news of the day and his love of golf was shown by being Vice Captain of the Glenelg Golf Club. He often shared Anzac Day with members of the 43 Bn. Arthur Howes Guymer died on the 15th December 1962 aged 69 years, at Somerton Park. He was survived by his daughter Joan and son, Dr Max Guymer.

Sources:
http://recordsearch.naa.gov.au/scripts/Imagine.asp?B=436202.
Photo: AWM A03389;
Photo brothers from Robert Likeman;
NLA Trove
The Register (Adelaide) 8th April 1922
Adelaide Advertiser 17th October 1916

The Psychological Effect of War

It has been asserted by more than one authority that in war the side will win which can hold out a quarter of an hour longer that the other side. This saying not only pithily expresses the fundamental importance of *moral* in warfare but it lays bare impassionately, indeed almost cynically, the kind of *moral*... The State demands of its fighting men the ability to suffer and to go on suffering the terrific and nerve-shattering onslaught of modern gun-fire and still retain in their depleted ranks an effect and alert organization.

BMJ, 13 March 1915, p. 475

GUYMER Ernest Albert

MB BS FRCS(Ed)

1891 - 1982

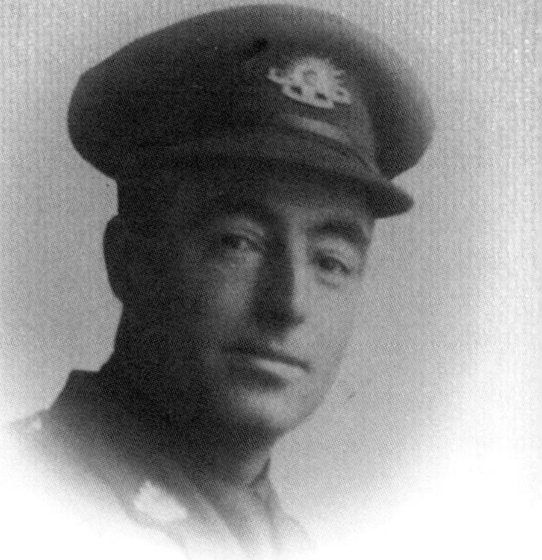

Ernest Albert Guymer was born on the 10th February 1891 in Adelaide. He was the eldest of three sons of George Huften Guymer of Kilkenny, South Australia. He was educated at Prince Alfred College and was prominent in athletics and tennis. He rowed in a school eight at the Henley on Torrens race and played Amateur League Football whilst at University. He partnered his brother Arthur in local and interstate tennis. He studied medicine at the University of Adelaide graduating in 1914. He then completed his residency at the Adelaide Hospital and was a house surgeon for 6 months before enlisting in the AIF.

Guymer joined the AIF on 19th September 1915 and was commissioned as a captain for general duties in the AAMC. He was single, 24 years old, 5ft 9ins, weighed 11st, of dark complexion, with brown hair and eyes. Shortly after enlisting in October 1915 he became engaged to Blanche Perry of Wilpena Terrace, Kilkenny. He embarked on 11th October 1915 with reinforcements for 2 AGH and proceeded to Gallipoli on 23 November 1915, but within a week was posted to 3 AGH on Lemnos. After the evacuation from the Dardanelles he remained with 3 AGH. He was detached to 4 LHR. When 3 AGH moved to England, Guymer went to France as RMO of 17 Bn. The Bn was then at Flers, bogged down in mud and suffering badly from trench foot. Guymer was transferred to 4 AFA Bde in April 1917, but was sick for several weeks with mumps, and did not return to the Bde until the beginning of June. Guymer was Mentioned in Despatches on the 9th September 1917 whilst attached to the 4th Field Artillery Brigade Headquarters. He was promoted major in February 1918, posted to 5 FdAmb for a short time, but was unwell again and sent back to England. During this time he had several bouts of pyrexia of unknown origin seemingly as a result of his illness with mumps. After recovering he did not return to France, but was posted to the Overseas Training Bde in England, where he remained until the end of the war. He used his accrued leave to gain surgical experience at Norwich Hospital, and in November 1919 he resigned from his AIF appointment. He returned to Australia the following year after passing the FRCS Edinburgh examination and his appointment was terminated at 4 MD, Adelaide on 20th August 1920. Guymer was issued with the 1914-15 Star, the British War Medal and the Victory Medal with Oak Leaves.

Guymer set up a surgical practice in Ballarat on return to Australia and began a family with the birth of a son, Len Farrer, on the 23rd November 1923 at "Muiravon", 9 Drummond St, South Ballarat. He was appointed Honorary surgeon at the Ballarat Base Hospital in 1937 and informed them that he was going to the Coronation in England and then for post graduate work in surgery in England, Vienna and United States. Guymer was often mentioned in the local press until 1947 as a Club golfer. The family left Ballarat in August 1960 and had address of Golightly St, Port Lonsdale Victoria. Ernest Albert Guymer died on the 2nd July 1982, aged 91 years, at Queenscliff, Victoria, and was buried at Ballarat, Victoria. His son Rex, a Melbourne Radiologist, died in Melbourne on the 20th February 2006.

Sources:

Likeman R., Gallipoli Doctors, Slouch Hat Publications Melbourne, 2010
http://recordsearch.naa.gov.au/scripts/Imagine.asp?B=4362026;
Photo: PAC, WW1 Doctors
http://www.awm.gov.au/collection/records/awm28/1/awm28-1-91-0045.pdf
The Mail Adelaide 16th October 1915.

HAINS Ivan Coronel

MB BS

1889 - 1952

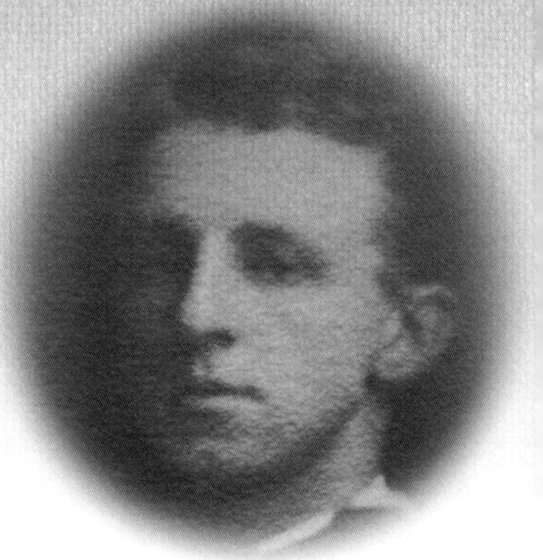

Ivan Coronel Hains was born on the 15th June 1889 at Portland Estate, SA. He was the son of John Hains and his wife Julia Louisa, nee Coronel. Hains was educated at Prince Alfred College and studied medicine at the University of Adelaide, graduating in 1911. He then completed his residency at the Adelaide Hospital in 1912. He first entered general practice in Adelaide, and then moved to Gilgandra, NSW.

Hains enlisted in the AIF on 10th August 1915 in Dubbo NSW. He was commissioned in October 1915 aged 26 years and spoke German moderately well. He was 5ft 8ins tall, weighed 10st, and his wife, Mrs Maud Jean Hains was named as his next of kin with his address given as care of PO Box 55 GPO, Adelaide. He sailed for the Middle East on the 10th November on HMAT *Orsova*. He served briefly with 1 Remount Unit on arrival in Egypt, and then in April 1916 was posted as RMO of 12 FdAmb. He went to France with the unit, and served until the 22nd July 1917, when he returned to Australia with his appointment terminated on the 8th October 1917. He was issued with the 1914-15 Star, the British War Medal and the Victory Medal.

Hains moved to Queensland and was an anaesthetist at the Bundaberg Hospital from 1920-22, and Medical Superintendent from 1922-24. During his latter period of office in Bundaberg, there occurred a local tragedy when twelve children died following inoculation against diphtheria. A Royal Commission found that the serum had been contaminated with staphylococcus by the use of a multi-dose vial. The Chairman of the Royal Commission, Dr Charles Kellaway, and one of the other Commissioners, Dr Arthur Tebbutt, had served abroad with the AAMC in WW1. Hains was appointed as an honorary Medical Officer at Bundaberg Hospital in 1934, and also at the Lady Chelmsford Hospital, Bundaberg. He was the GMO and also the CMO. He was in Bundaberg from 1925 to 1949. He moved back to New South Wales. Ivan Coronel Hains died suddenly at Mosman, NSW on the 18th April 1952 and was privately cremated.

Sources:
http://recordsearch.naa.gov.au/scripts/Imagine.asp?B=4266529
Photo, Adelaide University Archives 1911 graduates.
http://www.mytrees.com/ancestry/Australia/Died-1952/Ha/Hains-family/Ivan-Hains-fo001339-385.html
Adelaide Advertiser 6th May 1952
Townsville Daily Bulletin 2nd February 1928.

War Deafness

Otologists have given a great deal of careful thought and observation to the cases of deafness which occur in great numbers among our troops on active service. It has been estimated that about 16% of the men admitted to evacuation hospitals in the French *Zone des Armees* on account of illness show aural affections. The great difficulty experienced has been to distinguish between neuroses and actual ear lesions. This difficulty was accentuated by the fact that the affections were officially classified as shell shock, a term which suggest a central nervous commotion rather than an actual trauma. Concussion deafness is common in the present war, because the explosive force of the modern shell is terrific. At times the effects of the concussion are complicated by wounds, either in the neighbourhood of the ear or in some other part of the body. A careful investigation had revealed that many of the wounded, who were quite unaware of any interference with hearing, were found to be deaf.

MJA, 26 October 1918, p. 351

HALL Norman Bruce

MB BS

1893 - 1970

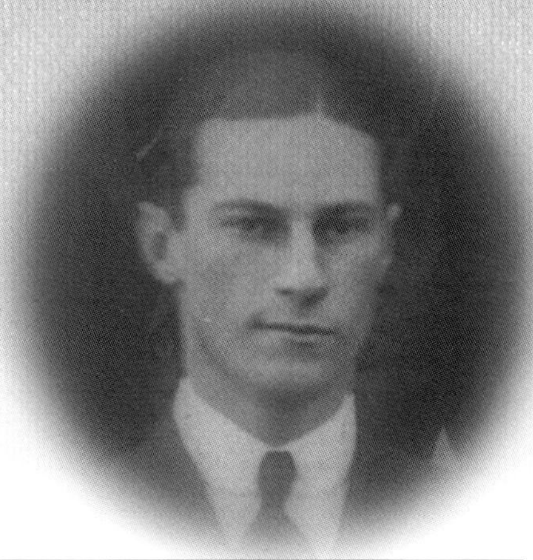

Norman Bruce Hall was born on the 31st July 1893 in Norwood South Australia, the son of James Hall, the Chairman of the South Australian Racing Club. He was educated at Prince Alfred College and studied medicine at the University of Adelaide graduating in 1917.

Hall enlisted in the AIF and was commissioned on the 7th August 1917. He was 27 years old, single, no previous military experience and with his father of Beulah Road, Norwood as next of kin. He was 5ft 8ins tall and weighed 10st 5lbs. He could ride and was proficient in German. He was posted for General Duties. He embarked from Melbourne for the Middle East on 2nd November 1917. After two months at 14 AGH he was detached to the LH Details Camp at Moascar. He was posted to 1 LHFA in April 1918. He was detached to 3 LHR in the Jordan Valley in June and in July posted to 1 LHR. He did not return to 1 LHFA until February 1919. He was attached to 14 AGH in May 1919 until he sailed from Port Said for England via Taranto in July. He was give study leave from 21st July 1919 to 25th March 1920 to attend Queen Mary's Hospital, Stratford in London's East End, and the Chelsea Hospital for women, and Queen Charlotte's Hospital. His appointment was terminated in 4 MD on the 18th June 1920. He was issued with the British War Medal and the Victory Medal.

He returned to Australia in March 1920. Hall did not settle down in Australia, and in 1923 he returned to London and established a practice in obstetrics and gynaecology in the West End. In 1927 he married society authoress Viola Bankes. Norman Bruce Hall died in 1970 whilst living at Eton Place in London.

Sources:

http://recordsearch.naa.gov.au/scripts/Imagine.asp?B=3007800.
Photo: The Adelaide University Archives, Graduates of July 1917.
Likeman R., "From the Jungle to the Desert"
Slouch Hat Publications, Port Melbourne Aus., 2012

The AAMC

For many months responsible and irresponsible critics have raised their voices to point out the defects of the Australian Army Medical Corps. The critics have emphasised what appeared to them to be the wastage of energy, the wrong application of material and the want of prominence given to the functions in which they were most interested. The authorities have apparently not been moved by the vapouring's of these malcontents....without exception these young men had proved themselves to be "extremely good and capable, not only at their professional work, but by their adaptability and by their willingness to go wherever ordered without demur." In the early stages of the war there were admittedly defects in the organization in the Australian Army Medical Corps directly traceable to unsuitable material... We may therefore assume that we have the very best material for the machine in these young men, who have completed their studies rapidly in order to do their duty to their country.

MJA, 25 November 1916, p. 455

HAMILTON James Alexander Greer

MB (Dublin) LRCS Ed LMRCSI LMRCPI

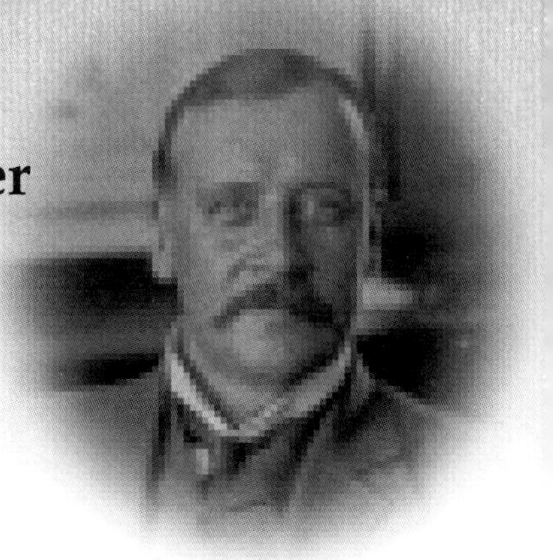

1854 - 1925

James Alexander Greer Hamilton was born in January 1854 in Castle Caulfield, Co Tyrone, Ireland, the third son of a family of thirteen of Rev Robert Hamilton and his wife Emily, nee Kinley. He was educated at Trinity College, Dublin with an arts and medical degree in 1870 followed by a licentiate of the Royal College of Surgeons, Edinburgh. He came to South Australia and was first registered in Adelaide in 1876 and received an appointment at Walloroo Hospital. He went to Kapunda after two years and stayed there for twelve years as a respected general practitioner and a skilful surgeon. Whilst at Kapunda he became a foundation member of the newly formed South Australian branch of the BMA and in 1890 was its President. This influenced his decision to come to Adelaide. He joined the practice of Dr Way and was appointed to the Adelaide Hospital where he became a leading gynaecologist and the Head of Gynaecology at the Adelaide Hospital. He was a member of the Council of Adelaide University from 1897-1911 and at one stage was on the Medical Board of South Australia. His love of horses was shared with his brother Dr T K Hamilton who bred race horses and he bet on them. Both had a long and unsuccessful career with their hobby. It was said that: *"He was a man of magnificent physique; his genial character revealed him as a characteristic Irishman. He was a great sportsman and a fine judge of horses, his love of them causing him to associate with the SAJC as honorary surgeon."* Drs T. K. Hamilton, C. W. Hamilton and R. H. Hamilton were his brothers; all practised in Adelaide.

Hamilton was commissioned as an honorary major in 1909 in the AAMC. He volunteered for the AIF in July 1915 and was posted to the No2 Hospital Ship. He was married, 61 years old, 6ft 1ins, and weighed 14st. He nominated his wife Helen Ketmnis Hamilton of Jeffcott St, North Adelaide as his next of kin. Hamilton made one voyage only, sailing in the *Orsova* in July 1915, and joining the *Kanowna* in Egypt. Hamilton was discharged in December 1915, with his appointment terminated on the 30th November 1915 and transferred to the Home Service staff of 7 AGH with the rank of honorary lieutenant colonel. Hamilton was issued with the British War Medal and the Victory Medal.

Troubled by increasing deafness and declining health in 1920, Hamilton retired to a farm worked by his son in Katanning, Western Australia. After the death of his son Robert, in Katanning in 1922 he and his wife returned to South Australia. In June 1923 he settled in Glenelg where he indulged in his hobby of gardening. James Alexander Greer Hamilton died on the 8th October 1925 at the North Adelaide Sisters' Private Hospital, aged 72 years. He was survived by his son, Reginald of Perth, one daughter Miss L Hamilton and six grandchildren. He is buried in the North Road Cemetery.

Sources:
http://recordsearch.naa.gov.au/scripts/Imagine.asp?B=4265576
Photo: ACH Cup Book.
MJA Dec 12th 1925 p 688
Adelaide Advertiser 9th October 1925

HARBISON Ernest John Keith

MB BS

1898 - 1945

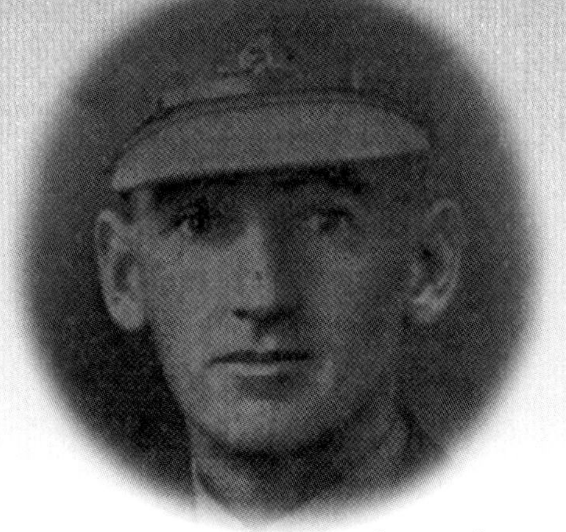

Ernest John Keith Harbison was born in Gladstone, South Australia on the 2nd September 1898. His parents were Dr William Henry and Nellie Adelaide Harbison. He had served for four years as a senior school cadet. He was educated at Prince Alfred College and studied medicine at the University of Adelaide.

Harbison was a medical student at the time of his enlistment on 13 September 1918. His father was given as his next of kin and his address was Lydia Terrace, Wallaroo South Australia. He was 5ft 6ins and weighed 145lbs. He was described as having a medium complexion with brown eyes and dark hair and gave his religion as Methodist. He was posted to B Company at Mitcham Camp from where he was discharged on 18th November 1918 due to the ending of hostilities.

Harbison returned to his medical studies at the University of Adelaide and graduated MB BS in 1924. He married Violet Mary Richards on the 1st July 1925 whilst he was still living in Wallaroo. They later lived at Toorak Gardens, South Australia. He re-joined the AAMC in WW2 at the rank of major and was posted to 4 Camp Hospital in Brisbane Queensland. Ernest John Keith Harbison was a casualty of WW2 and died from illness on the 5th March 1945. His name is on the honour roll at the Australian War Memorial and is located at panel 87 in the Commemorative Area. He is buried at Brisbane (Lutwyche) Cemetery. He was survived by his wife Violet.

Sources:

The Adelaide Advertiser 3rd Jan 1914
The Register Adelaide 16th Dec 1924
The Register Adelaide 1st July 1925
http://recordsearch.naa.gov.au/NameSearch/Interface/ItemDetail.aspx?Barcode=4245454
http://world-war-2-casualties.findthebest.com.au/l/9934/Ernest-John-Keith-Harbison
http://www.awm.gov.au/research/people/roll_of_honour/person/R1704586/

Industrial Training of Disabled Soldiers

The Department of Repatriation is fathering a National Economy exhibition in which the Department of Technical Education of New south wales is demonstrating the working capacity of returned disabled soldiers. This exhibition is at present to be seen at the Town hall, Sydney, and all who are interested in the training of disabled men should spend a half an hour or so in it. There is a small section divided into a number of compartments. In each compartment men are working at a special trade. These include joinery and cabinet-making, band-saw work, lathe work, pottery and boot making. In each case the men have learnt the work as a new trade since their discharge from the army, and the visitor is struck by the manner in which the training has neutralized the physical war disability. The exhibition is an eloquent testimonial to the admirable methods of Mr J. Nangle, Director of the Technical College Sydney.

MJA, 16 November 1918, p. 410

† HARVEY Gilbert Aberdein

MB BS

1886 - 1917

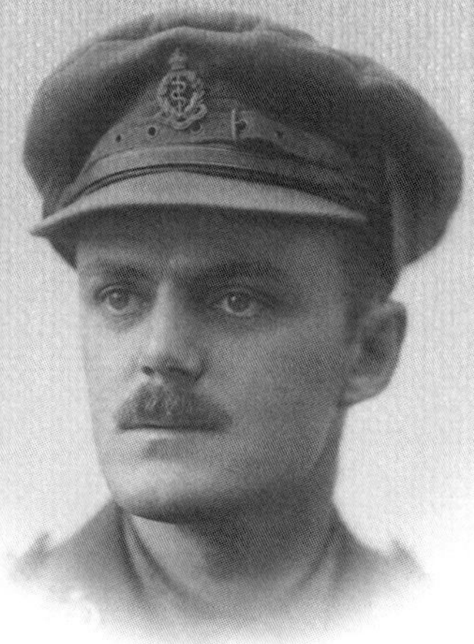

Gilbert Aberdein Harvey was born in Adelaide on the 22nd June 1886. He was the son of James Harvey of Adelaide and his wife Jessie Matilda (Maud). James Harvey came from Aberdeen in Scotland and immigrated to Australia when he was 18 years old. He moved to South Australia about 1864 and in 1872, acted as attorney for Sir Walter Hughes until Hughes' death in 1888. James Harvey became a leading businessman in Adelaide for many years. He was a director of Messrs. Elder, Smith, and Co., and at the time of his death he was also chairman of directors of the Adelaide Steamship Company, the Bank of Adelaide, the Commercial Union Assurance Company, the Adelaide Steam Tug Company, and the Wallaroo and Moonta Mining and Smelting Company. Gilbert Aberdein Harvey was educated at Queens School, North Adelaide in 1903 and studied medicine at the University of Adelaide, graduating in 1911. He then became a resident medical officer at the Adelaide Children's Hospital.

Harvey joined the RAMC in England at the outbreak of WW1. He was attached to the 1st Battalion, Kings Own Royal Lancaster Regiment. Harvey married Elspeth, eldest daughter of Mr George Young and the Hon. Mrs. Young, of Bude, Cornwall on the 29th September 1917. Two months later on 25th November 1917 Gilbert Aberdein Harvey was wounded and died on the Western Front. He is buried at Duisans British Cemetery, Etrun, France.

It was recorded in the Adelaide Register on 3rd September 1918 that the will of Gilbert Aberdein Harvey, who died in France, has been admitted to probate in England. The estate was left for the benefit of the widow after the payment of three small legacies. The bequests were given in November 1919 to the Adelaide Children's Hospital which received £500. It was presented by his widow Elspeth Harvey; 800 guineas also endowed a cot in his memory, and the balance of £185 entitled Mrs Harvey to a life governorship of the hospital. Gilbert Harvey's younger brother Leslie Morison Harvey, born on the 6th February 1888, also served in France.

Sources:

Photo IWM England

Reference: WO339/13525, the National Archives Kew, London. Former references: in its original department: 29234, Legal status: Public Record."

Adelaide Register 11th October 1917

Adelaide Register 3rd September 1918

German Experiences of War Surgery

Wounds of the Skull

At a meeting of the Hamburg Medical Society Dr Oehlecker discussed the treatment of wounds of the skull. In almost every case in which recovery ensued the patients had been taken straight by train to Germany, where they were operated on within a few days of the infliction of the wounds. After the relief of compression and the removal of fragments of the bone, the patients did well. It was astonishing to find how often extensive unilateral wounds of the cerebrum and cerebellum were unaccompanied by functional disturbances.

BMJ, 2 October 1915, p. 517

HASTE Reginald Arthur

MB BS BSc

1891 - 1968

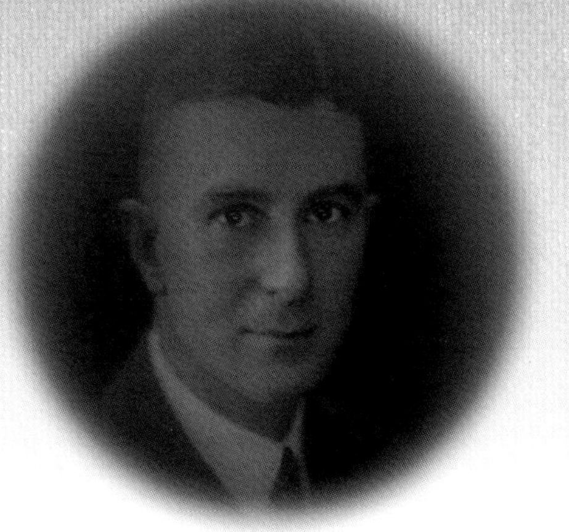

Reginald Arthur Haste was born on the 20th July 1891 at Rose Park, South Australia son of Dr. Arthur Reginald Haste and Minnie, nee Elliott. He was educated at Prince Alfred College and was Dux in his final year. He spent 1 year in the school Cadets before studying medicine at the University of Adelaide graduating in science in 1911 and medicine in 1914. He completed his residency at the Adelaide Hospital.

Haste enlisted in the AIF on the 15th October 1915. He was single, 24 years old, 5ft 10ins, and weighed 144lbs. He stated he could ride a horse and was slightly proficient in German. His father of "Roslyn", Kensington Rd, Rose Park was named as his next of kin. He embarked for the Middle East in March 1916. Haste like many young medical officers was attached to a unit for only one or two months at a time. He was posted initially to 3 Trg Bn on arrival in Egypt, and from there he was posted after a month to Ras el Tin, but fell ill with influenza. He moved between Ras el Tin, 3 AGH at Abbassia and 2 ASH at Tel el Kebir, before finally being taken on the strength of 3 AGH in August 1916. After a brief stay at the RAMC Base Depot at Mustapha, he left for England in October 1916, and rejoined 3 AGH at Brighton. He went to France in January 1917 to join 1 AGH at Rouen. This posting however only lasted a month, and he was then transferred to 3 Div Base Depot at Etaples. He was posted to 3 FdAmb in March, but it is unclear if he actually joined the unit before developing laryngitis and being admitted to 24th General Hospital. He was sent to the Canadian Con Depot at Dieppe to convalesce. Haste then received news that his father had suffered a stroke and died. As a result of his father's death he returned to Australia on the 2nd May 1917. His appointment in the AIF was terminated on the 8th August 1917. He was issued with the British War Medal and the Victory Medal.

Haste married Dorothy Edith Holden in 1919; they had 2 sons and a daughter. His mother Minnie died in December 1919. Haste became an Obstetrician and Gynaecologist and served on the Honorary Staff of the Queen's Maternity Home and the Adelaide Hospital for many years. His professional address was 175 Nth Terrace, Adelaide. Haste lived on Magill Rd, Maylands South Australia in 1929 and it was reported in the local paper that he was the owner of a new 1924 model Buick four passenger coupe. He gave the council land at the corner of Magill Road and Wellington Road in 1936 to ensure greater safety for vehicular traffic. In 1936 he was an examiner with the Royal Life Saving Society. His garden at Maylands featured in the Advertiser as the "Garden of the Week" in 1954. Reginald Arthur Haste died at Toorak Gardens, South Australia in 1968. His son Pilot Officer James Arthur Haste of 61 Squadron RAAF was shot down over Belgium in 1944 and is buried at Heverlee War Cemetery. His sister Edna Minnie enlisted as a nurse during WW1 and was posted to 7 AGH at Keswick.

Sources:
http://recordsearch.naa.gov.au/NameSearch/Interface/ItemDetail.aspx?Barcode=4738664. NLA Trove,
Likeman R., "From the Tropics to the Desert", Slouch Hat Publications 2012.
Photo: Family Collection, from Margot Maitland.
Adelaide Advertiser December 1919.

HAYWARD Lancelot Alfred

MB BS

1891 - 1964

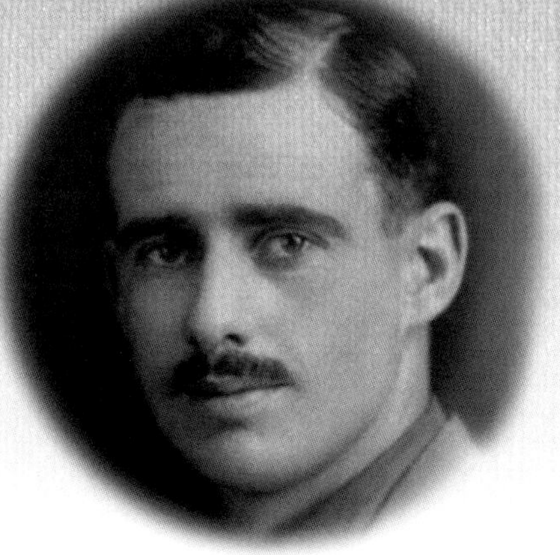

Lancelot Alfred Hayward was born in Norwood, South Australia, on 12th August 1891, the son of William Thornborough Hayward and his wife Florence. He attended St Peter's College and was prominent in newspaper reports of school cricket and swimming sports. He graduated MB BS from Adelaide University in 1914. Prior to the outbreak of war he was a 2nd lieutenant in the school cadets in 1909.

Hayward enlisted in the AIF on 19th April 1915. He was 23 years of age, single, 6ft, tall, and weighed 150lbs. His father was named as his next of kin. He was posted as a captain to 3 AGH at Mudros in August. He was evacuated sick to England in November on the *Mauretania,* and then sent back to Australia for a month. He had short attachments to 1 LHFA and 2 ASH on his return to Egypt, until he was sent to France to join 1 Div Engineers. He was promoted major in May 1917, and remained with the Engineers until September 1918. He was posted to 1 FdAmb and served with the FdAmb until I Aust Corps was withdrawn in October following the breaking of the Hindenburg Line. After the Armistice and during the Spanish 'flu epidemic Hayward was attached to 2 FdAmb. His appointment was terminated on the 2nd September 1919. Hayward was issued with the 1914-15 Star, the British War Medal and the Victory Medal

Hayward was appointed medical officer at the Barmera Hospital, South Australia in 1922. Hayward then moved to Perth where he worked as a Physician and Anaesthetist at the Perth Hospital. He was a Member of the Board of Health Western Australia in 1923. He had a younger brother living also in Perth and Hayward and his family, were often reported in the local newspapers for social events and their travel by rail and sea from Perth to Adelaide and back again visiting their large extended family. The family was living at St Georges Terrace, Perth in 1930 and in 1936 his family resided at Birdwood Parade, Dalkeith. He was President of the WA Branch of the BMA from 1938-9. He played golf at the Karrinyup Club. Hayward served with Home Forces from 1941-45 as DADMS 13 Bde, Western Command, and attained the rank of lieutenant colonel during WW2. Lancelot Alfred Hayward died on 5th September 1964.

Sources:

http://recordsearch.naa.gov.au/scripts/Imagine.asp?B=4749300
Photo: tumblr_lugyhwdmCJ1qz99gro1_4001] Mapping our Anzacs
The Daily News Perth 3rd July 1930
Chronicle Adelaide 26 August 1922

Military Life and Physical Health

The extraordinary improvement in the physical fitness of men who joined the new armies in this country is a commonplace observation, and most of us have had the opportunity of watching the improvement from month to month in personal friends or relations...The podgy shopkeeper has lost his *embonpoint* and pasty complexion. He is smart, his eyes are bright, his skin tanned, and his movements alert and manly. The fond wife is on the verge of disappointment, for she was expecting to play the nurse to a worn-out, debilitated husband, instead of which, he has regained the jollity of his early married days and, far from complaining, he boisterously describes his strenuous days and disturbed nights.

BMJ, 14 August 1915, p. 267

HAYWARD William Thornborough

CMG OBE LLD MRCS LRCPI

1854 - 1928

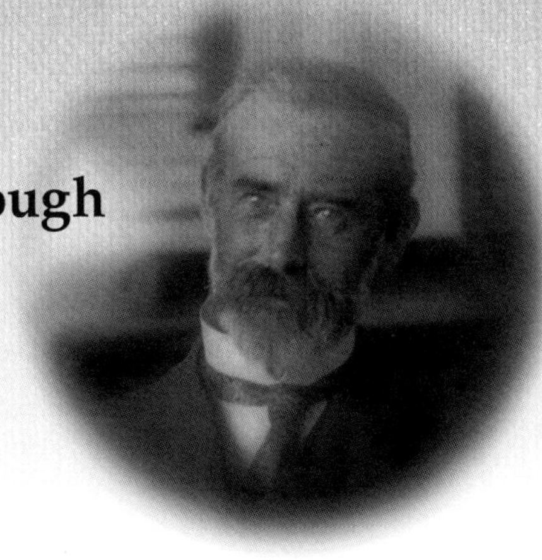

William Thornborough Hayward was born in Reading, Berkshire on 26th January 1854. At the age of 15 he entered the Royal Infirmary School of Medicine at Liverpool. He succeeded as a student with distinction and progressed to King's and Queen's College of Ireland. He came to Australia in 1878 as a ship's surgeon, and the following year set up practice in Riverton. He moved to Norwood in 1882 and became a lecturer at the University. He was made an honorary physician to the Adelaide Hospital in 1885 and in 1889 honorary medical officer to the Adelaide Children's Hospital. He was a forthright opponent to the Government over the Adelaide Hospital dispute that closed the medical school for 5 years. He was a member of the University of Adelaide Council from 1900-24. He was elected President of the SA Branch of the BMA in 1911, and was the first President of the Federal Committee of the BMA. William Hayward had served in the SA Militia for ten years and held the rank of surgeon major. He was presented with the gold medal of honour by the British Medical Association for distinguished service in 1914.

At the age of 61 years on the outbreak of war he volunteered for the AIF on the 12th August 1915 at Adelaide. His wife Florence was named as his next of kin. They were living at Ruthven Mansions, Pulteney Street, Adelaide. He was 5ft 10ins, and weighed 11st 9lbs. He was appointed to 10 AGH with the rank of lieutenant colonel. He embarked from Adelaide in August 1915 for England. The 10 AGH in England was never formally raised, and on arrival in England Hayward was posted to command 1 AAH at Harefield. He held this command for two years. He was appointed CMG and Mentioned in Dispatches for distinguished service in June 1917. He was sent to France to 2 AGH at Wimereux for a month in November. He was promoted Colonel and appointed OBE in January 1918 and returned to Australia in February 1918. He had requested a return to Australia due to age, (63 years) with approval from Surgeon General Neville Howse VC, DMS AIF *Climatic conditions are generally against an officer of his age and prejudicial to his health.* His appointment terminated on the 6th April 1918. Hayward was issued the British War Medal and the Victory Medal with Oak Leaves.

He continued his work at the Adelaide and Adelaide Children's Hospitals. He believed that alcohol had been considered too important in treatment and, in the last ten years of his practice, he spent much of his time encouraging the reduction of prescribing of alcohol in Australia. He was the author of many clinical papers in the Australian Medical Gazette. Hayward had married Australian-born Florence Burden, who made a considerable reputation for herself as an author and journalist, sometimes using the nom-de-plume 'Firenze'. Florence's mother was the widow of the Honourable J H Barrow the founder of "The Advertiser" in 1879. They had four sons and two daughters; Harold Thornborough Hayward, who served as a private in WW1 and a Corporal in WW2; Lancelot Alfred Hayward who also served as a MO in WW1; GB Hayward; JH Hayward; Mrs RM Steele and Mrs H Kay. William Thornborough Hayward died on 21st December 1928 with his address as 20 Alexandra Ave, Rose Park, SA. His obituary states *he belonged to that age both in his external appearance and his courteous bearing and his passing is a sign of the mode of manners of one generation differ from those of the next.*

Sources:

http://recordsearch.naa.gov.au/scripts/Imagine.asp?B=4749516

BMJ 5th January 1929

MJA, Vol. 1 No. 8 February 16th 1929 p 225.

Photo: ACH Cup Book, May 1904.

The Register Adelaide 8 Jan 1918

The Register Adelaide 7 Feb 1929

HEGGATON Rupert Dufty

MB BS

1873 - 1958

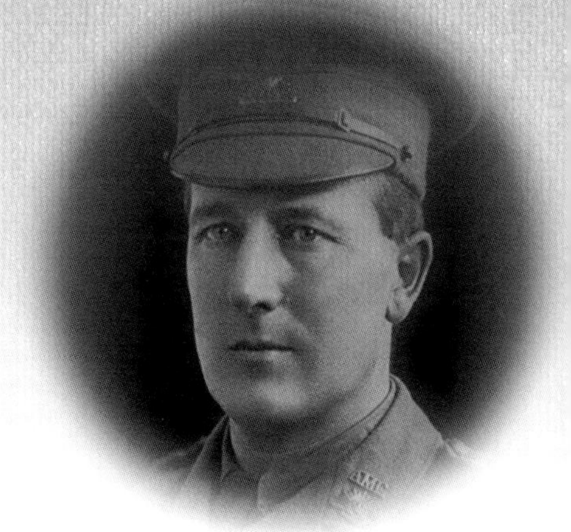

Rupert Dufty Heggaton was born 11th March 1873 at Middleton, South Australia and was the youngest son of William and Mary Heggaton. They later moved to Mitcham, South Australia. Rupert attended Prince Alfred College. He started his medical degree at the University of Adelaide but completed the degree at Sydney University in 1901 due to the 'Adelaide Hospital Row'. Like others affected by this dispute Heggaton did not to return to South Australia. He was a resident medical officer at the Royal Prince Alfred Hospital, Sydney in 1900 and moved to Harden-Murrumburrah south west of Sydney where he married Elizabeth Louise Burgess in 1902.

Heggaton enlisted in the AIF as a captain on 17th October 1915 at the age of 42 years and 11 months. He was 5ft 8ins tall, weighed 174 lbs, of fair complexion, grey eyes and black hair and able to ride. His wife Elizabeth of Albury Street, Murrumburrah was nominated as his next of kin. He was posted immediately to the headquarters 1 Mining Corps as a medical officer and spent the next few months at the Casula Camp, Liverpool. He embarked on the HMAT *Ulysses* on 20th February and arrived in Marseilles 5th May 1916. He was posted as RMO to the 3rd Australian Tunnelling Company from HQ 1 Mining Corps on the 2nd December 1916. Soon after on 19th December 1916 he was transferred to 2 AGH. Eight days later he was temporarily detached to the 14 General Hospital returning to 2 AGH in January 1917. He was struck off strength of 2 AGH on the 20th June 1917 and proceeded to England for duty. Heggaton then embarked for Australia on 2nd July 1917 and his appointment was terminated from the AIF on 3rd October 1917. He was entitled to the 1914-15 Star, the British War Medal and the Victory Medal. However, despite assurances from base records that his medals were issued on 21st July 1922 and sent to the Harden RSL they were not received by Heggaton. This problem continued until the 1930s and there is no indication that he ever received his war medals.

Heggaton remained in Harden-Murrumburrah after the war and was a much respected citizen for over 50 years. He became the Mayor of Murrumburrah in 1930 and lived at 19 Vernon Street, Murrumburrah. Heggaton had much tragedy in his life; his daughter Lorraine Madge Heggaton died as a result of a fire in 1928 at the age of 21 years and two of his sons were killed in WW2. Flt SGT Knox William Heggaton and Lance Corporal Vaudan Dufty Heggaton. Rupert Dufty Heggaton died in Murrumburrah on 9th August 1958 aged 85 years.

Sources:

http://recordsearch.naa.gov.au/scripts/Imagine.asp?B=5310039
Aldous Anthony M, Halm Helen, personal notes.
http://anzacsonline.net.au/tunnellers@bigpond.com
Photo from Family

Abortive Treatment of Infection

Dr Carrel began by quoting Professor Tuffier's statement that of 1,000 amputations at Maison-Blanche, the operations had to be done in about 800, not on account of the gravity of the wound, but owing to complicating infection.

BMJ, 23 October 1915, p. 609

HILL Alfred William

MD MRCS (Eng) LRCP (Lond) LSA

1863 - 1933

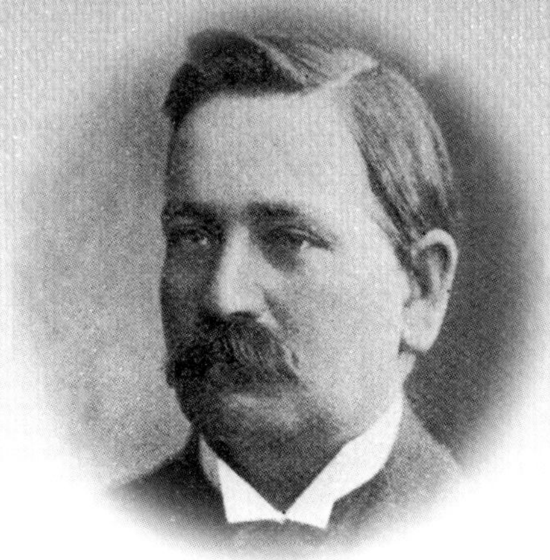

Alfred William Hill was born on 9th December 1863 in Rundle Street, Adelaide South Australia. He was the son of John Drake Hill (1831-1899) and Emma Elizabeth, nee Robjohns (1829-1920). He was educated at Prince Alfred College and studied medicine at Birmingham University and London University. He married Kate Alexandra Robjohns on 15 July 1888 on return to Australia. He had a practice in Terowie, South Australia for six years and travelled to London to undertake a postgraduate course. He returned to Adelaide in 1895 and was, in 1898, appointed honorary ophthalmic surgeon at the Adelaide Hospital.

Before WW1 Hill served in the AAMC reserve and in 1910 he was the sanitary officer at the rank of captain. During WW1 Hill continued to be a member of the AAMC reserve and served, at the rank of lieutenant colonel, as PMO for the South Australian Army Camps. He became interested in making walking sticks from the boxthorns which were plentiful at Semaphore, South Australia in the early 1920s. He became well known for his fine walking sticks and by 1930 he had made nearly 350 walking sticks. He travelled extensively during his lifetime. Alfred William Hill died on June 29th 1933 and was survived by his wife, his two daughters, Kate and Kitty, and son Wilfred.

Sources:

Prince Alfred College Archives

http://histfam.familysearch.org/getperson.php?personID=I279218&tree=SouthAustralia

http://www.rah.sa.gov.au/heritage/index.php for Photo and Hospital appointments.

South Australian Register 26 July 1888

Kalgoorlie Miner 27 Jan 1898

The News Adelaide 08 Dec 1930

Excerpts from the Medical experience of the action between HMAS *Sydney* and SMS *Emden* Cocos Isle 9th November 1914. Recorded by Leonard Darby MB ChB SMO Surgeon RAN

The stations for the surgical party are...two theatres, one for each Surgeon and his assistants, are prepared in well separated stokers bathrooms...10ft x 8ft x 7ft in size.... The *Emden* soon hit us and within 5 to 10 minutes the first wounded man was brought below... The second case was Sharp AB RN shot through the chest and bleeding freely, with the apex of the heart beating through a gaping hole in the chest, loud inrush of air into the chest and air hunger being marked. Pads were rapidly applied to the wounds with tight bandages and a large dose of morphia was given...Most of the wounded were got below by man-handling which was found to be quicker and less awkward ...The state of things on board the *Emden* was truly awful. Men were lying killed and mutilated in heaps with large blackened flesh wounds. The ship was riddled with gaping holes and it was with difficulty one could walk about the decks...Some of the men who were brought off to the *Sydney* presented horrible sights and by this time the wounds were practically all foul and stinking and maggots ¼ inch long were crawling over them i.e. only 24 to 30 hours after injury...After being blown overboard the [German] surgeon managed to get ashore...helpless and exhausted, dying of thirst... After much persuasion he got a sailor to bring him some salt water, of which he drank a large quantity and straightway became raving and died...It would be very difficult to imagine a more trying set of circumstances for the medical staff of a cruiser, and an action where so many wounded would be rescued. Had the Emden sunk before she reached the beach, our work would have just halved itself, as many wounded must have drowned.

Source: AWM

HOLDER Sydney Ernest

MB BS

1890 - 1953

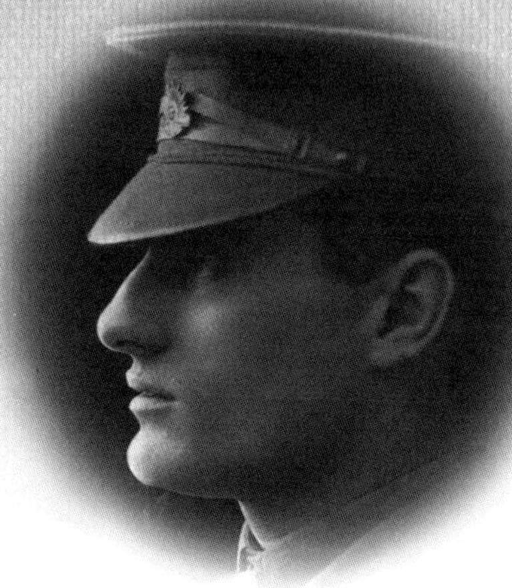

Sydney Ernest Holder was born on the 22nd February 1890 at Kooringa near Burra, SA. He was the sixth child and third son of Sir Frederick William Holder and his wife Julia Maria nee Stephens. Sir Frederick was twice Premier of South Australia and the first Speaker of the House of Representatives. They lived at 50 Sydenham Rd, Norwood. Holder was educated at Prince Alfred College. He won a South Australian Scholarship to study medicine at the University of Adelaide in 1907 and was awarded Blues for tennis and lacrosse. He was also a devout member of the Methodist Church. After his graduation in 1913 Holder completed his residency at Adelaide Hospital.

Holder enlisted in the AIF on the 7th July 1916. He was commissioned as a captain in the AAMC on the 13th September 1916. He married Dorothy Lillian Godlee at Kent Town Methodist Church, on the 28th September 1916. His wife of 38 Marlborough St, College Park, was named as his next of kin. He was 5ft 10ins, weighed 12st 8lbs, and could ride a horse. After 3 months of Camp Duty in 4 MD, he embarked for the Middle East in January 1917. After spending two months with 1 LH Training Regiment, he was posted to 3 LHFA at Marakeb in April 1917. He was transferred to 12 LHR at Belah in January 1918 and served with this unit until the end of the war. He contracted malaria and was evacuated to the 14 AGH. He returned to Australia in July 1919 with his appointment terminated at the 4 MD on the 30th September 1919. He was issued with the British War Medal and the Victory Medal.

Holder practised with Dr F L Thyer (SA Rhodes Scholar 1924) in Kadina, South Australia for about 25 years after the war. He became a town councillor, Medical Health Officer for the Kadina Corporation, and HMO for the Wallaroo Hospital. He was a prominent Prince Alfred College Old Collegian. He loved golf, tennis bowls and cricket. He was a member of the Repatriation Commission. Holder, in WW2, served as a major at 54 Camp Hospital, Loveday, South Australia and at 10 CCS in the Northern Territory. Sydney Ernest Holder died on Monday the 9th February 1953 at the Repatriation General Hospital, Daw Park aged 62 years and was survived by his 3 daughters. His son, Sydney John Holder, served in WW2 as a Flying Officer in the RAAF. He was killed in a flying accident in England in December 1944 while on secondment to 271 Sqn RAF. He is buried at Cirencester, Gloucestershire. Holder had two brothers who also served in WW1 Lieutenant Evan Morecott Holder and Lieutenant Clement Gladstone Holder.

Sources:

http://recordsearch.naa.gov.au/scripts/Imagine.asp?B=5844023

Likeman R., "From the Jungle to the Desert" Slouch Hat Publications 2012.

Photo, PAC Collection. NLA Trove.

HORNABROOK Rupert Walter

MB BS MRCS (Eng) LRCP (Lond)

1871 - 1951

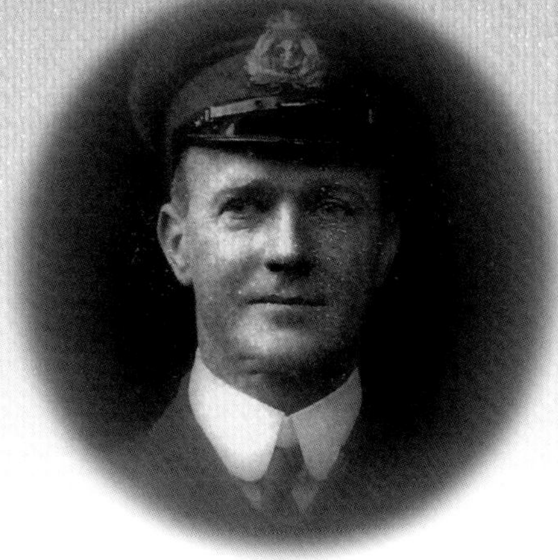

Rupert Walker Hornabrook was born in Kent Town, SA on 3rd August 1871 the son of Charles A Hornabrook and Eliza, nee Soward. This pioneer, well connected family included Charles' father John, of the York Hotel, at the corner of Pultney and Rundle Streets, uncle Archdeacon C S Hornabrook and brother- in- law G K Soward (Colonial Architect) and half-sister Alice married to Sir John Cox Bray, later Premier of South Australia (1881-1884). Hornabrook commenced his degree at the University of Adelaide however due to the 'Adelaide Hospital Row' completed his degree in London in 1899. Shortly after graduation he went to Bombay, India with a medical team to combat the bubonic plague. During the Boer War 1899-1901, as captain in the RAMC, was Mentioned in Despatches and awarded the Queen's South Africa Medal with 6 clasps. *On January 10th 1900, as medical officer of my regiment, the Natal Mounted Rifles, Dr. Hornabrook dashed across to the Gordon Highlanders on our right when the Scots had lost most of their officers at a critical stage of the battle. He saved the day and his orderly got the D.C.M., but though the Doctor was recommended for the V.C, he seems to have been lucky to escape court-martial- for exceeding orders! I honestly think that but for his action the Boers would have taken Ladysmith.* He joined the AAMC in February 1904 with rank of lieutenant, attached to No 1 Battery and was promoted Captain in Oct 1905. He transferred to the unattached list and moved to Melbourne where he married Winifred Emma Sargood of "Ripponlea" in Elsternwick on 10th May 1902. He was appointed to the Melbourne General Hospital in 1909 and he popularised the use of ethyl chloride-ether sequence in anaesthesia early in the 1900s.

He was appointed temporary surgeon on the 3rd of August 1914 at the age of 43 years in the Permanent Naval Force on HMAS *Australia* to serve with Alexander Ruan Caw. During this year he saw service in the AN&MEF which captured the German colonies in the southern Pacific. The AN&MEF was formed following a request by the British government on 6th August 1914 and was separate from the AIF. HMAS *Australia* led the force and proceeded to the UK and, on 8th February 1915, became flagship of the 2nd Battle-Cruiser Squadron of the Royal Navy's Grand Fleet. Hornabrook resigned from his naval commission, in Melbourne, on 7th August 1915. He enlisted in the AIF, in the army, in 1916. He was 45 years old, 5ft 8ins, and weighed 11st 7lbs, with a large scar 4ins long over the right crest of his pelvis from an old bullet wound. He sailed to England on the *Medic* in December 1916. During 1917 he served in 1 AGH, 11 Surgical Team, and 12 CCS. He was promoted to major in September. He requested to return to Melbourne to take up anaesthetic work at Melbourne University in November, with his appointment terminated on 5th December 1917. He was issued with the 1914-15 Star (Navy Issue), British War Medal and the Victory Medal.

Hornabrook followed his anaesthetic career after the war. He was the first Chairman of the Victorian Branch, Section of Anaesthetics, of the BMA and, with Gilbert Brown in 1934, a Foundation member of the Australian Society of Anaesthetists. He led a busy social and non-medical professional life. Rupert Walker Hornabrook died on May 7th 1951 at 10 Toorak Avenue, Toorak, Victoria.

Sources:

http://recordsearch.naa.gov.au/scripts/Imagine.asp?B=5831022;
http://recordsearch.naa.gov.au/scripts/Imagine.asp?B=225136
Photo from grandson.
The Torrens Park Estate. Preiss and Oborn, 1991.
Anesth Intensive Care: 1999. 27:519-522.
Med J Aust1914; 1:559-561.
The Argus Melbourne 19th May 1902
South Australian Register 22 February 1899.

HORWOOD Oswald Ryle

MA (Cantab) MRCS (Eng) LRCP (Lond)

1883 - 1930

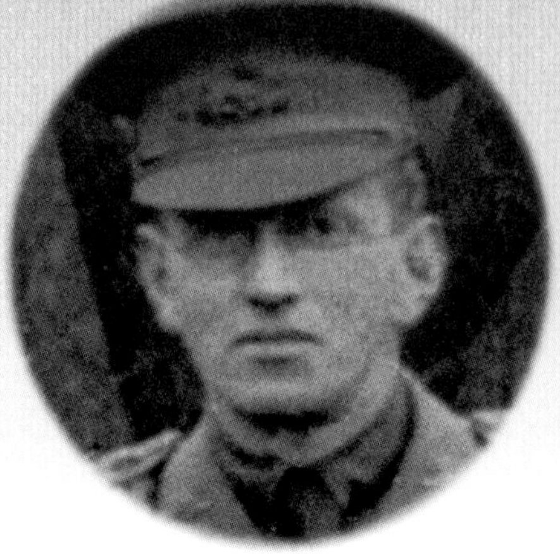

Oswald Ryle Horwood was born on the 23rd August 1883 in Tetbury, Gloucestershire. His father Thomas George Horwood was the Vicar of the Parish and his mother was Agnes, nee Whereat. He was educated at the Dean Close School in Cheltenham, the Philberds School, Maidenhead, Eton College and Corpus Christi College, Cambridge where he gained his BA in 1905. He served in the Cambridge Volunteer Rifles while at University. After graduating, Horwood went to India, where he was commissioned as a 2nd lieutenant in the Simla Volunteer Rifles in 1907. He returned to England in 1907. He was ordained as a deacon in the Church of England in 1910, and gained his MA in the same year, and served as a priest in 1911. Between 1910 and 1913 he was a curate in parishes in Canning Town, East Finchley, and Stepney England. At the same time he was studying medicine at The London Hospital Medical College, and passed the conjoint exams in 1913. Horwood completed his residency at St Mary's Hospital, Plaistow, the Hampstead, North West London Hospital, and Scarborough General Hospital. He was curate from 1913-14 to his father who at this time was Rector of Tunstall in Suffolk. He came to Australia in late 1914, allegedly to earn money, and was registered in SA in January 1915. He took up practice with Dr Dawes as a "physician and surgeon "in Hawker, South Australia.

Horwood volunteered for the AIF in August 1915. He was single, 31 years old, 5ft 10ins tall, and weighed 11st, His father, in England, was named as his next of kin. He stated he was familiar with all forms of anaesthesia, and could speak German and Hindustani well, with some French, Latin and Greek. He was posted to 1 AAH at Harefield England and later to the Bostal Heath Con Depot at Abbey Wood. He did not go to France until July 1916. After arriving at 5 ADBD at Étaples, he was sent briefly to 2 AGH at Wimereux, then on to 2 FdAmb, and was finally posted RMO of 10 Bn in August. He returned to England in November and requested his discharge in England on the grounds that his father was close to death. It was stated that the parish living at Tunstall Suffolk where his father was the incumbent belonged to the Horwood family, and that if Horwood did not take it up promptly, it would lapse. Horwood's request for discharge was supported by General Howse, and he did take up the parish on his father's death. He was awarded the Medaille du Roi Albert in June 1920; this was a war medal for Belgian citizens and foreign nationals for humanitarian assistance to Belgians during World War 1. He did not remain at Tunstall Suffolk for long. He had two periods of service with the RAMC in 1917-18 and 1920-21. In Australia he was issued with the British War Medal and the Victory Medal.

Horwood was appointed Chaplain to the Bishop of Zululand after the war. He returned to Zululand again from 1921-22. In 1924 the British Government, London enquired about the suitability of Horwood for a post in the Colonial Service. Whether a position was forthcoming remains unclear. The regimental history of 10 Bn contains an unconfirmed report that Horwood was working with a Christian Mission in China. Horwood seems to have been well connected and generally held in high esteem. He married Elizabeth Marguerite Hansford, in Warwickshire in 1929; they have no recorded children. He was acting curate of Sulhamstead near Reading Berkshire in 1929. Oswald Ryle Horwood died on the 16th November 1929 at Tunstall, Suffolk. He was 46 years old.

Sources:

http://recordsearch.naa.gov.au/scripts/Imagine.asp?B=5831660.

Lock Cecil Bert Lovell, 'The Fighting Tenth,' Webb and Son, Adelaide, 1936.

Photo: AWM 4058

JAMES William Abel

MRCS (Eng) LRCP (Lond)

1880 - 1938

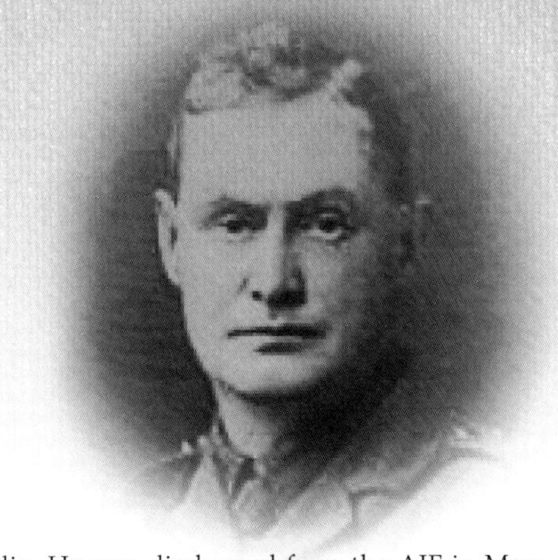

William Abel James was born on the 5th October 1880 at Cumbran, Monmouthshire, Wales. The son of a schoolmaster, William John James and his wife Elizabeth Ann, nee Brown. While studying medicine, James served for seven years in 3 Bn South Wales Borderers, and reached the rank of lieutenant. After graduation in 1906 James obtained a position as a ship's surgeon with the White Star Line. In the course of his service on the *Olympic*, he met a 28 year old Australian woman, Evelyn Marsden (1883-1938) who was employed by the Company as a stewardess and nurse. Marsden had been born at Stockyard Creek, Dalkey SA and was the daughter of the stationmaster there. Evelyn Marsden was working on the *Titanic* on her maiden voyage. After the ship sank, Marsden spent the night in a lifeboat until being picked up by the liner *Carpathia* next morning. She was the only Australian female survivor. Marsden and James were married on her return to England and left for South Australia, arriving at Semaphore in November 1912. James obtained the position of medical officer at the Adelaide Hospital, and they moved into a new apartment in Ruthven Mansions on Pulteney Street, Adelaide. Later they moved to Wallaroo, South Australia, living and working there for 15 months before finally moving to Newcastle and then Bondi in New South Wales where James set up practice.

James enlisted on the 1st March 1915 at Mitcham and named his wife as his next of kin care of W H Marsden of Yacka, South Australia. He was 34 years old, 5ft 7ins, and weighed 184lbs, and was of fair complexion, fair hair and brown eyes. He was commissioned and sailed from Sydney for the Middle East on the 11th February 1915 with the reinforcements for 1 AGH. He was transferred to 1 AAH on arrival. He served until May 1916, at which time he contracted amoebic dysentery, and was admitted to 3 AGH. He was twice discharged to convalescence, and twice re-admitted. He was sent back to Australia for three months rest in July. He was declared fit for home duty in November, and posted to 7 AGH at Keswick South Australia. He was discharged from the AIF in May 1917, but remained in the AAMC. He was promoted major in March 1918. Notwithstanding all that had happened, James volunteered a second time in June 1918, and was passed fit for overseas service. He reached England in September 1918, and was posted to 2 AAH at Southall. He returned to Australia in May 1919, with his appointment terminated on the 28th August 1919 in the 4 MD. He was issued with the 1914-1915 Star, the British War Medal and the Victory Medal.

James resumed his practice in New South Wales and lived in Bondi. William Abel James and his wife Evelyn both died in September 1938 and were buried in the Waverley Cemetery. They had no children.

Sources:
Likeman R., 2012, From the Tropics to the Desert, Slouch Hat Publications, Port Melbourne.
http://recordsearch.naa.gov.au/scripts/Imagine.asp?B=7336403
Photo; SLSA
Recorder Port Pirie 24 April 1937 'Personal Reminiscences'.
The Sydney Morning Herald 08 and 10 Sep 1938

Britain's Call

Britain has need of her medical sons, and will certainly not call in vain. In her hour of trial, with a possibility, nay probability, of numberless citizens of the empire lying wounded or sick on the field of battle, she looks to the medical profession in all parts of the world, and especially in her own dominions and territories, to volunteer to bring succour to the wounded and those affected by contagious diseases which always abound when armies oppose one another in warfare…No sacrifice it too great for the profession it is continuous struggle against trauma, disease and death….Volunteers are required at once, and we feel sure that a large number of practitioners will respond.

MJA, 15th August 1915, p. 155

JEFFRIES Lewis Wibmer

DSO OBE MB BS

1884 - 1971

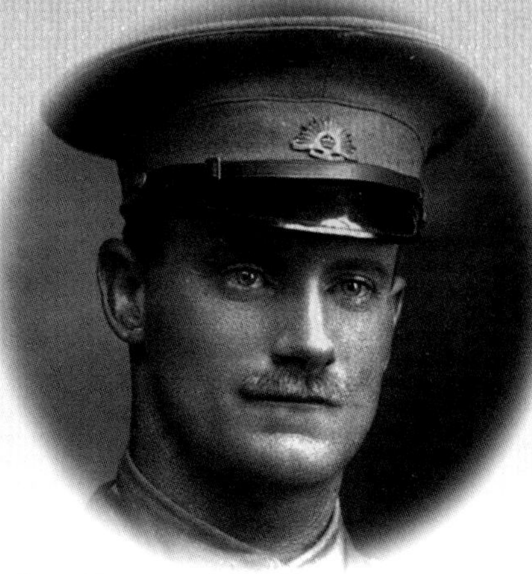

Lewis Wibmer Jeffries was born on 9th August 1884 in Derby, England. He was the son of Rev William Jeffries and his wife Mercy, nee Wibmer. He was educated in schools in Toowoomba and Broken Hill before completing his secondary education at Prince Alfred College. He completed his medical degree at The University of Adelaide in 1907. He was awarded a Blue for lacrosse while at the university. After graduation he assisted Dr Arthur Powell in Kadina before obtaining post-graduate experience by travelling to Johns Hopkins in Baltimore where he worked with Harvey Cushing, the Children's Hospital in Great Ormond Street, and Breslau in Germany prior to a year in Kashmir in a Church Missionary Society Hospital. At Great Ormond Street the famous surgeon John Percy Lockhart-Mummery described him as *"tactful, courteous and considerate for his patients."* He returned to Australia in 1914 and, there, after the declaration of war, joined the 1st AIF.

Jeffries enlisted in the AIF on 14th October 1914. He was 30 years old, 5ft 10ins tall and 156lb. He was posted to 4 FdAmb and travelled to Egypt and with his unit to Gallipoli where he landed on the first day of the campaign on 25th April 1915. He was to remain there for the entire campaign. He was wounded on 9th May 1915, unconscious with an obvious entry and exit wound in his chest had been 'red-tagged' as dead. He had been saved by his cigarette case. Subsequently he was posted to 50 Bn and promoted to major. It was with this unit on 13th to 15th August 1916 in the region of Mouquet Farm, that he exhibited *'great devotion to duty when he left his dressing station and went to the front line at great risk to attend to wounded and to re-organize the stretcher bearers. When only a few bearers were left he took parties of men out himself and assisted to carry back our wounded after having dressed them under very heavy fire'*. The DSO was awarded for conspicuous gallantry and devotion to duty during operations and gazetted on 14th November 1916. He was twice Mentioned in Despatches for his services in France and Belgium. He served as DADMS for the 4th Australian Division from December 1916 to January 1918. He was promoted to lieutenant colonel and, from January 1918 was DADMS for AIF Headquarters in London. He was issued with the 1914-15 Star, the British War Medal and the Victory Medal with Oak Leaves. He was appointed OBE in 1919.

Jeffries married Shirley Frances Singleton on 20th December 1917 in St Georges, Bloomsbury. He returned to SA in 1920 and to general practice where he was in partnership Dean Dawson, Charles Turner and Charles Yeatman. He performed his own surgery and confined up to 200 women annually, many in their own homes. He was appointed Inspector General of Hospitals in SA in 1933, an appointment he held until 1947. He was chairman of the board of the Adelaide Hospital, a member of the Medical Board of SA and the Faculty of Medicine of the University of Adelaide. Subsequently he returned to clinical practice performing relieving work in country SA as well as working as a medical officer with the Red Cross Transfusion Service until his death. Lewis Wibmer Jeffries died in Adelaide on 6th October 1971. A sister, Eleanor, a nurse with the AANC in WW1, was twice decorated with the Royal Red Cross and Mentioned in Dispatches and a brother, Sir Shirley Jeffries was a solicitor, and politician. Jeffries had three sons all of whom served in different services in WW2. Dr John S Jeffries served with the RAAMC and, his son Dr Lewis Peter Jeffries joined the Australian Defence Force Reserve.

Sources:

National Archives
http://recordsearch.naa.gov.au/NameSearch/Interface/ItemDetail.aspx?Barcode=7372302
Personal history Jeffries family
Gurner C. M, 'Jeffries, Lewis Wibmer (1884–1971)', Australian Dictionary of Biography, National Centre of Biography, Australian National University, http://adb.anu.edu.au/biography/jeffries-lewis-wibmer-6833/text11827.

JERMYN Frederick David

VD MB BS (Melb)

1865 - 1948

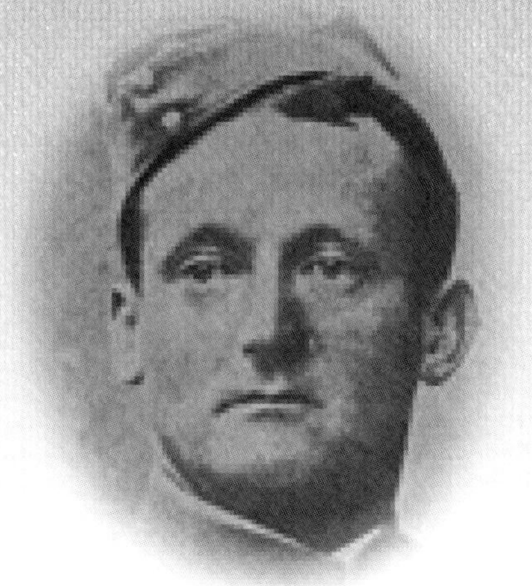

Frederick David Jermyn was born on 4th June 1865 at Port Fairy, Victoria. He was the second son of Dr Cosmo David Jermyn from Co Kerry and Josephine, nee Dittmar from Co Cork, who married in Melbourne in 1857. He studied medicine at the University of Melbourne graduating in 1887/8. He served as a surgeon captain in G Coy of the Victorian Mtd Rifles from 1890-95, when he was practising at Koroit, near Warrnambool. He moved to Mount Gambier in 1895 and was commissioned as a lieutenant in the South Australian Mounted Rifles in 1898. He served in the Second South Australian Contingent in the South African War from 1900-1902, and was promoted captain in April 1900. He received the QSM with 5 clasps, having seen service in the Cape and Orange River Colonies and the Transvaal, and having been present at the actions at Johannesburg, Pretoria, and Diamond Hill. He was invalided to England with an eye problem in 1902, and while recovering pursued post-graduate studies in London. On his return to Australia he joined the AAMC as a Captain in 1903, and was promoted major in 1910 and was appointed as RMO of 22 LHR. He received the VD in 1913. Jermyn's brother moved to Mount Gambier in 1904 and went into partnership with him in general practice. He married Bertha Jessie Belle Newberry in Victoria in 1909.

Jermyn volunteered for the AIF on the 30th October 1914 at Adelaide in 4 MD. He was 49 years old, 5ft 8ins, and weighed 12st. He was posted as OC B Section of 4 FdAmb. He proceeded to join the MEF on 12th April 1915. He was evacuated from Gallipoli to Mudros in June 1915 and from there to Egypt in June with glaucoma of the left eye. He was subsequently reported as having dysentery as well. He returned to Australia in September 1915 and worked at Keswick Hospital until his appointment was terminated on the 10th February 1916. He was issued with the 1914-15 Star, the British War Medal and the Victory Medal.

After the war Jermyn decided to move back to Victoria and was Medical Officer to the Queenscliff Garrison from 1917 to 1936, and was also the Public Vaccinator for the South Western District from 1917. The local newspaper the Border Watch, Mount Gambier, said of his leaving; *"During the 22 years he had been a resident of the town he had proved himself a worthy citizen, and had taken an interest in all kinds of sports. Many people would feel deep regret at his departure, especially his patients, whom he had attended with care and consideration."* Frederick David Jermyn died in Wandin, Victoria in 1948.

Sources:
Likeman R., "Gallipoli Doctors" Slouch Hat Publications, 2010.
http://recordsearch.naa.gov.au/scripts/Imagine.asp?B=7336618
Photo SLSA,
Adelaide Observer Feb 3rd 1900.
Boar War departures.
http://www.bwm.org.au/site/Doctors_and_Vets.asp
Border Watch Mount Gambier April 1917.
Ancestry.com

The War Emergency

The people of this country [Britain] are accused of not taking the war seriously enough, and not realizing the calls which it makes on our resources in men, energy, and material. Germany is determined, ruthless, and unscrupulous in her methods, and still confident of success.

BMJ, 15 May 1915, p. 853

JERMYN Walter Herbert

MB BS (Melb)

1867 - 1946

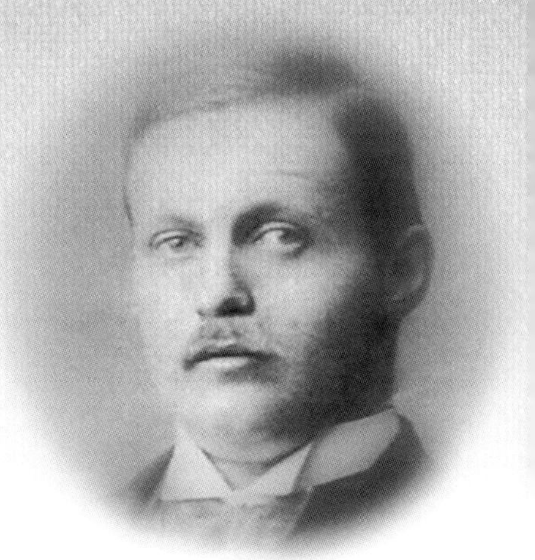

Walter Herbert Jermyn was born on the 16th March 1867 in Port Fairy, Victoria the son of Dr Cosmo David Jermyn, a practising doctor in Port Fairy and Josephine, nee Dittmar. He was the brother of Frederick David Jermyn. Jermyn studied medicine at the University of Melbourne graduating in 1889. Jermyn worked as a RMO in the Melbourne Hospital in 1889 and House Surgeon in Launceston Hospital 1890-93 before going to Mount Gambier to a general practice in partnership with his brother Frederick. They erected the residence at the corner of Ferrers and Sturt Streets later occupied by Dr. C. E. King and Dr. G. N. Lorimer. Jermyn married Miss Euphemia (Tot) Williams, youngest daughter of the late Mr. and Mrs. Thomas. H., Williams, of "Llandovery," Penola Road. Jermyn and his wife moved to Guandaring, Western Australia to undertake farming. However, they returned to South Australia which may have been due to his wife's illness as on the 25th September 1916 his wife 'Tot' died at Konetta Private Hospital, North Adelaide.

Jermyn enlisted in the AIF on the 4th March 1917 after the death of his wife. He had, since March 1916, worked in 4 MD in the AAMC Reserve both as SMO and CO of the 6 AIDH, North Adelaide. He was 5ft 5ins, and weighed 12st 6lbs, and he was able to ride a horse and had limited proficiency in French. His age was overlooked *"as he was otherwise fit and has much active experience in the AAMC Reserve and is particularly fit for general Duty aboard"*. His next of kin was named as his brother Frederick David Jermyn. He embarked from Melbourne on the 12th May 1917 for England where he worked in various AIF Training, Depot and hospital facilities. He had several bouts of bronchitis and in April 1918 he was admitted to the Military Hospital in Fovant and then transferred to 3rd London General Hospital with influenza, senility and bronchitis, his medical records stating that he *looks his age. Has a constant and distressing cough.* He returned to Australia in June 1918 and despite the unusual diagnosis of senility he served as the ships SMO on the return journey. He was struck off strength with his appointment terminated on the 2nd October 1918. He was issued with the British War Medal.

He took up residence in Nelson, Victoria where he continued to live until his death. He did not continue as a doctor but participated in community life and a presentation was made to him of a fly fishing rod, in appreciation of his contribution to the Nelson community. Jermyn played cricket for the Mt. Gambier Club from 1897 to 1931. He was a prolific scorer as a left hand batsman and a superb fieldsman. He was a fine tennis player, and occupied high administrative positions in the Mount Gambier Tennis Club. He was a keen member of the Mt. Gambier Gun Club and had few equals in his best days as a trap shot. Walter Herbert Jermyn died in April 1946 at Nelson, aged 79 years.

Sources:
http://recordsearch.naa.gov.au/scripts/Imagine.asp?B=7336621
Border Watch April 9th1946.
Adelaide Register 27th September 1916
The Adelaide Advertiser 13th April 1946
http://www.launcestonfamilyalbum.org.au/detail/1030622/walter-herbert-jermyn

Medical News from Germany

In Berlin twenty-five hospitals have been improvised with accommodation for about 20,000 wounded...German surgeons with experiences of the war of 1870 express boundless praise of the improved conditions to which ambulance have contributed.

BMJ, 28 November 1914, p. 944

JOHNSON Edward Angas

JP MB BS (Melb) MD Gottingen

1873 - 1951

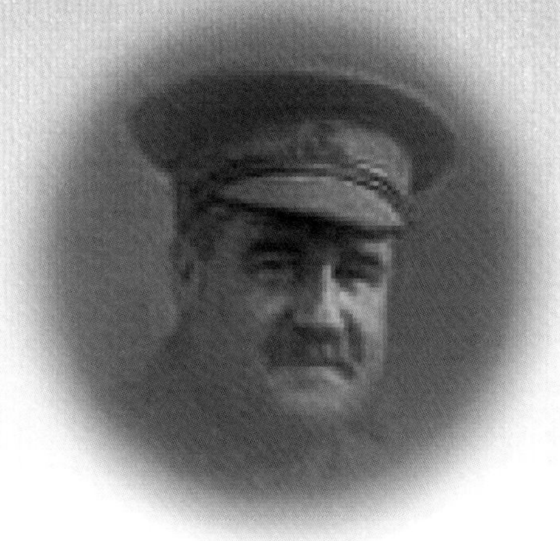

Edward Angas Johnson, was born on the 15th January 1873 and was the second son of James Angas Johnson and Catharine, nee Williams. They lived at Lindsay Villa on the Lindsay Park estate at Angaston. Lindsay Park was the home of his great-grandfather George Fife Angas, one of the founders of South Australia. Angas had built Lindsay Villa for his grandson James so that James may assist him to manage his affairs. James's father had died at sea enroute to South Australia. Lindsay Villa was a short walk from Lindsay Park House. The Johnson family were industrialists from Manchester where the family made wire products. They had made the first undersea cable connecting England with Ireland and had the initial expertise in making barbed wire. The first overland cable across Australia had been made of Johnson's wire. Johnson, always known as Angas, was educated at Whinham College in North Adelaide and St Peter's College. He studied medicine at the University of Adelaide and, because of the 'Adelaide Hospital Row', completed his final year in Melbourne graduating in 1897, before returning to Adelaide. After a house surgeon appointment at the Children's Hospital he travelled overseas in 1898 to undertake postgraduate studies in pathology and bacteriology at the University of Gottingen and gained his MD 1899. Further experience was gained in Berlin, Strasburg, at the Pasteur Institute in Paris and, in London and Cambridge. Johnson was made a Justice of the Peace in Adelaide in 1902. He was appointed honorary assistant physician at the Adelaide Hospital in 1902 and from 1909-1924 honorary physician. He was the honorary sanitary advisor from 1926-1942.

Johnson was commissioned in the AAMC in 1902 and served until 1920 reaching the rank of major. During WW1 he served as an MO to the Adelaide military camps and undertook the initial enlistment medical examinations for the AIF.

Johnson sat on the Adelaide City Council in 1903 and again after he returned from further study at the London School of Hygiene and Tropical Medicine 1907-1924. He resigned from the council in 1924 when he became the medical officer of health for Adelaide, a post he held until 1938. At this time he was chairman of the Adelaide Board of Health and represented the Government on the Central Board of Health. He was a governor and benefactor of the Botanic Gardens and published many papers on the history of plants. He was also the South Australian editor of Virchow's Jahresbericht (Berlin). He was an avid collector of early South Australia memorabilia, including personal belongings of Queen Adelaide and Colonel Light, much of which was donated to the Adelaide City Council and which makes up a large part of The City of Adelaide Civic Collection. He married Margarethe Friedericke Charlotte Klevesahl, in September 1900 in London, the sister-in-law of Charles Rasp, of Broken Hill fame. Margarethe died in 1936 and they had one son. He married Dorothy Muriel Brandt in January 1939. Edward Angas Johnson died 19th June 1951 at his home in Glenelg South Australia. He was survived by his second wife and son from his first marriage.

Sources:

Escourt Hughes J., 'Johnson, Edward Angas (1873–1951)', Australian Dictionary of Biography, National Centre of Biography, Australian National University. http://adb.anu.edu.au/biography/johnson-edward-angas-6852/text11867

Image No B 6324 SLSA

Adelaide Advertiser 20 November 1902

Adelaide Advertiser 21st June 1951

JOSE Sir Ivan Bede

MC MS FRCS FRCS(Ed) FRACS

1893 - 1969

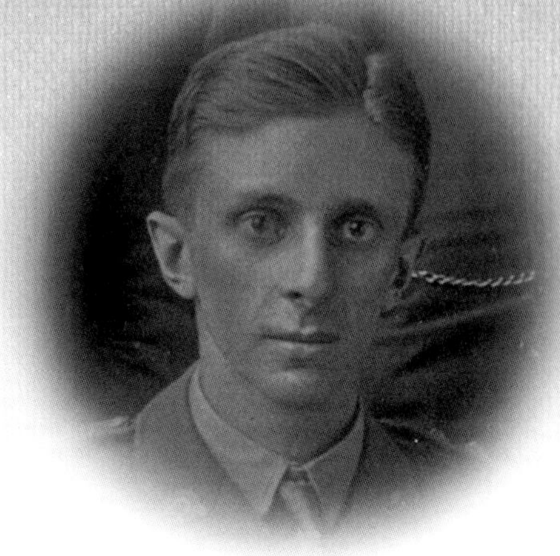

Ivan Bede Jose was born in Ningpo, China, the eldest of three sons of George Herbert Jose, an English Anglican missionary, and his wife Clara Ellen, nee Sturt from South Australia. George took his family to England in 1899 where he studied in Oxford before relocating to Adelaide in 1903. Ivan was educated at the Queen's School in North Adelaide and then, from 1905-1910, St Peter's College. At school he served in the cadets. He studied medicine at the University of Adelaide and graduated in 1915.

Jose joined the AIF as a medical student on 27th November 1914 at the age of 21 and nine months. He was 5'10" tall and weighed 154lbs, of fair complexion with brown eyes and 'medium' hair. He was to join the second reinforcements of 1ASH and achieved the rank of acting Sergeant. He was discharged on 1st March 1915 to complete his medical studies which he did, re-joining the Army as a captain on 5th February 1916 when he was an inch taller and 4lbs lighter. He embarked from Australia on 17th November 1916. He was posted initially to 2FdAmb and later served with distinction in 14FdAmb in France. He was Mentioned in Despatches for 'distinguished and gallant service and devotion to duty in the field' from 22nd February 1917 to 20th September 1917. He was later decorated with a Military Cross for conspicuous gallantry and devotion to duty during the period 25th September 1917 and 25th February 1918 near Polygon Wood, east of Ypres; *'at great personal risk he supervised and insured splendid communication with the RAPs. To his coolness and organization despite extremely heavy shelling.....successful evacuation of the heavy casualties sustained during the operation'.* He was promoted to major in 1918. He spent some time in hospital in February 1918 with enteritis. His appointment was terminated on 10th December 1918. He was issued with the British War Medal and the Victory Medal. His younger brother Lieutenant Wilfred Oswald Jose of 50 Bn was killed in action in 1917. His surviving younger brother, Gilbert Edgar, who had also served as a soldier in WW1, graduated from medicine in 1924 and was later to die in Changi Jail, a prisoner of war of the Japanese.

Jose married Imogen Mervyn (Jean) Hawkes at Christ Church, North Adelaide in May 1919 and subsequently travelled to England for postgraduate study in Surgery. He qualified FRCS (Eng) and FRCS (Edin) in 1922, MS (Adel) 1923 and FRACS in 1929. He was appointed a medical and surgical registrar at the Adelaide Hospital in 1923 and was described as an enthusiastic teacher. At the Adelaide Hospital he was appointed honorary assistant surgeon from 1924 and honorary surgeon, with a particular interest in urological surgery, from 1930-1950. He was the foundation director of surgical studies from 1936 and by the age of 40 was the hospital's senior surgeon. He restructured surgical teaching and, at the University of Adelaide, was the Dean of Medicine in 1948. He had remained a member of the AAMC reserve from 1921 and in WW2 served at home in the RAAF with the rank of group captain. Jose was an RACS councillor from 1946-1948 and president 1955-57. He gave a great deal of his time to the Australian Red Cross in South Australia. He was SA branch president of the British Medical Association. He was knighted in 1963. He was a member of the Adelaide Club and in addition to his many other activities developed a grazing property. Ivan Bede Jose died in 1969 at his North Adelaide home and was survived by his wife, two sons and a daughter. One of his sons followed his interest in urology.

Sources:

Hunter R: "Jose Sir Ivan Bede (1893-1969)" ADB

Photo; Adelaide University Archives, Graduates 1915

National Archives

http://recordsearch.naa.gov.au/NameSearch/Interface/ItemDetail.aspx?Barcode=11545731

JUETT Alexander

MB BCh BA FRACS

1886 - 1953

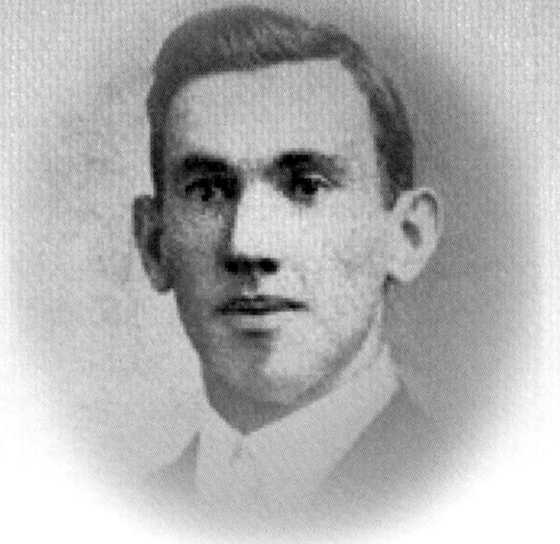

Alexander Juett was born in Adelaide on 12th November 1886. His father, John Duncan Juett was the owner of Great Fingall Mine near Day Dawn, Western Australia and his mother was Clara Jane, nee Smith. He was educated in Adelaide until 1902 when his family moved to Perth where he was educated at Christian Brothers College in Perth Western Australia. Alexander was awarded a Rhodes Scholarship in 1906. He studied medicine and arts at Brasenose College, Oxford, and graduated in 1912 with a BA, MB BCh. He was said to be proficient in field sports as well as academically. Following graduation in 1913 he worked as a Casualty Officer in Heidelberg Hospital and as House Officer in the Middlesex Hospital. He returned to Australia and was a medical officer at Cue-Day Dawn Hospital and a District Medical Officer for the next 2 years. He married, Miss Ida Grierson from London, in Perth on 3rd March 1914.

Juett enlisted on 4th January 1916. He was described as 29 years old 6ft tall, and weighed 200lbs. His next of kin was recorded as his wife Ida, and gave her address as 84 Warwick Road, Ealing, London; he gave his postal address as Day Dawn, Western Australia. He could ride a horse and had some French language. Juett was initially posted to the 44 Bn. He embarked for overseas from Fremantle on 6th June 1916 on the *Lydia* disembarking in Plymouth on 21st July 1916. He was transferred to 11 FdAmb on 9th February 1917 and on the 17th April 1917 he was transferred to 1 ACCS; he returned to his unit on 29th April. He was wounded in action with a gunshot wound and was admitted to 30th General Hospital at Calais on the 5th June 1917. However within three day he was back in the field and was gassed on the 8th June and transferred, on 13th June 1917, to the 3rd London General Hospital. He was attached for duty to 3 AAH in Dartford on 24th July. He was Mentioned in Despatches by Sir Douglas Haig on 7th November 1917 and was brought to the notice of the Secretary of State for his valuable work. He transferred to 2nd Convalescent Depot on 24th Aug 1918. He attended Mundesley Neurological Hospital for education purposes on 12th February 1919. He embarked for Australia on 16th March 1919. He was transhipped to the *Dunluce Castle* at Alexandria on 7th April 1919. His appointment was terminated on 8th August 1919. He was issued the British War Medal and Victory Medal with Oak Leaves.

Juett had a medical practice in Perth after the war and became "one of the most prominent" and "selfless" of orthopaedic surgeons. He established orthopaedic clinics at the Children's Hospital and Perth Hospital. He was a foundation Fellow of the Royal Australasian College of Surgeons. He gave free services to the Fairbridge Farm School and he was Honorary Surgeon to the Maimed and Limbless Ex-Servicemen's Association. He was a consultant with the rank of major during the WW2. Alexander Juett died on 19th May 1953. He was survived by his wife Ida. When Ida died she left a bequest to the University of Western Australia in memory of her husband to enable graduates of the Faculty of Natural and Agricultural Sciences to gain additional knowledge outside of Australia.

Sources:

National Archives of Australia
http://recordsearch.naa.gov.au/NameSearch/Interface/ItemDetail.aspx?Barcode=7366367
Official Publications of the University of Western Australia
The West Australian (Perth) 22nd May 1953
The Bone and Joint Journal, Vol. 3413, No 3, August 1954.
Photo:https://www.google.com.au/search?q=alexander+juett&tbm=isch&tbo=u&source=univ&sa=X&ei=gEB3UvmqM4LukQX6loAg&ved=0CDAQsAQ&biw=1536&bih=747

KEIPERT Leslie James

MB BS

1895 - 1942

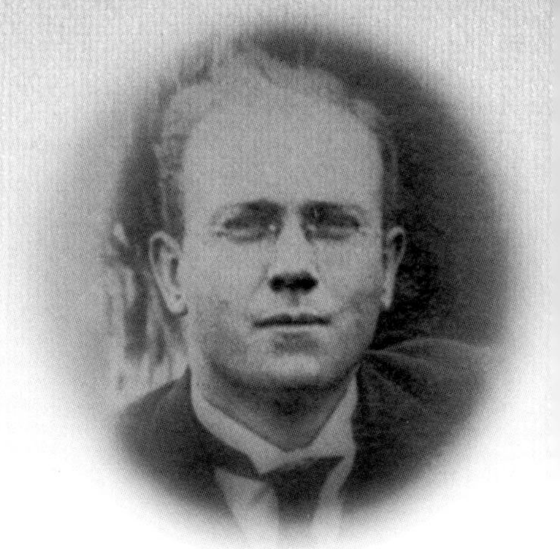

Leslie James Keipert was born in 16th May 1895 in Laura, South Australia (see note) to Heinrich Johann Keipert, born in Zweibrucken Bavaria, and Esther Louisa, nee Harry. He was one of eight children, four brothers and three sisters. He was educated at Laura High School and won an Exhibition in December 1908 to attend Adelaide High School. He studied medicine at the University of Adelaide and graduated in 1918.

Keipert enlisted in the AIF on 18th June 1918 when he was waiting for his final year medical results. His father (now called Henry John) was given as his next of kin and living in Laura. He had eight years of service experience in the cadet and citizen forces. He was living in Kyre Avenue, Kingswood. He was 23 years old and single and was 5ft 10ins tall, and weighed 155lbs with fair hair, blue eyes and a fair complexion. He was not called up for duty and his enlistment was terminated on 18th November 1918 after 50 days of war service. His appointment as an officer terminated on 6th August 1919.

Keipert was married to Annie (Juddy) Charlotte Browning, daughter of Mr W. Browning, of North Carlton, Victoria in Maitland, South Australia on 15th September 1919. He moved to Victoria and had a practice in Rupanyup, Victoria. Leslie James Keipert died in Melbourne on 8th March 1942. He was survived by his wife and his son James, a medical student, and his daughter Lesley.

Note: Several records incorrectly state Keipert was born in Laura Queensland.

Sources:

National Archives of Australia
Biographical Index of South Australians 1836-1885
The Register 23rd December 1908, 26th November 1918
The Argus 10th March 1942
The Advertiser 14th October 1919
Chronicle 3rd July 1920
http://histfam.familysearch.org/getperson.php?personID=I123001&tree=SouthAustralia
Photo: Adelaide University Archives; Medical Graduates 1918.

Alcohol and Military Efficiency

The facts are that all but the smallest quantities of alcohol impair the efficiency of the soldier, diminish his powers of resistance both moral and bodily, and render him more readily to venereal infection. Secondly, drunkenness among the soldiers has been and still is common.... The very strongest opposition to the continuation of wet canteens throughout the Commonwealth was voiced by... the Temperance Alliance...While we sympathize with the Temperance Alliance... we recognize that expediency must be considered before ideals, and that any measure which promises a practical result is to be preferred to a more efficient but less radical proposal.

MJA, 15 January 1915, p. 58

KENIHAN Raphael Leo

MC MB BS MRACP

1890 - 1964

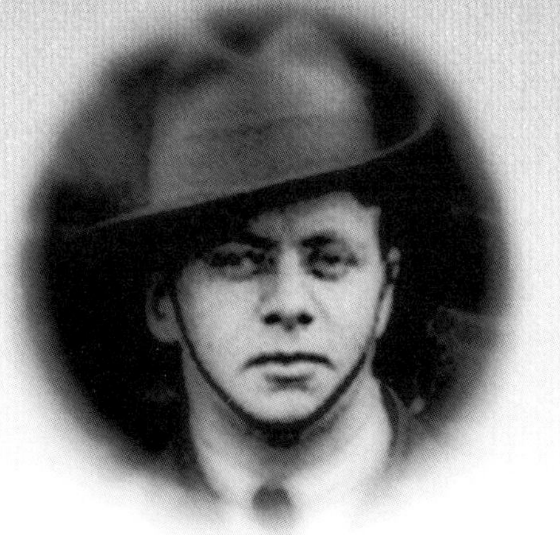

Raphael Leo 'Ken' Kenihan was born on the 23rd October 1890 at O'Halloran Hill, South Australia. He was the youngest of the ten children of Michael Joseph Kenihan, a farmer, and his wife Elizabeth, nee Pearson. He was educated at the Christian Brothers College where he was a keen athlete maintaining interest in all sporting activities. He studied medicine at the University of Adelaide graduating in 1915. He completed his residency at the Adelaide Hospital.

Kenihan enlisted in the AIF in November 1915. He was, single, aged 25 years, and his mother of "The Brae" Reynella was named as his next of kin. He was 5ft 9ins tall, weighed 10st and of fair complexion and hair with blue eyes. He had previous military experience of 3 years as a lieutenant in the cadets and could ride a horse. Kenihan was commissioned as a captain in the AAMC for general duty. He sailed from Adelaide in July 1916 and reached Plymouth in September. After training at the AAMC Depot at Parkhouse he was attached to 13 Trg Bn at Rollestone until he was sent to France in January 1917. He was attached to 9 FdAmb at first, then in February posted as RMO of 44 Bn. He was awarded a Military Cross at the Battle of Messines. *'During the attack on the Green Line he established the most forward RAP in the Division, and although under heavy shell fire he carried on attending to the wounded. He had to move his RAP on two occasions on account of having been shelled out of his former places. He himself was wounded but would not relinquish his work.'* Kenihan was gassed in October 1917 during the Third Battle of Ypres, and was away from the Bn recovering until December. He was transferred to 9 FdAmb in September 1918, but also detached to 3 San Section and 11 FdAmb for short periods. He was granted study leave for three months in March 1919 and went to the Rotunda Hospital in Dublin for post-graduate training. His appointment was terminated on the 13th November 1919 after he had returned to Australia in July 1919. Kenihan was issued with the British War Medal and the Victory Medal.

After the war Kenihan had a general practice in Millswood, Adelaide; he also held hospital appointments. He was appointed as an honorary anaesthetist at the Repatriation General Hospital Keswick in 1921 and at the Adelaide Hospital where he was a tutor in anaesthetics from 1923 to 1933. He married Glen Hewitt, the daughter of IT Hewitt. Miss Glen Hewitt featured in the local Adelaide newspapers as a singer and piano player, giving many charitable performances. Kenihan had a long association with the Repatriation Hospital at Keswick in turn anaesthetist, physician and pathologist before his appointment as physician in charge of outpatients in 1946 which he held until his retirement. Kenihan continued to serve in the CMF; he was CO of 6 Cav FdAmb from 1926 to 1930 with the rank of lieutenant colonel, and from 1930 to 1932 was Assistant Director of Hygiene. In 1939 he was CO of 10 ACCS at Warradale. Kenihan served from 1940 to 1942 as OC Troops on 2/2 AHS, the *Wanganella,* which carried casualties from the Middle East and New Guinea. He was a regular attendee at the Adelaide Oval; he enjoyed gardening, the stock market and the company of his children and grandchildren. He returned to practice at Millswood in 1942 and continued to work until ill health over took him. Raphael Leo Kenihan died at Reynella on the 20th October 1964.

Sources:

http://recordsearch.naa.gov.au/scripts/Imagine.asp?B=7369000

Photo: AWM E01500

Sons Robert Kenihan's RACP article, and Michael Kenihan.

The Mail Adelaide 8th July 1916

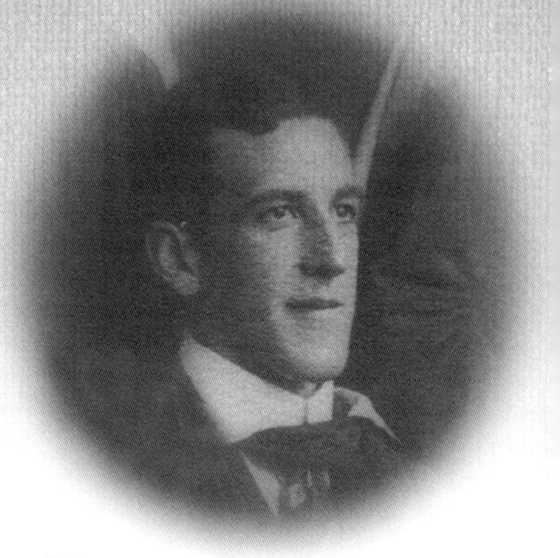

KNEEBONE John Le Messurier

MS MB FRCS FRACS

1890 - 1976

John Le Messurier Kneebone was born on 25th March 1890 in Adelaide, the eldest son of John Henry and Mary Matilda, nee Le Messurier. He was educated at Pulteney Grammar School and St Peter's College where he topped each year. As dux in his final year at St Peter's College he won the Young Exhibition and the DaCosta University Scholarship and the Farr special prizes in Greek, Latin, French and Chemistry. He had also won prizes in German and Geometry. He continued with the same academic success when studying medicine at the University of Adelaide, being awarded the Everard Scholarship in his final year. He represented his university at intervarsity Lacrosse winning a Blue. He was also a member of the University Rifle Club. He graduated at the age of 20 in 1911. He travelled to England in 1914 to pursue studies at St Mary's Hospital London and at the Middlesex Hospital for his surgical fellowship.

Whilst in England Kneebone joined the RAMC in 1914. He was reported as killed at the front in September 1914 and a detailed obituary, with, curiously, a splendid photograph of Captain Kneebone in an Australian uniform (he had joined the AAMC Reserve Volunteer in 1913), appeared in the Adelaide's 'The Mail'. Reports a few days later confirmed that he was alive and still in England. He served at Gallipoli where he was selected to be one of the last to leave and to remain with the wounded should the evacuation be discovered. Subsequently he served with Allenby's Army in the Middle East, and in France. He was Mentioned in Despatches on more than one occasion. He was issued with the 1914-15 Star, the British War Medal and Victory Medal with Oak Leaves.

Kneebone returned to England after the cessation of hostilities. From 1919 to 1921, he trained in surgery at The London Hospital and gained his FRCS. He married Eva Gladys Le Messurier on the 29th December 1920 in London. She was completing her medical degree in Manchester where she was dux in surgery following an honours arts degree from Reading. Their marriage united the two Le Messurier families from Guernsey. Returning to Australia he found surgical appointments filled so he went to Burra and Jamestown before accepting the post of surgeon superintendent at the Broken Hill Base Hospital. Here the demand for his surgical expertise was considerable and it was inevitable that he finally clashed with the hospital authorities in his requests for improvements in facilities and administration. Kneebone resigned and moved to Hamilton in Victoria, where he practiced surgery, particularly orthopaedic surgery for more than 30 years. He was President of the Orchestral Society, trustee of the YMCA and District Governor of the Hamilton Rotary Club. He was an enthusiastic member of the BMA represented the Western District Branch for many years. He was a perfectionist not only in surgery but also in photography, both still and cinematic. John Le Messurier Kneebone died on 19th July 1976, his wife predeceased him by two months and he was survived by a sister and his three daughters and their families.

Sources:
MJA 1976 (2) 696-7
Barrier Miner 30April 1923
Photo: Adelaide University Archives 1911 Graduates
The Mail (Adelaide) 16 Sept 14 p1
The Register Adelaide 24 February 1921
Ancestry.com

Uniforms and Outfits

At home and in peace time the authorities are esteemed worshippers of red tape, but in the field they are above all things practical, and the tendency is for both officers and men to fit themselves up in the way that seems to them best suited to the needs of their individual occupation....

BMJ, 2 January 1915, p. 31

LAMPHEE Alan Dunstan

MB BS DA FFARACS

1899 - 1981

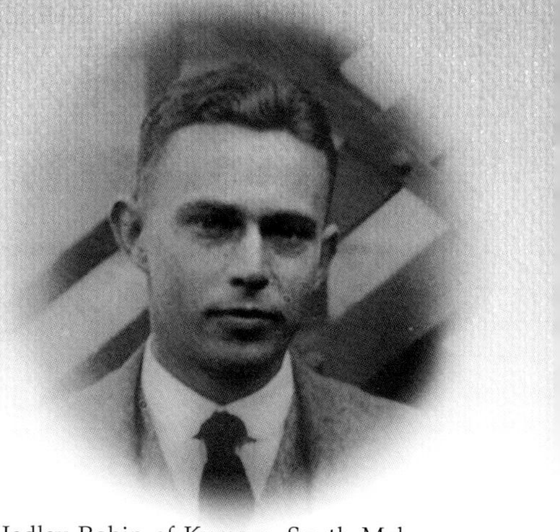

Alan Dunstan Lamphee was born in Adelaide on 3rd January 1899. He was the son of Phillip Lamphee, an accountant, and Clara, nee Dunstan and had two sisters. He was educated at St Peter's College. He had four years of Cadet Service and served in the citizens forces in the 22nd Signallers prior to enlisting. Lamphee was accepted as a medical student at the University of Adelaide but before commencing his medical studies he enlisted in the AIF in 1917.

Lamphee enlisted on 10th November 1917 with his parent's approval. He was living on Magill Road, Magill, South Australia. He was described as 18 years and 10 months old, 5ft 5ins tall and weighed 130lbs with a fresh complexion, hazel eyes and fair hair. Lamphee joined the AAMC reinforcements as a private soldier on 4th February 1918 and embarked on the *Gaika* in Adelaide on 6th August 1918. He disembarked in England on 13th October 1918 and was posted to an AAMC Training Depot. He served in 2 Clearing Hospital and Sanitary Section in Hurdcott Camp, near Fovant village, Salisbury England. He embarked on the *Karagola* for return to Australia on 30th April 1919. He disembarked in 4MD on 9th June 1919 and discharged on 24th June 1919. He was issued with the British War Medal.

Lamphee re-commenced his medical studies in 1920 at the University of Adelaide and graduated in 1924. At school he had formed a lasting relationship with Howard Florey. He spent a year as a resident medical officer at the Adelaide Hospital, followed by further postgraduate studies in England before he returned to Australia and entered General Practice in Walkerville. He married Inez Robin, the youngest daughter of Mr and Mrs Hedley Robin of Kumara, South Malvern, South Australia, on 29th May 1929 at St Peter's College Chapel. During WW2 he served again in the AAMC but this time as a doctor and reached the rank of lieutenant colonel. Eventually he took up full-time anaesthetic practice. He was considered to be an excellent anaesthetist especially in the days of ether anaesthetics. He was, however, quick to take up new techniques as they were developed. He was appointed an honorary anaesthetist at the Royal Adelaide Hospital and a lecturer of the University of Adelaide. He was a foundation member and State Vice President of the Australian Society of Anaesthetists and was elected a Fellow of the Faculty of Anaesthetists of the Royal Australasian College of Surgeons when it was formed in 1952. He was President of the South Australian Branch of the BMA 1948-1949 and elected a Fellow of the Association in 1970. He was a voluntary supporter of the Walkerville Boys Home amongst other philanthropic work. Alan Dunstan Lamphee died on 9th November 1981 and was survived by his two daughters and son.

Sources:

Escourt Hughes J, 'Obituary, Dr Alan Lamphee" Medical Journal of Australia 10th July 1982

National Archives

http://recordsearch.naa.gov.au/NameSearch/Interface/ItemDetail.aspx?Barcode=7376334

Biographical Index of South Australia 1836-1885

FIFTY YEARS. The Australian Society of Anaesthetists 1934-1984 by Gwen Wilson.

Photo: Adelaide University Graduates 1924

LE MESSURIER Frederick Neill

DSO MD

1891 - 1966

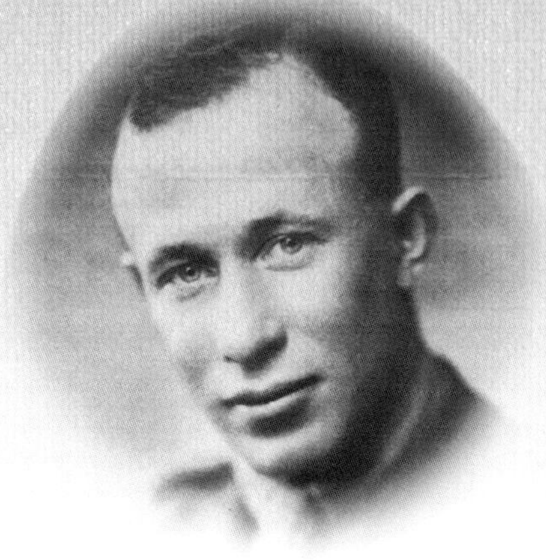

Frederick Neill Le Messurier was born on the 12th January 1891, the youngest son of Alfred and Jane, nee Neill. The Le Messurier family came from Guernsey; Captain Peter Le Messurier and his wife Betsy came to South Australia in 1853 and he established a business as shipowner, agent and merchant. The business was expanded in coastal shipping by his sons Alfred and Ernest. Le Messurier was educated at St Peter's College, where he excelled both academically and in sporting prowess. He played for the Port Adelaide Football Club during his last year. He was in the cadet corps rising to the rank of subaltern; he was the School captain in his last year and the top student. He was awarded a Blue for football in 1910. He studied medicine at the University of Adelaide and graduated in 1913 with first class honours.

Le Messurier joined 1 ASH as a captain on 7th October 1914. He was 5ft 6ins tall and weighed 150lbs. He travelled on the *Kyarra* to Egypt and subsequently to Lemnos (where he underwent an appendicectomy), Gallipoli and France. He was promoted to major in August 1916 and posted to 1AGH. Subsequent postings included 3 AAH, 13 FdAmb, 12 FdAmb and 48 Bn. He was Mentioned in Despatches of 7th April 1918. He was awarded the DSO which was gazetted on 7th November 1918, in recognition of his *"conspicuous gallantry and devotion to duty. He was continuously in the front line during both stages of an attack, assisting in collecting and arranging the prompt disposal of the wounded to the rear. He behaved splendidly, and by his untiring efforts and the complete disregard of his own safety he greatly assisted the brigade throughout."* He was promoted to lieutenant colonel and again Mentioned in Despatches on 8th November 1918. He returned to Australia in December 1918 with his appointment terminated on the 14th February 1919. He was issued with the 1914-1915 Star, the British War Medal and the Victory Medal with Oak Leaves.

He took up a resident medical officer post at the Adelaide Children's Hospital on return and a lifelong interest in paediatrics developed. He married Frieda Gwendoline James in the chapel of his old school in 1920 and they had one son. After a short period in general practice, in 1922 he was appointed to the post of Honorary Physician to the Mareeba Babies Hospital and in 1923 was joined by Dr Cyril Pitcher and Dr Helen Mayo. He subsequently was appointed an honorary assistant physician, and in 1926 honorary physician to the Adelaide Children's Hospital. He was the lecturer in medical diseases of children and a member of the Faculty of Medicine at the University of Adelaide for many years. He introduced lactic acid milk feeding of infants to Adelaide after a trip to St Louis (USA) in the mid-1920s. He practised as a specialist paediatrician and was the first to do so in Adelaide. He took a great interest in his old school and was the school doctor from 1927 until 1961. He served again in WW2 and was promoted to colonel and appointed commanding officer of 105 (Adelaide) Military Hospital in 1941 and remained in command until 1946. His task was to establish the unit and supervise the construction of what later became The Repatriation General Hospital on Daws Road. His personal contacts, including members of his family, were useful in obtaining building materials for the hospital. To make the hospital self sufficient and to provide a form of therapy staff and patients grew food and raised animals. Among his other achievements were the enclosures of eight sunrooms for the wards, the construction of a bowling green, bathing box and canteen. Gifted with a keen sense of humour, he inspired confidence, and could be considerate and kind. Frederick Neill Le Messurier died in Calvary Hospital, North Adelaide on the 20th May 1966, survived by his only son.

Sources:

http://recordsearch.naa.gov.au/scripts/Imagine.asp?B=8203275
http://adb.anu.edu.au/biography/le-messurier-alfred-roy-10812/text19179,
McKay DG Frederick Neill Le Messurier; MJA 1Oct66 p666
Photo from Le Messurier Family.

LEITCH Oliver

MB BS BSc

1875 - 1926

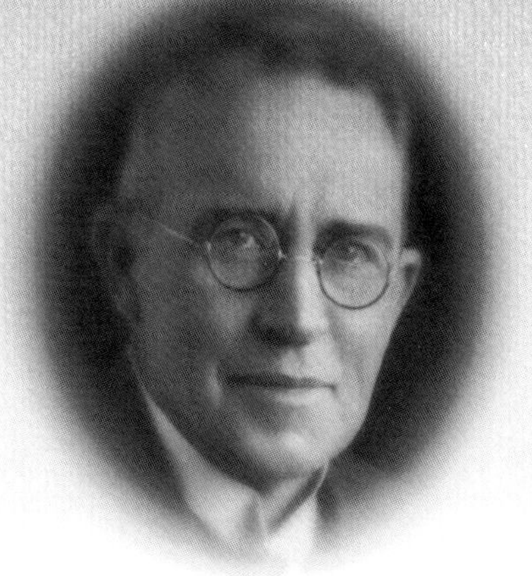

Oliver Leitch was born on the 19th April 1875, fourth son of John Leitch of Adelaide and Elizabeth, nee Westwood. His parents married at the residence of David Fowler of Mitcham South Australia on the 23rd June 1859. He was a younger brother of Dr J W Leitch (1867-1903) an early doctor on the York Peninsula who had died aged 27 years. He was educated at Sturt Street School and Prince Alfred College. He studied science and medicine at the University of Adelaide gaining his BSc in 1895. He then started a medical degree in the same year but after completing the first three years had to complete his degree at Melbourne University due to the closure of the Medical School in the 'Adelaide Hospital Row'. He graduated in 1901 and was registered as a Medical Practitioner in South Australia that year. He moved to Port Pirie and married Millicent Myrtle Grey on the 10th October 1906, with daughter Millicent (1908) and son Oliver W (1911) born in Port Pirie. He became Medical Superintendent at the Port Pirie Hospital in 1911.

Leitch enlisted in the AIF on the 27th April 1916 at the age of 41 years. He had previous service in the AAMC reserve. He was 5ft 9ins, and weighed 12st, with his wife named as his next of kin. He was recommended as a captain for sea transport duty. He was allocated for duty with Henry Gilbert on the Transport Ship *Geelong*, however he joined *Botanist* at Port Adelaide on the 24th April 1916. He returned to Australia from Egypt on duty in June 1916 and after arriving into the 4MD it was recommended that his and Gilberts appointments be terminated on the 23rd July 1916. He was issued with the British War Medal.

Leitch returned to Port Pirie and joined a partnership with Leslie Gemmel Tassie. He was the Health Officer of Port Pirie when he reported 6 cases of typhoid, 2 cases of diphtheria and a case of tuberculosis in 1918. His return was followed by the birth of two daughters, Joan (1922), who did not survive, and Elizabeth (1923) who did not survive. He went to England and Switzerland with daughter Millicent to study "Plumbism" and brain conditions in 1925. He was very concerned about the health issues of employees at the Port Pirie Lead Smelter works. On his return he presented a paper to the South Australian Government resulting in a change in the working conditions at the lead smelter at Port Pirie. Oliver Leitch, in 1926, decided to return to their new home at 29 Wood Street, Millswood, Adelaide and extend his career as a Thoracic Surgeon. The Town held a farewell function for him and his family on the 19th February 1926 at which he collapsed and later died at Sister Bray's private hospital. Both Drs Tassie and Yeatman attended him at the function. He was survived by his wife and children, a son and two daughters. His wife remarried in 1936 to Mr WB Carr. His son Dr O W Leitch also returned to Pt Pirie for a few years after WW2.

Sources:

Photo and story: Port Pirie Hospital and grandson Marcus Beresford.

http://recordsearch.naa.gov.au/scripts/Imagine.asp?B=8193442

Port. Pirie District Family History Group

South Australian Register 5 December 1893

The Argus Melbourne 19 March 1901

Port Pirie Recorder 20 February 1918

Port Pirie Recorder 18 February 1926

LENDON Guy Austin
MD BSc FRCP FRACP

1895 - 1970

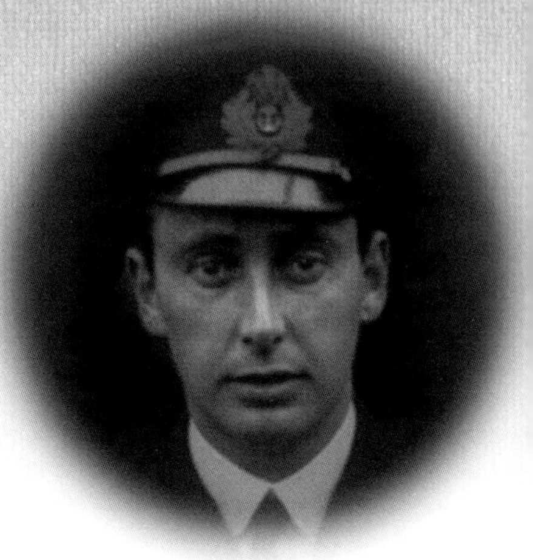

Guy Austin Lendon was born on 22nd January 1895, son of Dr. Alfred Austin Lendon, an eminent Adelaide physician, who founded the district nursing society in South Australia, and Lucy Isabel nee Rymill. Lendon had one brother Dr Alan Harding Lendon and a sister Dorothy. They lived at 117 Mills Terrace, North Adelaide. Lendon was educated at St Peter's College and studied science and medicine at the University of Adelaide graduating BSc in 1912, MB BS in July 1917 and MD in 1922. He joined the Cadet Corps in 1912.

Lendon enlisted in the Royal Australian Navy as temporary surgeon (SSC) on the 6th August 1917. He served in HMAS *Australia* with Fleet Surgeon Alexander Caw from 27th November 1917 until 17th August 1919. During his Commission HMAS *Australia* was deployed to the United Kingdom. She became flagship of the 2nd Battle-cruiser Squadron of the Royal Navy's Grand Fleet on 8th February 1915. At the end of his posting he was at HMAS *Cerberus* until the 9th November 1919 when he was transferred to the Emergency List.

Lendon married Mollie Burston the youngest daughter of deceased Brigadier General James Burston in Toorak Victoria on 24th September 1925 in a high society wedding. The Burstons were originally from South Australia. He subsequently undertook postgraduate training in Oxford, England; first at Magdalen College, which he disliked, and later at the Radcliffe Infirmary, which he enjoyed. He was a first-class scholar and an outstanding athlete, excelling in rifle shooting, tennis and golf. He was a formidable competitor in all his fields of endeavor. While studying anaesthesia at the Radcliffe Infirmary he graphically demonstrated, at a BMA meeting, the use of ethyl chloride. He was appointed honorary physician to the Adelaide Hospital in 1929, on his return to Adelaide. Lendon made his name as a consultant physician and particularly as a clinician, teacher and medical politician at the Royal Adelaide Hospital. He did not accept opposition or criticism graciously and his quick wit and sometimes acerbic repartee alienated many colleagues, some for long periods. One instance involved his own brother-in-law, Major-General Sir Samuel Burston, who received precedence in appointment to the honorary staff of the Royal Adelaide Hospital. They did not speak together for the latter half of Guy's life. On the other hand Lendon had many friends, brought together by his extensive interests. He was a keen and adventurous motorist-mechanic from his early days. He enjoyed tennis with a group of first-class players and was a very low handicap golfer who was captain of the Royal Adelaide Golf Club. A love of cats was a less widely known facet of his life. His daughter Elspeth, now Mrs Peter Wells, remembers when a dozen of them shared their home. He was a popular postgraduate teacher and devoted much time and energy to the young, would-be physicians who left the armed forces at the end of World War 2. He was living at Mills Terrace, North Adelaide in 1937. During WW2 Lendon was appointed a Captain in the AAMC. He was transferred to the Retired list of the RAN on the 22nd January 1955 with his appointment terminated on the 21st June 1962. It was unfortunate that illness in his later life, and particularly after the accidental death of his wife, led Lendon to become a recluse. Guy Austin Lendon died on 27th April 1970, he was survived by his daughter.

Sources:
http://recordsearch.naa.gov.au/NameSearch/Interface/ItemDetail.aspx?Barcode=5229022
J M McPhie Munk's Roll, 6, 281-3;
Med Journal Aust., 1970, 2, 426-7, 604;
Photo: AWM, EN 0003
The Adelaide Register 10 Jul 1917
The Mail 14th December 1940
The Advertiser 23 December 1909
The News Adelaide 5th July 1929
The Adelaide Register 3rd October 1925

LEWIS Eric Henry

ED MD

1884 - 1972

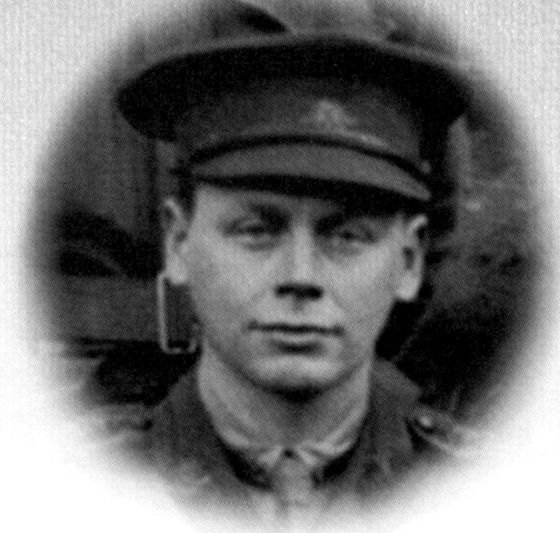

Eric Henry Lewis was born in May 1884 in Gawler, South Australia, son of a solicitor Frederick Henry Lewis and his wife Francis Maria, nee Smythe. He was educated at Gawler South Grammar School and studied medicine at the University of Adelaide graduating in 1906. He then undertook residency at the Adelaide Hospital in 1907. After his residency Lewis entered general practice in Gawler, and in 1913 was appointed Medical Officer of Health for Gawler and the Barossa District. He was commissioned as honorary captain in the AAMC Reserve in 1913 and appointed Area Medical Officer for Gawler. He married Winifred Letitia Bonython, the niece of Sir Langdon Bonython the proprietor and editor of the *Adelaide Advertiser,* in November 1916.

Lewis was commissioned in the AIF on 22nd January 1917. He was 32 years old and named his new wife of High St, Gawler as his next of kin. He embarked from Melbourne in May 1917, and landed at Devonport in July. After initial training at the AAMC Depot at Parkhouse, Lewis was posted to 1 ADH at Bulford Camp on the Salisbury Plain England. He received orders to proceed to France on October 1917. He passed briefly through 2 AGH and was posted to 11 FdAmb at the height of the third battle of Ypres. He began to suffer from fevers, assumed to be trench fever in December of 1917. He was posted as RMO of 42 Bn for several weeks, and then to 3 Pioneer Bn. in May 1918. The fevers returned and Lewis was evacuated to the British Red Cross Hospital at Rouen in September 1918. He was evidently very ill, although the diagnosis appears somewhat loose, septicaemia in one report, pleurisy in another. Tuberculosis seems to have been excluded, so the presentation may represent the complications of influenza. Lewis was returned to England, and within two weeks shipped back to Australia on the *AHS Karoola,* with his appointment terminated on the 11th October 1919. He was issued with the British War Medal and the Victory Medal.

He convalesced at Mt Lofty before returning to his practice in Gawler in 1919. Lewis became a staunch member of the community; he was a strong supporter of the Boy Scout Movement. His authority as Medical Officer of Health was extended to 'Greater Gawler' in 1933. He was recalled to duty to service 18 LH MG Regt in 1940, which was based on the Cheltenham Racecourse, and the same year was awarded the ED. He continued to serve until 1945. Eric Henry Lewis died at Walkerville in September 1972 and was cremated at Centennial Park.

Sources:

Photo: AWM E1535

http://recordsearch.naa.gov.au/scripts/Imagine.asp?B=8198461

Trove

Adelaide Advertiser 5th June 1913

Chronicle Adelaide 18 November 1916

Treatment of "Gunshot Wounds" of the knee-joint.

...the importance of certain factors in successful treatment were not grasped sufficiently: (1) that wounds of the knee-joint which are liable to become septic demand immobilization of the joint...(2) There existed quite a widespread notion that foreign bodies in the joint should be removed "only if they lead to trouble". Fortunately, the fallacy of this view has been demonstrated, and now only those which are imbedded in the bone outside the joint are left alone, if they are not causing trouble. (3) The good effect of excision of the wound of the skin and superficial tissues, or of the whole wound where possible, was not appreciated...Primary suture is, of course, out of the question in the wounds we are at present considering – free drainage must be provided, therefore, the wounds are left open – but secondary suture, when advisable, can certainly be performed at an earlier stage after excision has been made.

BMJ, 10 July 1915, p. 41

LEWIS James Brook

MB BS (Melb)

1877 - 1966

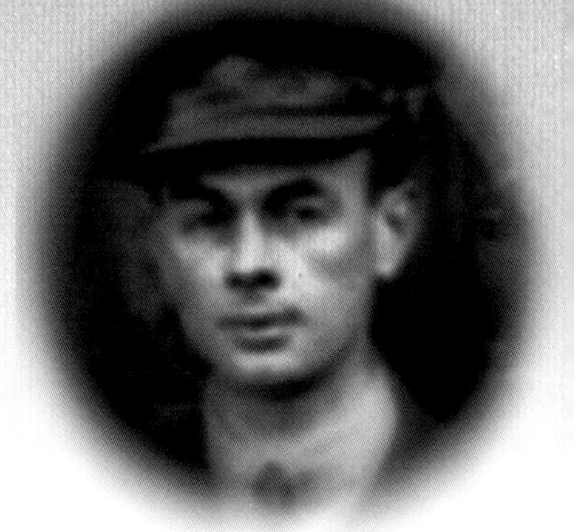

James Brook Lewis was born on 11th August 1877 in Kooringa, near Burra, South Australia. He was the eldest of six children of the Honourable John Lewis and Martha Ann, nee Brook. His mother died in 1894 and his father later remarried. His grandparents were early settlers having arrived in South Australia in 1836 on the Rapid. His father who was born in South Australia was pastoralist, explorer, miner and politician. A younger brother was Essington Lewis noted General Manager of BHP. Lewis was educated at Whinham College and St Peter's College. He studied medicine at the University of Adelaide and later at Melbourne University as a result of the 'Adelaide Hospital Row', graduating in 1901. After graduation he went to live in Menzies, Western Australia where he was District Medical Officer and Public Vaccinator. Lewis married Nancy Phillips prior to enlisting in the AIF and his address was Narrogin, Western Australia.

Lewis was appointed a captain in the AAMC on 16th June 1911. He enlisted in the AIF on 12th July 1915. He was 5ft 8ins tall, weighed 182lbs, of dark complexion with brown eyes and hair. His wife was named as his next of kin. He embarked from Fremantle on the *Karoola* on 11th November 1915 with the rank of temporary major while second in command of a hospital ship. He disembarked in Suez on 20th March 1916. He relinquished the rank of major on 4th July 1917 after his duty on *Karoola* was terminated. He proceeded overseas to France on 12th July 1917 and on 18th July was posted temporarily to 14th British General Hospital and later returning to 2 AGH. He was promoted to major on 24th August 1917. He was posted to 10 FdAmb on 16th October 1917. He returned to England on 13th March 1918. He was granted leave without pay from 2nd November 1919 until he was demobilised in England on 18th May 1920 *"for business purposes"* which was to study ophthalmology. His wife and children joined him in England. He was reported as having no disability at discharge. He was issued with the 1914-15 Star, but later return of the medal was requested, the British War Medal and Victory Medal.

After the WWI he worked at Moorfields Hospital, London and in Madras, India. He returned to Adelaide in 1922 and continued his practice as an eye specialist. There followed a number of honorary appointments at the Adelaide Hospital. He became a shareholder and Director of John Lewis and Company in 1925. In 1937 he was appointed as consulting ophthalmologist to the Adelaide Hospital. In WW2 he was appointed in the AAMC as a medical officer for the Artillery Militia with the rank of major in 1940. His son John Lewis, a private soldier in WW2, was killed in action in December 1942. John Brook Lewis died on 22nd September 1966.

Sources:

National Archives of Australia

http://recordsearch.naa.gov.au/NameSearch/Interface/ItemDetail.aspx?Barcode=8198725

Biographical Index of South Australians 1836-1885

State Library of South Australia, PRG 247 Series List

Burra record 4th July 1894

The News Adelaide 7 July 1937

Burra record 19th January 1943

The Medical Profession at Home

From all over the kingdom news has been received that the local medical profession is taking steps to safeguard the interests of the practitioners who are called in the service of their country and leave their practices. This means that those who remain at home will undertake between them to act in every respect as substitutes for the absentee, keeping a separate account of all attendances on his patients, and refusing to continue attendance on them when he is able to take up his practice once again.

BMJ, 22nd August 1914 p.368

LINDON Sir Leonard Charles Edward

MS MB FRCS FRACS

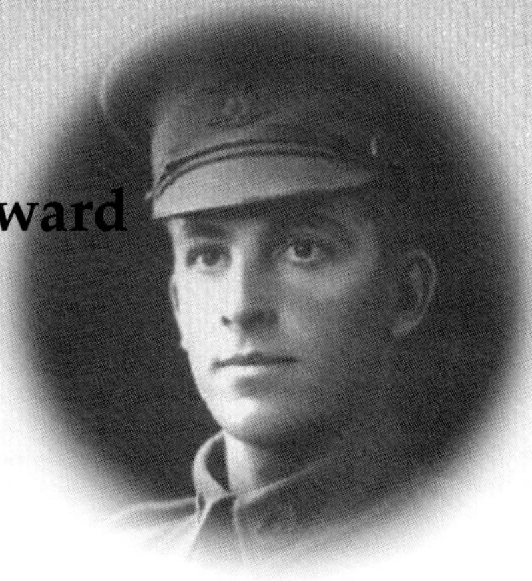

1896 - 1978

Leonard Charles Edward Lindon was born on 8th February 1896 in North Adelaide. He was the second son of James Hemery Lindon and his wife Mary Ellen, nee Cockburn. His father had founded the Queen's School in North Adelaide. Lindon was educated at Geelong Grammar School, St Peter's College and studied medicine at the University of Adelaide. He played cricket and tennis and rowed for his school and university. He entered the University of Adelaide as a medical student in 1914 but was to interrupt his studies to serve overseas with the AIF.

Lindon joined the Army on the 13th February 1915 as a private soldier. He had already joined 78 Infantry P Company reserve unit 6 months earlier. He was 19 years old, 5ft 7ins tall and weighed 154lbs. He joined 1ASH and served on Lemnos in Jun 1915 and with the same unit at Gallipoli. His brother in law, Major Henry Simpson Newland, who had married Lindon's older sister Mary, also served with this unit. Lindon was admitted with influenza and subsequently troubled with a whitlow during his service overseas. He returned to Australia on the *Argyllshire* working as a medical orderly/nurse. He transferred to 4MD and was discharged to complete his medical studies on 3rd March 1916. He was issued with the 1914-15 Star, the British War Medal and the Victory Medal

Lindon resumed his medical course on return to Adelaide and graduated MB BS in 1919. Lindon studied for his MS in 1923. He was awarded a Rhodes scholarship in 1918 which he took up in 1920 at Balliol College. His time in Oxford overlapped with that of his colleague and Rhodes Scholar predecessor Hugh Cairns who was to have a great influence over him and his choice of career. At Oxford he, like Cairns, worked with the great neurophysiologist, Charles Sherrington. He married Jean Monteith Marten, the only daughter of Dr and Mrs R Humphrey Marten of North Adelaide on 12th December 1921 in Brompton England. He took the FRCS in 1922 and returned to Adelaide as a general surgeon in association with his father-in-law and brother-in-law, Henry Newland. He was appointed honorary assistant surgeon at the Adelaide Hospital in 1925 and subsequently at the Adelaide Children's Hospital. He travelled overseas in 1929 where he spent time at the London Hospital with his colleague Cairns who was establishing neurosurgical services there, and visited neurosurgical centres elsewhere in Britain and Paris before spending time in Boston studying with famed neurosurgeon Harvey Cushing. He returned to Adelaide to establish a neurosurgical unit and drew up farsighted plans for this. He was appointed an honorary surgeon at the Adelaide Hospital in 1931 and, although this was a general surgical appointment he was able to concentrate on neurosurgery. He was to re-join the Army in WW2 and served in the Middle East as lieutenant colonel with 2/2 AGH. He served as a surgeon/neurosurgeon. After WW2 he held various appointments at the University of Adelaide, the SA branch of the BMA and the RACS (vice-president 1956-1958 and president 1959-1961). He was knighted in 1964. Predeceased by his wife in 1974 Sir Leonard Charles Edward Lindon died on 28th August 1978 in North Adelaide. He was survived by his daughter and two sons.

Sources:

http://recordsearch.naa.gov.au/scripts/Imagine.asp?B=8203796

Simpson D., "Neurosurgery in the age of Cushing: the achievement of Leonard Lindon" ANZ J Surg 82(2012) 311-317, 2012

Fraenkel G.J., 'Lindon, Sir Leonard Charles Edward (1896–1978)', Australian Dictionary of Biography, National Centre of Biography, Australian National University, http://adb.anu.edu.au/biography/lindon-sir-leonard-charles-edward-10832/text19219,

The Mail Adelaide 17th December 1921

LINN Leslie Wadmore

MB BS

1894 - 1974

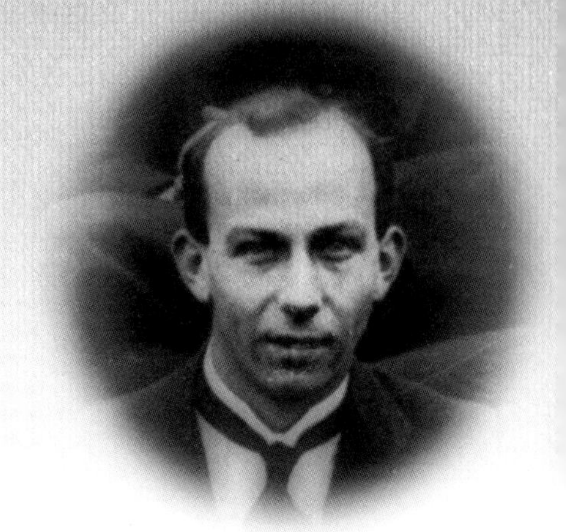

Leslie Wadmore Linn was born in Kensington, South Australia on 20th November 1894. He was the younger son of Matthew Edward Linn and Mary, nee Wadmore of Kensington Road, Leabrook, South Australia. He was educated at Prince Alfred College and studied medicine at the University of Adelaide.

He initially enlisted on the 26th November 1915 but, after 55 days in the AIF, was discharged to continue his studies. He re-enlisted on the 25th March 1918 when he was in his fifth year of his medical studies. At that time he had 5 years in the AAMC in the citizen forces and was credited with the 55 days of war service. He was 5ft 3½ins tall, weighed 129lbs, and of medium complexion with blue eyes and dark brown hair. He was not called up and was discharged on 18th November 1918.

He married Gladys Kathleen Saltmarsh, daughter of William Henry Saltmarsh, at the Parkside Baptist Church on the 27th March 1920. He practised in Tailem Bend and Woodside after the war. He was appointed to the Commission of the Peace as a Justice of Peace by the Governor in 1924. He was also appointed as honorary dermatologist at Parkside Mental Hospital in 1935. He was appointed as a surgical clinical assistant to the Adelaide Hospital in 1937. He was again appointed as an honorary captain to the Reserve of Officers AAMC in 1940. Leslie Wadmore Linn died on 26th September 1974 in Hawthorn, South Australia.

Sources:
National Archives of Australia
http://recordsearch.naa.gov.au/NameSearch/Interface/ItemDetail.aspx?Barcode=8195896
The Advertiser 21st October 1940
The Register 24th August 1924
News 21st March 1935
Chronicle 24th APRIL 1920
Photo: Adelaide University Archives: Medical Graduates 1918.

Uniforms and Outfits [cont]

He will also find it useful to possess a couple of linen overalls of his own in which to do his ward work, and perhaps a small surgical dressing case containing scissors, dressing forceps, and the like…a small writing case, a good stylograph or fountain pen, and an ordinary supply of toilet articles. His wardrobe will be best made up as follows: Two suits of pyjamas, and some bedroom slippers, two or three vests and drawers such as he usually wears in winter, half a dozen pairs of merino socks, a couple of khaki flannel shirts, four turn-down khaki flannel collars, two khaki-coloured silk ties, a gilt safety-pin, two or three tie-clips, a neutral coloured cardigan waistcoat, a lined khaki tunic, a Brodrick cap, a Sam Browne belt, without either sword or revolver attachments, a plain walking-stick with crook handle, a pair of dogskin gloves, two pairs of brown boots, and overcoat and leg gear.

BMJ, 2 January 1915, p. 31

LOVE John Alexander

MB BS

1894 - 1977

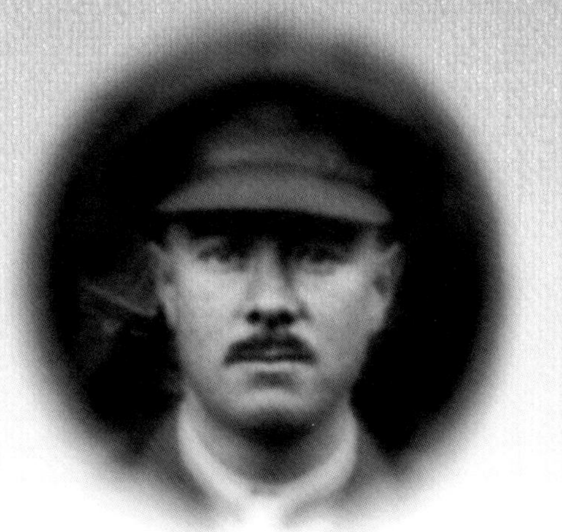

John Alexander Love was born in Strathalbyn, South Australia on 31st March 1894. He was the son of the Rev George Clarke Love and his wife Margaret Georgina, nee Beattie. He was educated at Strathalbyn School and Prince Alfred College. He studied medicine at the University of Adelaide and graduated in 1915. While in medical school in Adelaide he served for three years as a private in 31 LHFA.

Love enlisted in the AIF on the 15th September 1915 whilst he was a resident medical officer at the Adelaide Hospital. He was single, 21 years old, 5ft 9ins tall, 147lbs, and had a fair complexion, blue eyes, and light brown hair. His father was named as his next of kin. He was posted to 11 FdAmb. He embarked from Melbourne in June 1916 and arrived at Southampton in July. He took part in the unit training on the Salisbury Plain, but in October, prior to leaving for France, was transferred to 43 Bn for two months in the absence of Arthur Guymer. He was recommended for the Military Cross at Ypres in October 1917, when he was Bearer Captain in charge of the left sector of the Divisional front, but it was not awarded. He was transferred to 2 AGH at Wimereux in May 1918, and served there until the end of the year. He was Mentioned in Despatches in November 1918. He moved around the Divisional units as required in the first two months of 1919, and in March was granted six months study leave. Love was issued with the British War Medal and the Victory Medal with Oak Leaves.

Love married Winifred Mary Addis, who was from Melbourne, on 13th August 1918 whilst still in England. His appointment was terminated in Australia on the 6th November 1919. He practised at Booleroo Centre, South Australia until 1927, and then, after further postgraduate study in the USA, moved to Perth Western Australia. John Alexander Love died in Western Australia in 1977. James Robert Beattie Love, his older brother, served in the Camel Corps and 14 LHR. He was awarded the DCM and MC in the Sinai-Palestine Campaign. He was ordained after the war and became the Moderator of the General Assembly of the Presbyterian Church of South Australia.

Sources:

Photo: AWM E05135

http://recordsearch.naa.gov.au/scripts/On the 15th September 1915,Imagine.asp?B=8206496

Likeman R., '2013 No Time for Regrets: Australian Doctors of the Western Front', Rosenberg Press.

The Register Adelaide 17th August 1918.

Rum Ration [cont]

Sir – this discussion on this subject is decidedly interesting. In reasoning on it, it is well to bear in mind the following admitted facts:

1. The shooting in the English navy is first class. This has been proved in all the naval actions fought with the German fleet, and also by the excellent marksmanship shown at the Dardanelles and on the coast of Belgium, where our seaman gunners speedily demolished the guns and forts of the enemy
2. The rum ration is still being daily served out on board our men-of-war to the gunners.
3. It is these rum-drinking men who make this splendid shooting…

Plymouth March 4th - T.B.P. Wilkinson, MB

BMJ, 20 March 1915, p. 529

† LUCAS Reginald Blockley

MB BS

1889 - 1916

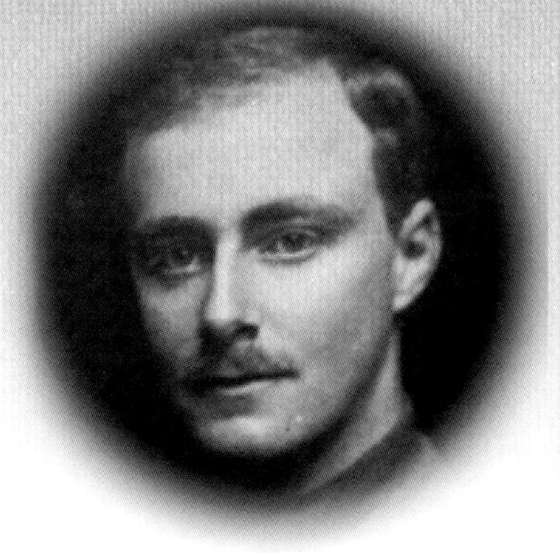

Reginald Blockley Lucas of Millswood, South Australia was born in September 1889, at Hyde Park the son of Alfred Robert Blockley Lucas and his wife Ellen, nee Chambers. He was educated at St Peter's College and Adelaide University graduating in medicine in 1913.

Lucas transferred from the AAMC Reserve, where he had been an honorary captain in the 4 MD, to the RAMC in January 1915. Shortly after he was posted to the Base Hospital at Rouen, France as a lieutenant. He remained there until March 1916 when attached to 7 Bn of the Norfolk Regiment as a temporary captain. The 7 Bn, was formed at Norwich, England in August 1914 as part of 35th Brigade, 12th Division in Kitchener's New Army. He married Cecily Helen McKail of North Adelaide on 3rd April 1916 at West Hampstead, London. During the night of 1 July 1916, the 12th Division relieved the badly knocked about 8th Division after its attempt to take German held Ovillers-la-Boisselle. Early on 3 July, the 35th and 37th Brigades advanced under the cover of their artillery and rushed forward the remaining short distance toward the German trenches once the barrage lifted. Heavy shelling however soon caused some of the attacking troops to lose direction and momentum; those units which made good progress and entered the German's trench lines were suddenly bogged down in titanic bomb fights. The highly trained and aggressive German troops fought bravely to hold their line and the 12th Division was unable to take the objective and later counted their casualties in the thousands. Captain Reginald Blockley Lucas was killed in action on 3 July 1916. He is commemorated on the Thiepval Memorial, on the WW1 Memorial at Unley, SA and in the Memorial Hall and the Memorial Plaque in the entrance to the large Quadrangle at his school, St Peter's College. His younger brother Alfred enlisted on 24 September 1915 and served with the Australian Engineers as well as the 3rd Light Horse Regiment; he returned to Australia in 1919.

Sources:

Kearney RS "Fallen Saints"

Likeman R "No Time for Regrets: Australian Doctors of the Western Front", in press, Rosenberg Press, 2013.

Photo; SRSA GRG 26/5/4/1745

The Advertiser Adelaide 19th December 1913

The Adelaide Register 13 May 1916

The Square Egg (A Badgers-Eye view of the War Mud in the Trenches)

…much more to be thought about than the enemy over yonder or the war all over Europe is the mud of the moment, the mud that at times engulfs you as cheese engulfs a cheese-mite. In Zoological Gardens one has gazed at an elk or a bison loitering at its pleasure more than knee-deep in a quagmire of greasy mud, and one has wondered what it would feel like to be soused and plastered hour long, in such a muck-bath. One knows now. In narrow-dug support-trenches, when thaw and heavy rain have come suddenly atop of frost, when everything is pitch-dark around you, and you can only stumble about and feel your way against streaming mud walls, when you have to go down on hands and knees in several inches of soup-like mud to creep into a dug-out, when you stand deep in mud, lean against mud, grasp mud-slimed objects with mud slimed fingers, wink mud away from your eyes, and shake it out your ears, bite muddy biscuits with muddy teeth, then at least you are in a position to understand thoroughly what it feels like to wallow – on the other hand the bison's idea of pleasure becomes more and more incomprehensible.

Saki (HH Munro)

MAGAREY Archibald Campbell

MS MB FRCS LRCP

1882 - 1919

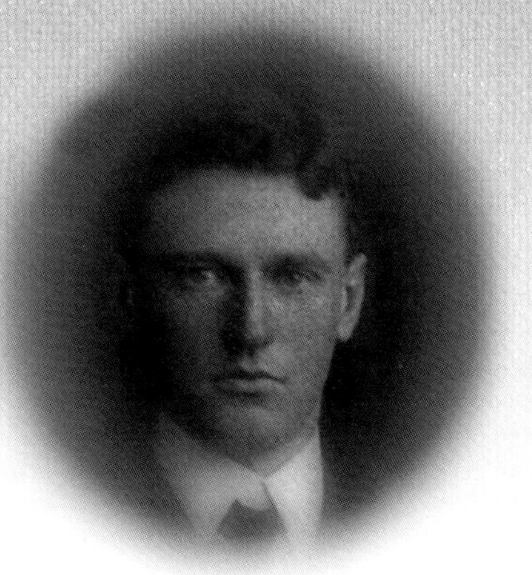

Archibald Campbell Magarey was born on 15th July 1882 in North Adelaide, South Australia the son of Alexander Thomas Magarey and Virginia, nee Campbell. He was the grandson of Thomas Magarey who, after unsuccessful migration to New Zealand subsequently migrated to South Australia in 1845. Thomas Magarey was one of the founders of the Church of Christ in Australia, a Member of the House of Assembly for West Torrens from 1860 to 1863 and a Member of the Legislative Council from 1863 to 1865. Archibald Campbell Magarey was educated at St Peter's College and studied medicine at the University of Adelaide, graduating in 1907. After completing his residency at the Adelaide Hospital he went to England in 1909 and studied surgery at St Mary's Hospital, Paddington. On his return to Australia he completed the MS at the University of Adelaide and was the second person to do so after Sir Henry Newland. He became a Fellow of the Royal College of Surgeons in 1911. Magarey married Edna Ling Stanton and they had three daughters, Constance, Virginia and Philippa and they lived at 'Gurrawarra', Mount Lofty in South Australia. Magarey was appointed as temporary assistant gynaecologist at the Adelaide Hospital from November 1914 until May 1915 then temporary assistant surgeon releasing Dr Wilson then Dr Cudmore for war duties.

Magarey enlisted in the AAMC Reserve in September 1915 where he served as an area medical officer for 6 years. He also retained the position of temporary surgeon at the Adelaide Hospital until his death in May 1919. He joined the Australian Naval and Military Expeditionary Forces (AN&MEF) on the 8th April 1918 and embarked on the SS *Marsina* on the 31st May 1918 from Sydney for Rabaul and returned to Australia on the *SS Melusia* for furlough his appointment was terminated on 19th January 1919. He was issued with the British War Medal.

Archibald Campbell Magarey contracted influenza on return to Australia and died on 20th May 1919. He was buried at Stirling Cemetery, Aldgate, South Australia and was survived by his wife and three daughters.

Sources:

http://recordsearch.naa.gov.au/scripts/Imagine.asp?B=8212469
Royal Adelaide Hospital Heritage Office
Photo: Adelaide University Archives; 1st Year Med Students 1903
The Adelaide Advertiser 17th January 1908.
The Adelaide Advertiser 26th July 1919

The German Use of Asphyxiating Gases.

Our correspondent in Northern France writes to us from Boulogne under date April 28th, stating that a considerable number of men who are suffering from the effects of the asphyxiating gas used by the enemy in the country near Ypres have reached the Boulogne hospitals...Among those that have arrived at Boulogne there have been several deaths, and in one case I was able to observe for myself some of the physical results. Around the larynx, including the epiglottis, was a band of acute inflammation, and the trachea was intensely irritated. The kidneys were cyanotic – that is to say, they presented the deep colour seen in cases of asphyxia from any cause. The clinical features are those of acute bronchopneumonia, and in grave cases there is pulmonary oedema.

BMJ, 1 May 1915, p. 774

MAGAREY Cromwell

MB BS

1864 - 1940

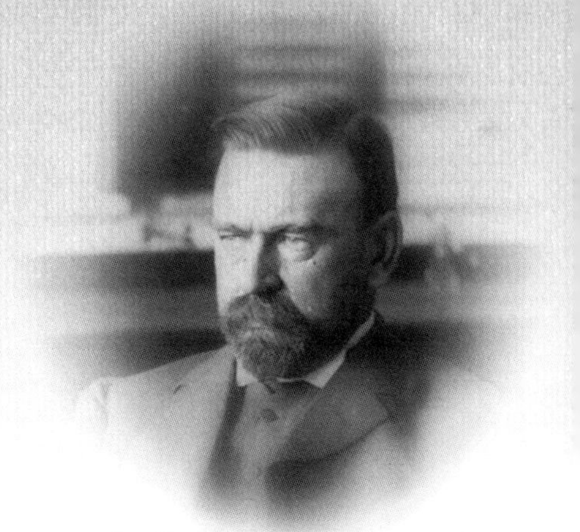

Cromwell Magarey was born on 5th June 1864 at Enfield, South Australia. He was the son of Thomas Magarey and Elizabeth, nee Verco, and the brother of Alexander Thomas Magarey and uncle of Archibald Campbell Magarey. He was educated at Prince Alfred College. Magarey was one of the first six students to study medicine at the Medical School of the University of Adelaide. The school opened at the beginning of 1885 and his fellow students were Charles Hope, A. F. Lynch, F. Goldsmith, A. F. Joyce, and James Robin. Magarey then went to England to further his studies. After completing his studies in London he married Sophia Mildred Sandilands at St Paul's, Newton Abbot, Devon, on 25th August 1891. He returned to Australia with his new wife within days of his marriage. He was a public vaccinator and medical examiner in 1892. Magarey became Chair of the Barrier Tramway Company Limited formed for the purpose of promoting the passage of a bill through the New South Wales Parliament for the construction of a railway from Cockburn to Broken Hill, via Thurkaringa and the Pinnacles. The select committee passed the Bill but it failed in the legislative council and the company was wound up voluntarily in October 1908.

Magarey enlisted to join the AIF on 3rd Dec 1915 at the age of 51 years and 6 months, his wife Sophia was named as his next of kin. They lived at that time at 62 Beulah Road, Norwood, South Australia. He was described as 5ft 8ins, and weighed 13st 8lb. He was appointed and assigned to a transport ship for one voyage only, he returned from the Suez on the *Ayrshire* with invalided soldiers from the war. His appointment was terminated on 31st March 1916. There is no record of any medals issued to him.

Magarey returned to his practice at Norwood on his return from the war, and he remained at his practice there for 40 years. Cromwell Magarey died 15th June 1940 at his home in Malvern and was buried at Magill. He was survived by his four daughters and a son, Ivan Sandilands Magarey. Magarey's 13 roomed house on the corner of Sydenham Road and Beulah Road, Norwood was bought by the government to be used as a centre for 'spastic' children in 1950. His daughter Mildred Kathleen Magarey was inducted as the first Deaconess in the Church of England at St Peter's Cathedral Adelaide on 1 May 1926. She was attached to the parish of St Mary Magdalene in Moore Street, Adelaide.

Sources:

http://digital.library.adelaide.edu.au/dspace/handle/2440/15029
http://recordsearch.naa.gov.au/NameSearch/Interface/ItemDetail.aspx?Barcode=8212470
Photo: The Children's Hospital "Cup Book" 1904
The News Adelaide 17th June 1940
The Adelaide Advertiser 17 November 1950.

Military Medicine [Infection]

It is, however, extremely probable, in spite of the precautions which are known to have been taken by the sanitary services and medical corps...that a considerable amount of epidemic sickness is present among the troops. It must be remembered that the gigantic German army has split itself into two great segments, and, together with Austria's large forces on the one side is opposing millions of Russian troops and on the other is struggling with the full strength of the French and Belgian armies and a considerable number of British regiments. These millions of soldiers, living and dying on the field, in trenches, under insanitary conditions...form a fruitful soil for the outbreak of diseases, such as cholera, typhus, dysentery, small-pox, enteric fever and plague.

MJA, 7 November 1914, p. 448

MAGAREY Rupert Eric

MB BS FRACS FRCOG

1880 - 1967

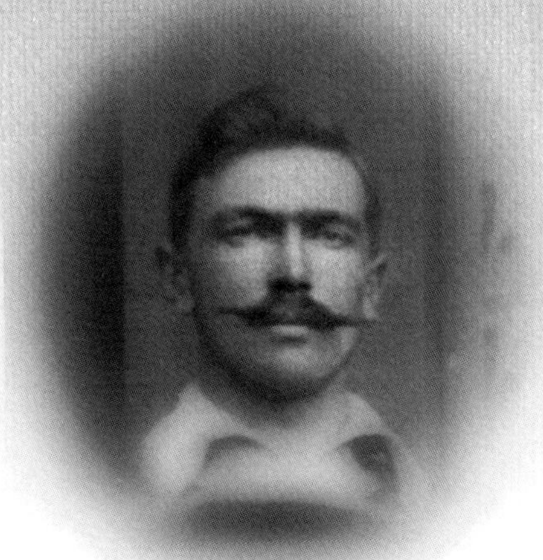

Rupert Eric Magarey was born at Glenelg in 1880 the eldest son of James W Magarey and grandson of Thomas, the original Magarey migrant who had arrived in South Australia in 1845. He settled in the original Naracoorte Station, after which the town was named, in 1886. Rupert Eric Magarey was educated at Prince Alfred College and was notable for his success in sport. He then studied medicine at the University of Adelaide. He graduated in medicine in 1905 but his registration was delayed because of illness. He became a resident medical officer at the Adelaide Hospital in 1906. His first appointment at the Adelaide Hospital was in 1915. He was a Temporary Honorary Assistant Gynaecologist from 1915-1918, and followed further postgraduate study in England mainly at the Great Ormond Street Hospital for Sick Children. He entered partnership, on returning home, with Dr F S Hone at Semaphore, South Australia. He married Elsie Emily Cowell at the home of her parents in Medindie, South Australia on 25th February 1913. Magarey joined the AAMC Reserve with the rank of honorary captain on 26th June 1915. He was the Port Adelaide Medical and Quarantine Officer where he served throughout the war. Magarey was appointed honorary assistant gynaecologist to William Alfred Verco, the Honorary Gynaecologist at the Adelaide Hospital after the war. Their professional practice address was at Verco Buildings on North Terrace. He was honorary assistant gynaecologist at the Adelaide Hospital from 1920 to 1927, honorary gynaecologist from 1927 to 1936 and 1939 to 1940. His final appointment there was honorary consulting gynaecologist from 1940 to 1943. He was also acting honorary obstetric surgeon at the Queen's Home. He lived at Stephen Terrace, Gilberton. Emily died in September 1950 and Rupert Eric Magarey died on the 25th June 1967. They were survived by their five children, four sons and a daughter. Their eldest son, Sir James Rupert (Bob) Magarey served during WW2 and was a noted surgeon in Adelaide.

Sources:
Heritage Office, Royal Adelaide Hospital
MJA 10th Feb 1968 p 240
Photo: Adelaide University Archives; 1902 Intervarsity Lacrosse team.
The Register Adelaide 27th March 1913
The Mail Adelaide 26th June 1915.

Terrorismus

Attila, it has been said, had to lament that his illiterate subjects were destitute of the art which could perpetuate the memory of his exploits... of which the professor of constitutional law in University College, London, has recently published a translation under the title, The German War Book. Thus we read that "a war conducted with energy cannot be directed merely against the combatants of the enemy state and the positions they occupy, but it will and must in like manner seek to destroy the total intellectual and material resources of the latter. Humanitarian claims such as the protection of men and their goods can only be taken into consideration in so far as the nature and object of the war permit"....The officer is told that he must avoid arriving at false views about the essential character of war by steeping himself in military history, and thus guarding himself "against excessive humanitarian notions; it will teach him that certain severities are indispensable to war; nay, more, that the only true humanity very often lies in a ruthless application of them."

BMJ, 6 February 1915, p. 257-8

MAKIN Frank Humphrey

MB ChB (Melb) LM (Dublin)

1875 - 1961

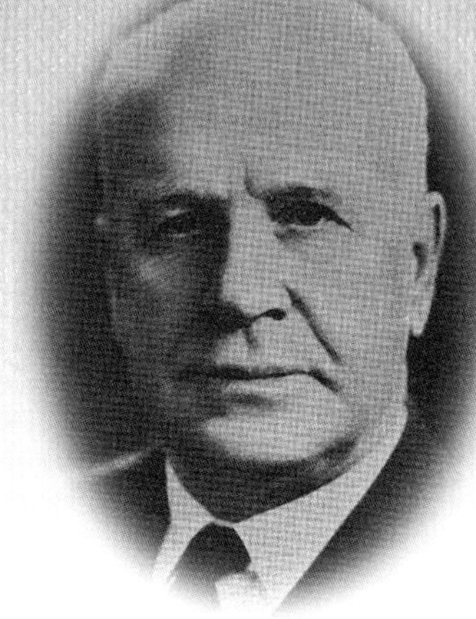

Frank Humphrey Makin was born on the 25th November 1875 at Gawler, SA, the son of Colonel Frank Makin VD, the Honorary Colonel of the 78th Infantry (Adelaide Rifles). Makin was educated at Geelong Grammar School and St Peter's College. He commenced his medical degree at the University of Adelaide in 1894 but interrupted his studies to serve as a trooper in the South African War with the Second South Australian Contingent (Mounted Rifles) and rose to the rank of Corporal. At this time he was living in Gawler, South Australia. Makin had to complete his medical studies at Melbourne University on return from South Africa likely due to 'Adelaide Hospital Row'. He graduated in 1901. After graduating he completed his residency in Melbourne. He gained his MB at the University of Adelaide in 1906. He then travelled to England where he worked in a number of hospitals around the country. He set up practice in Warrnambool, Victoria on his return to Australia, and worked there from 1907-14. He married Ivah Gladys Cuzen on 3rd June 1908 in Warrnambool. She was the younger daughter of Mr B Cuzen of Ely House, Warrnambool.

Makin volunteered for the AIF in March 1915. He was 39 years old, married, 5ft 9ins, 39ins chest and weighed 11st 7lbs. His wife, Ivah, was named as next of kin and gave his father's address at Palmer Place, North Adelaide for correspondence. He was posted to 6 FdAmb as a Major. The FdAmb arrived at Anzac at the beginning of September. He fell sick with dysentery and jaundice in October, and was evacuated first to Malta and then to London. He spent the next year working at the Parkhouse and Perham Downs Depots in England, narrowly avoiding being sent back to Australia. After being passed fit in February 1917 he went to France to rejoin his unit, but was instead transferred to 7 FdAmb. This unit was heavily engaged in the Second Battle of Bullecourt in May 1917. Makin's service with the unit included a month's detachment to 2 ACCS during August 1917 in the aftermath of the Battle of Messines, at which time the ACCS was at Trois Arbres, Steenwerck. He was promoted lieutenant colonel in September 1917 and given command of 8 FdAmb in place of Lieutenant Colonel Arthur Shepherd just before the Battle of Passchendaele. Unfortunately his tenure of command was brief, as he went down with trench fever two weeks later. He was sent back to the Red Cross Hospital at Rouen, and was not able to re-join his unit until 7th December, by which time the offensive was over. He went on leave to England in February 1918, and while there faced a medical board, which declared him unfit for overseas service. His appointment was terminated in the 3 MD Australia on the 15th June 1918. He was issued with the 1914-15 Star, the British War Medal and the Victory Medal.

Makin returned to Adelaide in 1918, and settled in Mile End, SA where he established a practice in dermatology. He was living at 198 North Terrace, Adelaide at the time. He was an honorary dermatologist at the Adelaide Hospital from 1925-35, with a private practice on North Terrace. He took an interest in local politics and was an Adelaide City Councillor from 1940-44. Frank Humphrey Makin died in 1961 at the age of 86 years.

Sources:

National Archives

http://recordsearch.naa.gov.au/NameSearch/Interface/ItemDetail.aspx?Barcode=8206726

Likeman R., "Gallipoli Doctors" Slouch Hat Publications, Melbourne Aust., 2010.

The Adelaide Advertiser 5th November 1900

The Chronicle Adelaide 11 December 1906

The Adelaide Advertiser 18 June 1908

The Recorder Port Pirie 4th July 1938

http://gawlerworldwar1.weebly.com/m.html

MARSHALL Charles Edward

MB ChB Ed LRCP LRCS Ed

1875 - 1967

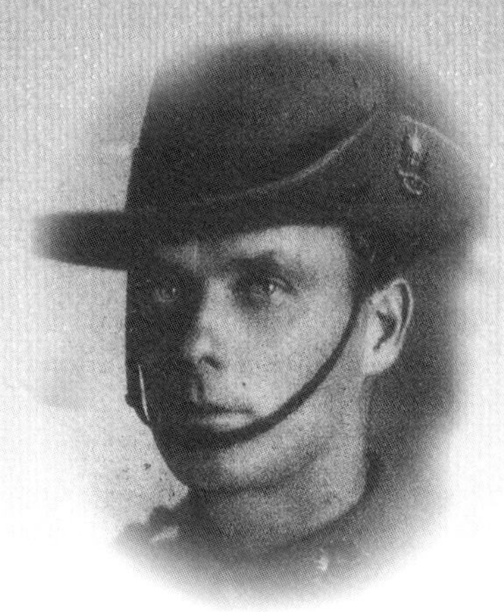

Charles Edward Marshall was born on the 5th April 1875 in Dunedin, New Zealand. He was the seventh of the nine children of William and Catherine Marshall. He studied medicine in Scotland. After graduating LRCP LRCS Ed in 1902 and MB ChB Ed in 1903 and obtaining a certificate in tropical medicine in 1903 he worked for a time in India. Here he was commissioned as a lieutenant in the volunteer Kolar Goldfields Bn in Mysore with promotion to captain in 1904. He arrived in South Australia in 1907, he settled in Coolcha on the Murray River near Mannum. He moved to Cowell and became medical health officer for the Franklin Harbour District. This occurred because there was no doctor in the district and it was serviced by a doctor from Wallaroo. This entailed crossing the Spencer Gulf by boat which caused much delay in bad weather or by horse and buggy around the gulf which took three days. The Franklin Harbour Council engaged Marshall for £400 ($800) per year in 1906. He bought a block of land in Cowell and built a cottage hospital on the South Bank facing the harbour. He married Edith Jane Gillespie and they had three children. A son died at fourteen days old in 1909.

Marshall enlisted in the AIF on the 28th April 1915. He was 40 years old, 5ft 11ins, weighed 165lbs, and was commissioned into 27 Bn that month. He arrived at ANZAC Cove with the Bn in September 1915. He was evacuated to Egypt with jaundice in early November and, after recuperation, transferred to 5 Div Arty and went to France with 14 AFA Bde in June 1916. He was posted to 8 FdAmb in February 1917 and was promoted to major. He served with the FdAmb through the Second Battle of Bullecourt. He was transferred to 1 ACCS in July 1917 in time for the unit's move from Bailleul to Oultersteene. It remained in that location through the Third Battle of Ypres, and he remained with them until the end of the war. Marshall was issued with the 1914-1915 Star, the British War Medal and the Victory Medal. His appointment was terminated in Adelaide on the 11th November 1919.

After taking study leave in Scotland Marshall returned to Australia. He returned to practice in Franklin Harbour, but later moved to the United Kingdom. Charles Edward Marshall died in South Australia on 24th May 1967. His son Dr Charles Edward Marshall (1912-2005) served in WW2 and was a renowned pathologist in Seattle, America.

Sources:
http://recordsearch.naa.gov.au/scripts/Imagine.asp?B=8216327
Likeman R., Gallipoli Doctors, Slouch Hat Publications 2010
District Council of Franklin Harbour
Med J Aust. 2006; 184 (9): 471.
The Register Adelaide Tues 7th July 1925
http://www.franklinharbour.sa.gov.au/page.aspx?c=346
'Radius' the Newsletter of Sydney's Medical Graduates Association March 2006.
Ancestry.com

Wanted Immediately

J. R. Kaye, Lieutenant Colonel
Div. san. Officer WR Div. TF

Your doing and acting, not thinking only.
Your co-operation, not grumbling
Clean bodies, clean hands, feet, and teeth.
Clean tent-floors, and a clean camp surface, not polluted with urine or excrement.
Clean food, not fly-poisoned
All refuse and filth rendered harmless by fire, burial, or disinfection.
Open tents, to let in the sunshine and fresh air, and keep away the doctor.

BMJ, 19 September 1914, p. 517

MATTERS Sir Reginald Francis

MD MS FRCS FRACS FRCOG

1892 - 1975

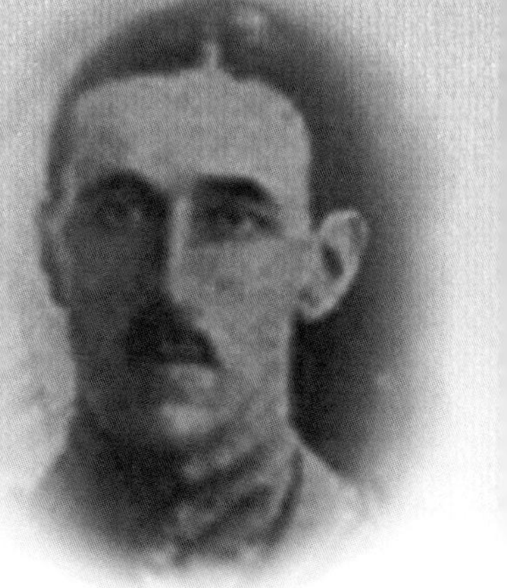

Reginald Francis Matters was born on 23 July 1892 at Malvern, South Australia. He was the son of Thomas James Matters and Jane, nee Waterhouse of Unley Park. He was educated at Prince Alfred College, and studied medicine at Sydney University graduating in 1917. Prior to WW1 Matters served with the 4th Infantry Service in South Australia from 1904 to 1912 and with the 29th Infantry in Sydney from 1913 to 1914.

Matters enlisted in the AIF as a Captain and medical officer on 28th January 1918. He was 30 years of age, 6ft ½ in tall, weighing 175lbs of dark complexion, brown eyes and black hair. He embarked on the HMAT *Osterley* on 9th May 1918 for France via Folkstone, England. He was originally posted to the 3 AGH 11th September 1918 but was then immediately reposted to 11 FdAmb on the 15th September 1918. He was wounded in action on 29th September 1918 and discharged back to duty on 7th November 1918. The extent of his injuries and the cause is not recorded. He returned to Australia on 30th November 1919. He was issued with the British War Medal and the Victory Medal.

Matters was registered to practice medicine in Adelaide in 1919. He married Elbe Cornwall aged 26 years from Burwood, New South Wales. He subsequently became a noted obstetrician and gynaecologist in Adelaide. He had several interests and was a member of two anthropological expeditions to Central Australia studying the metabolism of nomadic Aboriginal people. He was living in College Park, Adelaide in 1933. During WW2 he served with the Royal Australian Navy as a surgeon commander. After the war he became the President of the Navy League of South Australia and of the Naval Officers Association and led the naval contingent in the Anzac Day March in Adelaide each year. He was knighted for his service to medicine on the 10th June 1961. Sir Reginald Francis Matters died on 14th October 1975.

Sources:
http://recordsearch.naa.gov.au/scripts/Imagine.asp?B=8039575
http://www.geni.com/people/Reginald-Matters6000000019984599491
The Medical Journal of Australia, March 13, 1976, p 365.
Sydney Morning Herald 5th September 1917
The News Adelaide 4th April 1933
Canberra Times 10th June 1961

The Mentality of the Kaiser.

A question much debated at the present time is the mentality of the Kaiser... in the *North American Review* for October, 1904, the well-known psychologist, Dr McLane Hamilton, wrote that in the history of the Hohenzollerns, "it is not difficult to find a distinct insane trace, which in times more remote found expression in cruelty, oppression, and unmistakable insanity of other kinds"...Dr McLane Hamilton ...declares the Kaiser to be "a menace to the world, for the reason that he not only has shown the exceedingly bad judgement that belongs to those who are mentally inferior , but has delusive ideas of grandeur and consequent power of persecution and conspiracy".

BMJ, 28 August 1915, p. 331

MAYO John Christian

MB BS FRCS(Ed) FRACS FRCRA

1891 - 1955

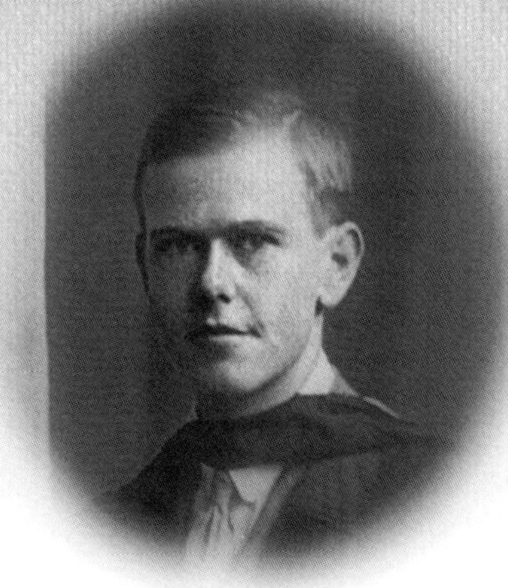

John Christian Mayo was born on the 4th August 1891 in Adelaide, South Australia. He was the youngest of the seven children of a civil engineer George Gibbes Mayo and his wife Henrietta Mary, nee Donaldson. Mayo was grandson of Dr George Mayo, the first South Australian to receive the FRCS, who had arrived in Australia in 1837. His grandmother was Maria Gandy, the mistress of Colonel William Light, who married George Mayo after Light's death in 1839. Mayo attended St Peter's College and was in the School Cadets from 1907. He studied medicine at the University of Adelaide and graduated in 1913. He completed his residency from 1914-15 at the Adelaide Hospital.

Mayo was commissioned in the AMF in November 1914 and allotted to the 76 Inf Bn. He enlisted in the AIF on the 4th March 1915 and posted as a captain in the AAMC. He was 23 years old, single, 5ft 10ins, 154lbs and his father, of 47 Melbourne St, North Adelaide, was named as his next of kin. He was posted to the Sea Transport Service and embarked on the *Orsova* in July 1915 with the other MOs posted to the *Kanowna,* and joined the ship at Alexandria. Mayo sailed with her for the round trip to Australia and back. After arriving in Cairo in February 1916 he was posted to 2 AGH. He went to France with the Hospital in March 1916, and served at Wimereux until August 1916, at which time he was detached to 2 FdAmb, which was then heavily engaged on the Somme. He returned to 2 AGH in October, only to be sent back to 2 FdAmb in December after a short leave. At the beginning of 1917 he spent three months as RMO of 6 Bn, and then a month with 5 Bn. He was promoted major in February 1917, and attached briefly to 1 Div Train and 56 CCS. He was recalled to England in July 1917 and appointed SMO of No 1 Command Depot at Parkhouse. He moved to Sutton Veny in October. At the end of the war he was 'Brought to Notice', and granted three months study leave, which he managed to stretch to six. His appointment in the AIF was terminated on the 14th January 1920 in the 4th MD. Mayo was issued with the 1914-15 Star, the British War Medal and the Victory Medal.

Mayo returned to Australia in September, and he entered general practice at Lameroo; later working in Moonta and Glen Osmond. He then decided on a surgical career. He was appointed an honorary surgeon at the Adelaide Children's Hospital in 1928. However his interest soon turned towards radiology, and he became an honorary assistant radiologist and radiotherapist at the Adelaide Hospital in 1933. He held this position until his death in 1955. He set up a private radiology practice on North Terrace in the mid-thirties. He was a Foundation member of the College of Radiologists of Australia and New Zealand in 1949 (since 1998 titled the RANZCR). John Christian Mayo died 27th September 1955. Mayo's eldest sister Helen was the second woman to study medicine at the University of Adelaide, although she was required to complete her studies at the University of Melbourne due to the 'Adelaide Hospital Row'. She became an eminent paediatrician. His brother Herbert became a Judge of the Supreme Court of South Australia. Another brother George Elton Mayo was the famous industrial psychologist and organisation theorist. His nephew Lieutenant Eric Mayo was killed during WW2 when he went down with the HMAS *Sydney* in 1941.

Sources:

http://recordsearch.naa.gov.au/scripts/Imagine.asp?B=8030504

Likeman R., "From the Tropics to the Desert" Slouch Hat Publications, 2012.

SLSA State Government

http://www.slsa.sa.gov.au/archivaldocs/PRG/PRG127_Mayofamily_serieslist.pdf

Adelaide Advertiser 29th September 1955

McGLASHAN John Eric

MC MB BS

1888 - 1942

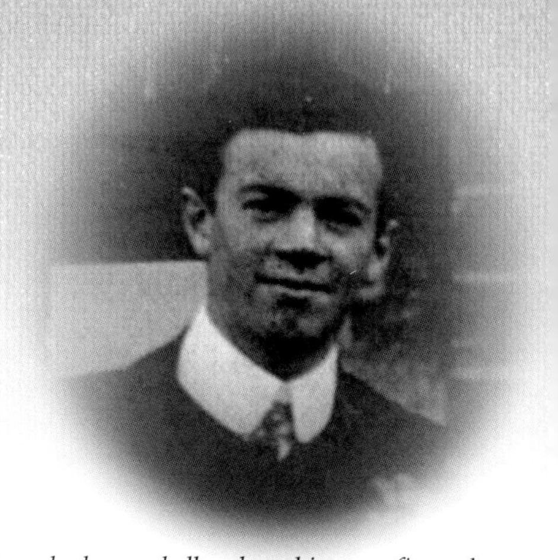

John Eric "Ricky" McGlashan was born at Orroroo, SA on the 31st August 1888. He was the eldest son of John McGlashan of Salisbury. He was educated at Carrieton Public School and studied medicine at the University of Adelaide graduating in 1909. He married Mary Beatrice Gardner on 16th February 1915 at the St Peter's College Chapel. He took up a general practice at Booleroo Centre, South Australia.

McGlashan enlisted in the AAMC on the 17th April 1916. He was 29 years old, with his wife named as next of kin. He had previous experience in the AAMC Reserve. He was 5ft 8ins tall, weighed 140lbs, with a ruddy complexion, brown hair and eyes. He embarked from Melbourne on the 11th September 1916 and arrived in Plymouth, England on the 26th October and was posted to 3 AAH. He spent most of April 1917 in France, with 2 AGH, seconded to 32 Stationary Hospital until September, then in October to 14 FdAmb. He was detached to 56 Bn for a month in February 1918. At Mericourt on the Somme in July he was awarded the Military Cross because *'he visited his various posts under heavy shell and machine-gun fire and was largely responsible for the successful evacuation of the wounded, in the open under the observation of the enemy'* He was granted study leave from March to June 1919, with return to Australia in June 1919 onboard the *Boonah.* His appointment was terminated on the 8th August. He was issued with the British War Medal and the Victory Medal.

After the war McGlashan returned to Adelaide and moved to Perth in 1924. He took positions as a dermatologist at the Perth Hospital and Children's Hospital. John Eric McGlashan died in Perth on 16th October 1942 of a ruptured aortic aneurism. He was survived by his wife, Mary.

Sources:
http://recordsearch.naa.gov.au/scripts/Imagine.asp?B=1944434
Photo: Adelaide University Archives, Medical Students 1906
http://members.iinet.net.au/~dodd/gail/publications/trengrouse/family_tree/11.htm

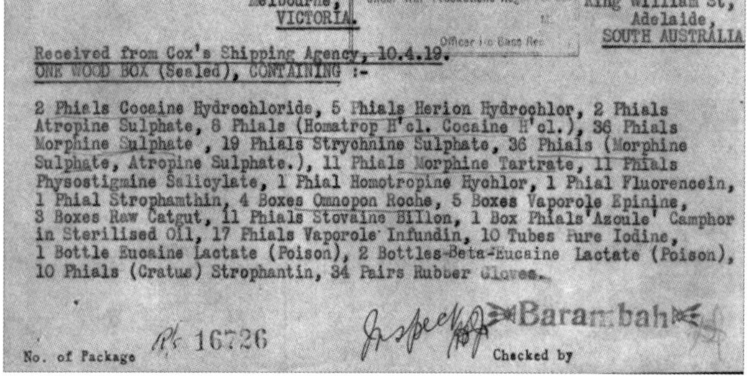

Australian Imperial Force.

FDJ. 23.

A.I.F. KIT STORE.
110. GREYHOUND ROAD,
HAMMERSMITH,
LONDON, W.6

Inventory of ~~Effects of~~ Property of :- Captain J.E. McGlashan, MC. A.A.M.C.

Forwarded to - Returned to Australia.

HOME ADDRESS :-
c/o G.F. Gardiner,
Royal Exchange,
King William St,
Adelaide,
SOUTH AUSTRALIA

The Secretary,
Department of Defence,
Melbourne,
VICTORIA.

Received from Cox's Shipping Agency, 10.4.19.
ONE WOOD BOX (Sealed), CONTAINING :-

2 Phials Cocaine Hydrochloride, 5 Phials Herion Hydrochlor, 2 Phials Atropine Sulphate, 8 Phials (Homatrop H'cl. Cocaine H'cl.), 36 Phials Morphine Sulphate , 19 Phials Strychnine Sulphate, 36 Phials (Morphine Sulphate, Atropine Sulphate.), 11 Phials Morphine Tartrate, 11 Phials Physostigmine Salicylate, 1 Phial Homotropine Hychlor, 1 Phial Fluorencein, 1 Phial Strophamthin, 4 Boxes Omnopon Roche, 5 Boxes Vaporole Epinine, 3 Boxes Raw Catgut, 11 Phials Stovaine Billon, 1 Box Phials 'Azoule' Camphor in Sterilised Oil, 17 Phials Vaporole Infundin, 10 Tubes Pure Iodine, 1 Bottle Eucaine Lactate (Poison), 2 Bottles Beta-Eucaine Lactate (Poison), 10 Phials (Cratus) Strophantin, 34 Pairs Rubber Gloves.

No. of Package Pk 16726 Checked by Baranbah

McNEIL John (Ian)

MB BS

1893 - 1976

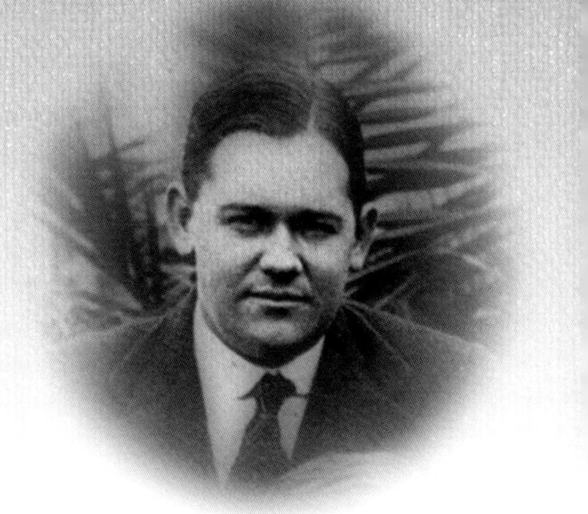

John (Ian) McNeil was born in Fairfield Park, Victoria in 25th January 1893. He was the son of William James McNeil and Helen Leis, nee Hilson. At some time during his childhood they moved to South Australia where he was educated at Prince Alfred College and studied medicine at the University of Adelaide graduating in 1918. During his school, university and enlistment years he was known at John McNeil, however he adopted the Christian name of Ian after the war.

McNeil enlisted on 18th June 1915. He was a medical student and single. He had four years of cadet service at school. He named his father as his next of kin and gave their address as Payneham Road, St Peters, South Australia. He was 5ft 6ins tall, and weighed 164lbs, of fair complexion with blue eyes and dark hair. He had a right sided abdominal surgical scar. He was sent to Mitcham Camp but was discharged on 24th July 1915 to complete his medical studies. He next sought to enlist on 4th July 1918. Again he went to Mitcham but was discharged on 18th November 1918.

McNeil married Miss Lulu Hylton daughter of Mr and Mrs Cyril G Hylton of Zinc Corporation at St Peters Church in Broken Hill on 19th August 1919. They had a daughter Judith. McNeil had a GP practice in Pinnaroo, South Australia in 1920. He was in Ballarat where he was the city health officer by 1926. Whilst in Ballarat he offered the Pinnaroo community a 14 acre parcel of land to establish a bowling green for the town. He stood for election as a councillor in the council election in Smith Ward Melbourne in 1939 and again in 1941 in Albert Ward Melbourne; he was unsuccessful on both occasions. He and his wife returned to Adelaide on several occasions to follow his interest in horse racing. At one stage he was the President of the Pinnaroo Racing Club. He was a member of the Victorian Racing Club and owned a gelding called 'Night Life'. It was reported that he had some drugs and surgical instruments stolen from his car overnight outside his practice at 81 Collins Street, Melbourne in 1945. He was still living in Victoria in 1949. Ian McNeil died in 1976.

Sources:

The Adelaide Advertiser 26 September 1923
The Argus Melbourne 8th July 1939
The Argus Melbourne 7th June 1941
The Argus Melbourne 6th November 1945
Adelaide Advertiser 11th May 1948
National Archives
http://recordsearch.naa.gov.au/NameSearch/Interface/ItemDetail.aspx?Barcode=1957827
Photo: Adelaide University Archives, Medical Graduates 1918.
http://www.genealogysa.org.au/resources/onlinedatabases.html?option=com_search&ref=search

The War

The response of the country to the great emergency has been worthy of our traditions. Men of all ranks and classes and occupations have come forward quietly and promptly to fill their places in the Royal Naval Volunteer Reserve and in the Territorial Force. We are proud to know that the members of the medical profession have been not less ready than the rest, and that the special responsibilities thrown upon the profession in every town and district have been met by prompt concerted action. Within the last week many hundred medical officers have left their civil practise to do military duty with the divisions of the Territorial Force, and many others are busily engaged in organizing, in all the great centres, the general hospitals of this force as provided by the scheme worked out when it was established.

BMJ, 15th August 1914, p.336

MEIKLE Alexander Jamieson

VD MD LRCPS Ed LRCP Ed

1869 - 1954

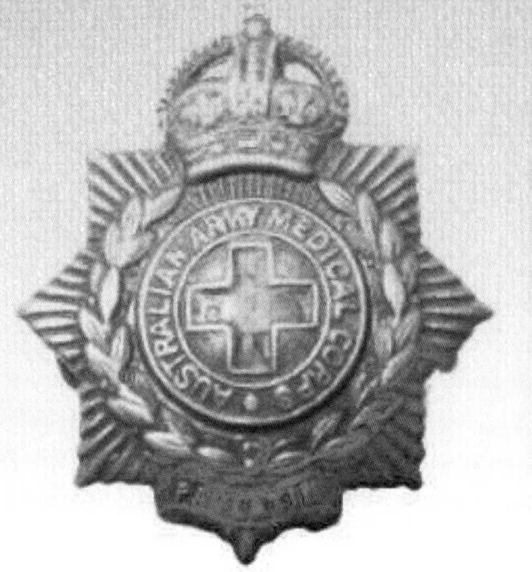

Alexander Jamieson Meikle was born on the 20th April 1869 in Inverary, Argyllshire, son of Rev Gilbert Meikle, a minister of the United Presbyterian Church. He was educated at George Watson's College, and studied medicine at Edinburgh University. He graduated MBChM in 1892 and MD in 1894. He came to Australia soon after his graduation and registered as a medical practitioner in South Australia in December 1894. He was living in Yankalilla by July 1895 when he was appointed as public vaccinator. He spent 12 years at Yankalilla, and then a further six years at Port Lincoln, where he was the medical officer of the Government Hospital. He was commissioned in the AAMC reserve in August 1900 as a captain, and served until 1903 and served again in the AAMC from 1906-10. He married Ellen Amelia from Port Lincoln and they had three children.

Meikle volunteered for the AIF on the 28th October 1914 at the age of 44 years and his wife was named as his next of kin. He was 5ft 8ins tall, and weighed 10st 7lbs. He was promoted to major in February 1915 and replaced Major James Stewart, who had been left behind at Colombo with suspected typhoid. He took temporary command of 4 FdAmb with the Medical Unit at Anzac Cove, Gallipoli. A letter home on the 7th July 1915 records: *"The first few days ashore were perfect Hell. The Turks did give us a hot reception, what with a constant downpour of shrapnel & snipers at work everywhere; you never knew when you'd be hit. We know we're going to win alright. So far as the Turks are concerned, we've got the upper hand. The Turks are darn good soldiers and play the game... On the whole, we have nothing much to complain of, one doesn't expect too much comfort or any luxury in the firing line."* He was promoted lieutenant colonel and his command of 4 FdAmb was confirmed in January 1916. He took the unit to France in June 1916 with 4th Div joined the attacks on Pozières Heights and Mouquet Farm in the first week of August 1916. Meikle was Mentioned in Despatches for his service between June and October 1916. He went on leave in Scotland after Pozières, and in September was admitted to hospital with bronchitis and emphysema. Meikle did not return to France. He remained in England until January 1917 and then returned to Australia. His appointment was terminated on the 21st August 1917 as *"medically unfit for further Service"* with his address at 27 Marlborough Street, College Park, South Australia. The same year he received the Volunteer Decoration. After he was invalided home he was on continuous home service, commanding 15th AGH, first at North Adelaide and then Torrens Park. He remained at the Mitcham Hospital until it was disbanded. He was issued with the 1914-15 Star, the British War Medal and the Victory Medal with Oak Leaves.

Meikle was appointed Deputy Superintendent of the 'Mental Hospital' in 1919 as he had considerable experience in connection with shell shock and mental cases. Alexander Jamieson Meikle died at 23 Bakewell Street, Tusmore, SA on 23rd March 1954. His wife, Ellen, died one month later on 21st April 1954. They were survived by two of their children Kathleen and George; their son Colin predeceased them.

Sources:

http://recordsearch.naa.gov.au/scripts/Imagine.asp?B=8039821;
SLSA; Mr Graham Jenkin
Adelaide Advertiser 17th October 1919
Advertiser Adelaide 26th March 1954
Adelaide Advertiser 23 April 1954

War Deafness

It has been estimate that about 16% of the men admitted to evacuation hospitals in the French *Zone des Armeés*...showed aural affections. The great difficulty has been to distinguish between neuroses and actual ear lesions.

MJA, 26 October 1918, p. 351

MESSENT Sir Philip Santo

MS FRACS

1895 - 1976

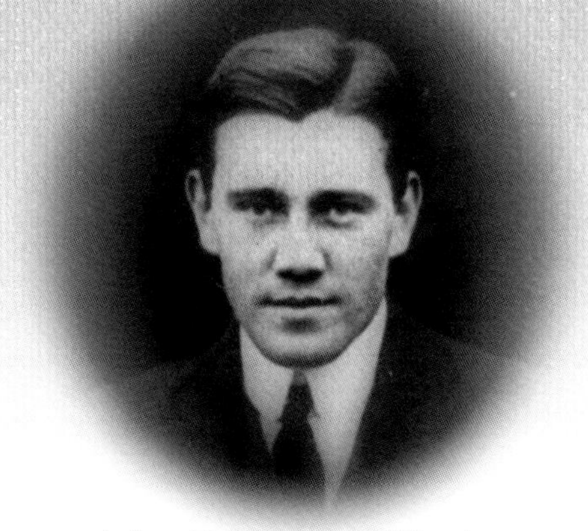

Philip Santo Messent was born in Hyde Park, South Australia on 22 February 1895. He was the son of Philip Messent and Amelia Elizabeth, nee Santo. He was educated at Kyre College and the University of Adelaide gaining his MB BS in 1918, and Master of Surgery in 1923. He became a Fellow of the Royal Australasian College of Surgeons in 1927.

Messent enlisted in the AIF in Adelaide, South Australia on 17th June 1918 whilst he was a final year medical student at the University of Adelaide. Messent had tried to enlist in Melbourne two years earlier. He also had 4 years' experience in the Citizen Forces Medical Corps in South Australia. He was recorded as 22 years old and single. He was 6ft 4ins and weighed 165lbs of medium complexion with brown eyes and brown hair. He had a scar on the back of his right calf and was slightly flat footed, but this was not sufficient to be rejected. His father was named as his next of kin and they still resided at Hyde Park, South Australia. He was not called up for duty and was discharged on 18th November 1918.

Messent was married on 4th September 1920 to Agnes May Newberry 1895-1967. They had three daughters and one son. He also served as a Captain in World War II and was discharged on 31st July 1942. He was knighted on 7th June 1951. At that time he was the Director of Surgical Studies at The University of Adelaide. Philip Santo Messent died on 5th February 1976 in Hyde Park, South Australia.

Sources:
National Archives of Australia
http://recordsearch.naa.gov.au/NameSearch/Interface/ItemDetail.aspx?Barcode=8012427
Homepages.rootsweb.ancestry.com
Supplement to the London Gazette, 7 June 1951
http://www.itsanhonour.gov.au/honours/honour_roll/search.cfm?aus_award_id=1083592&search_type=quick&showInd=true
Photo: Adelaide University Archives Med Graduates 1918

Extract from a letter of an Australian Lieutenant to his Father

31st May 1915

The ship was under the control of Australian Medical Officers, who show much better attention compared with the English. The English RAMC has evidently not availed itself of the South African war, and Australia and New Zealand are miles and miles ahead in every detail…All the wounded officers, who were with me, held the same opinion. Don't imagine that even the Australian medical arrangements are all they ought to be… Once a wounded soldier is landed in Egypt he is well looked after…but it is the getting there – and some troops never do. I told you…our brigade is with the British troops at the southern end of the Peninsula, and we are doing very well, and have been congratulated for our good work. We are the only Australians there…We always find time for some fun of some sort, and thoroughly enjoy ourselves…

MJA, 17 July 1915, p. 60

MITCHELL James Thomas

MD (Aberdeen) MRCS (Eng)

1856 - 1945

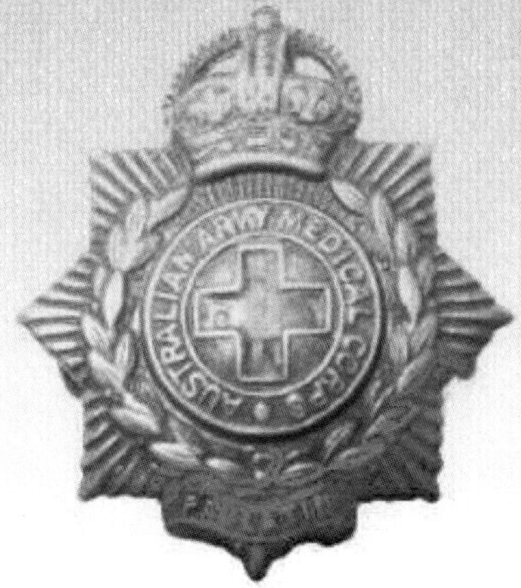

James Thomas Mitchell was born on 1st March 1856 in North Adelaide, South Australia, the son of Thomas James Mitchell, who was the Manager of Bank of South Australia and his second wife Thyrza Lucy, nee Cole. He was a foundation student of Prince Alfred College being one of four boys to enrol on the first day the College opened in1869. He was awarded the Longbotttom Scholarship and studied medicine at University College, London and Aberdeen University graduating in 1879. He returned to South Australia in 1880 and practised in Port Adelaide and remained in this practice until 1890. He married Edith Mary Dunn, daughter of John Dunn, on 9th July 1884 in Kent Town. They had two children a son, Dr Leonard Mitchell, and a daughter, Mrs Pulsford. He gained his MD from Aberdeen in 1885. He moved to Ballarat practising as a senior surgeon there for 25 years in 1890.

During WW1 Mitchell served in the AAMC as the Principal Medical Officer in 3 MD in Victoria at the rank of Lieutenant Colonel.

Mitchell lived in Malvern, Victoria following the war. He travelled extensively. He had started first aid classes for women whilst living in South Australia, this later merged into the St John Society. Throughout his time in Ballarat he was associated with classes for young men in the Methodist Church. James Thomas Mitchell died in Northbridge, Sydney on 14th September 1945.

Sources:

Advocate, Burnie Tasmania 17th sep1945.
The Advertiser 21st July 1937
South Australian Indexes of Birth Deaths and Marriages
PAC School Chronical

Extracts from the Gallipoli Landing. Recorded by Harry Carew Nott

We sailed out of harbour [Mudros] at 2pm, 6 battleships in line, and proceed round the west of the island and were still steaming at 8pm…I was awakened at 12.45 am on 25-4-15; put on my equipment and had a hurried meal in the wardroom…eventually we filed down a wooden gangway…into small open boats....As we neared the shore, the first glimmer of dawn was appearing in the sky ahead of us… my most constant thought was "will we get ashore before it is light enough for the Turks to see us?"… We must have been some hundreds of yards from shore when the first shot broke the stillness of the dawn…we felt the boat ground, and we all jumped over the side into the water and scrambled ashore and lay flat on the sand, surrounded by similar prone forms… I looked around for my bearers and collected 4 of them…the units were all mixed up and I couldn't ascertain what the Bn was in front of us: but I thought it a good place to establish an RAP…I sent 2 of my bearers forward to direct the casualties back to me and to bring any back the best way they could – all the stretchers had been left on the beach or in the boats…My 3 bearers got lost and I didn't find them again that day... that night a bad habit of calling out for a doctor became popular; the word would be passed along up and down the line "Doctor wanted on the right". …I would scramble and crawl in the direction indicated only to find eventually that no one knew exactly where the doctor was wanted!

Source: AWM

MOODIE Charles George Gordon

MB BS (Melb)

1885 - 1927

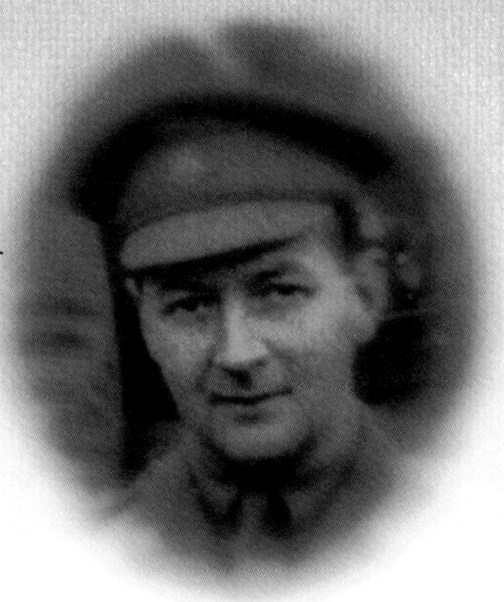

Charles George Gordon Moodie was born on 24th February 1885 in Portland, Victoria. He was the second youngest of the 12 children of William Moodie (1830-1914) from Scotland and Elizabeth Ann, nee Owens from Wales. He graduated from the University of Melbourne in 1913. He was registered with the Medical Board of South Australia in 1915 with his address given as Nailsworth.

Moodie enlisted in Adelaide on 1st September 1914. He was single and he had previously 16 months with AAMC with the rank of captain. He gave his address as Main North Road, Medindie, South Australia. His next of kin was his mother whose address was Coleraine, Victoria. He was 5ft 10ins tall, weighed 159lbs. He was posted to 3 FdAmb but was transferred to 2 AGH. He departed Australia on the *Port Lincoln* on 21st October 1914. A Medical Board conducted on 6th February 1915 declared him unfit for duty for not more than three months in Egypt. He returned to Australia on 3rd March 1915 on the *Ulysses*. He was posted to Gallipoli on 26th August 1915. He was ill from 30th October to 7th November 1915 and was evacuated to Malta and later Gibraltar. He was sent to England to 3rd London General Hospital on 14th December 1915. He was promoted to major on 1st January 1916 and on 14th February he was posted to the 5 FdAmb. He was again in hospital from 23rd September to 2nd October 1917. He was posted to the Australian Division Base Depot on 1st May 1916 and transferred to England to 1st Division Base Depot on 2nd February 1917. After working in the Training Depot he returned to France and to 1 AGH on 18th May 1917. After further appointments back in England he returned to the 2 AGH in France on 1st September 1918. He returned to England before leaving for Australia on 2nd Jan 1919 on the *Karmala*, disembarking in Fremantle before returning to Adelaide on *Morvada*. His appointment was terminated on 6th May 1919. He was issued with the 1914-1915 Star, British War Medal and Victory Medal.

Moodie married Diane Wells on 20th January 1923 but they were divorced in 1926. Charles George Gordon Moodie died in 2nd June 1927 in Darlinghurst, New South Wales from an accidental overdose of morphine.

Sources:
National Archives of Australia
http://recordsearch.naa.gov.au/NameSearch/Interface/ItemDetail.aspx?Barcode=11547345
Profiles and Historical Records - Ancestry.com
http://www.swvic.org/digby/fami;y/moodie.htm
Sydney Morning Herald 16th September 1926

Medical Students and the War

During the past few weeks occasional letters have been appearing in the local newspaper press of Edinburgh in which it has been hinted that the medical student is among the shirkers. It is therefore interesting to find that the great majority of the candidates now sitting for the final examination of the University are pledged to give their aid in bringing to an end the stupendous struggle in which the nations are engaged… Any suggestion that medical students are showing any tendency to shirk their duties to the country to-day is utterly unfounded.

BMJ, 5 June 1915, p. 977

MOORE Brian Formby

MB BS FRACS DOMS (Lond)

1894 - 1943

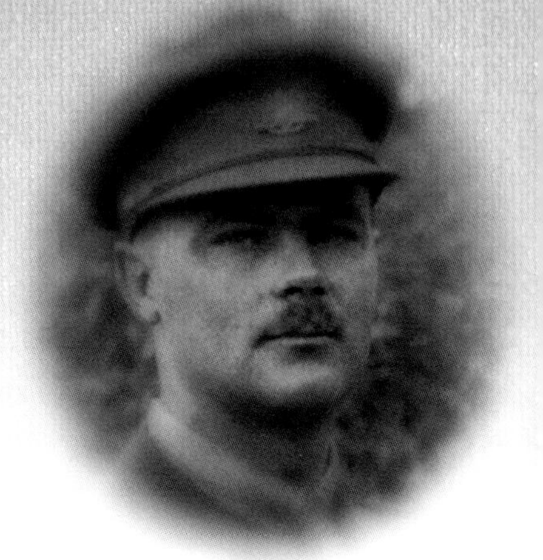

Brian Formby Moore was born in Mount Barker, South Australia on the 9th July 1894, son of Henry Percival Moore. He had two brothers and a sister. He was educated at St Peter's College and studied medicine at the University of Adelaide graduating in 1917. He was a sergeant in 79th Infantry CMF and, after graduating, spent 3 months as a house surgeon at the Adelaide Hospital before enlisting.

Moore enlisted into the AIF on the 7th August 1917. He was single and his father of 70 Buxton St, North Adelaide was named as his next of kin. He was 5ft 10ins, and weighed 168lbs. He embarked in November 1917 for Suez and then on to Taranto, Southampton, Parkhouse and Codford. He was sent to France in March 1918 and over the next 8 months served with the RAMC in several units and then returned to the 2 AGH, and 1 and 2 FdAmb until his return to Australia in September 1919. His service aboard was noted as 14 days with pleurisy in France and a gunshot wound in the left leg and foot. His appointment was terminated on the 27th September 1919 and he was issued with the British War Medal and the Victory Medal.

Moore became one of South Australia's leading ophthalmologists. He gained his FRACS in 1932 and DOMS in London in 1936. He was appointed an honorary ophthalmologist at the Adelaide Children's Hospital and Queen's Home Adelaide, and at the time of his death, was in partnership with Geoffrey Howard Barham Black and living at Buxton Street, North Adelaide. Brian Formby Moore died at the age of 48 years at Victor Harbor on 11th April 1943 after a short illness. He was survived by his wife Joyce. His brother Captain Harry Formby Moore served in WW1 in Egypt and France, and he died in 1927.

Sources:

http://recordsearch.naa.gov.au/NameSearch/Interface/ItemDetail.aspx?Barcode=3005621

The chronicle Adelaide 19 November 1927

The Adelaide Advertiser 13 April 1943

Photo in uniform: unknown source

The Final Stages

The signing of the armistice, the termination of hostilities...have given the people of Australia a feeling of a task completed...While the war lasted the director General of Medical Services experienced much difficulty in supplying the Australian Imperial Force and other expeditionary forces with a sufficient number of medical officers. The remembrance is still fresh of the opposition raised to the enlistment of medical students as combatants. This expedient adopted to ensure a constant supply of medical officers for the army. Many of the men who are now graduating, were prevented from enlisting for this purpose....The Director-General looks to these young graduates to place their service at his disposal now... and it is their duty to undertake service at home...We therefore appeal to the younger members of the medical profession to enlist in the Australian Army Medical Corps for home service without loss of time.

MJA, 5 April 1919, p. 279-280

† MOREY Alan Wilson,

MC Medical Student

1893 - 1918

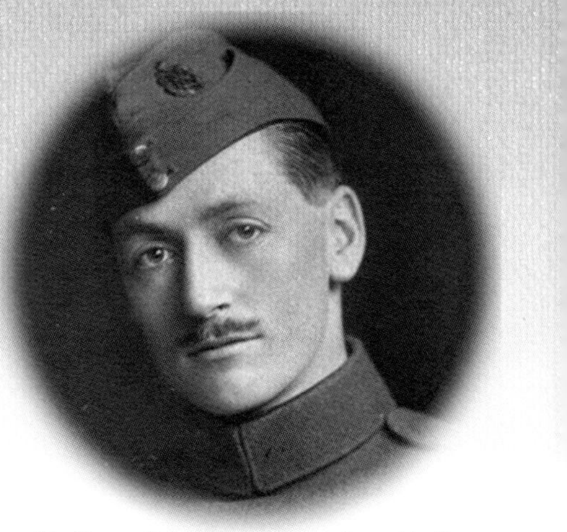

Alan Wilson Morey was born on the 1st March 1893 at 215 Hunter St, Newcastle, NSW, son of Henry Augustus Morey (1859-1907), bank manager, and Mary Morey, nee Collier (1867-1926). He was educated at Queen's College and St Peter's College. He was an all-round sportsman and gained a Government Bursary to enable him to study medicine at the University of Adelaide from 1912. At the end of his first and second years he achieved the first place in the medical examinations and won a (tied) Elder Scholarship for outstanding performance in 1912. He was awarded a Rhodes scholarship in 1913. Magdalen accepted him as a Commoner to read Medicine. Morey, his brother and his mother left Adelaide on 14 July 1914, travelled to England and arrived in London on the 20th August 1914.

Morey paid a brief visit to Oxford before joining the recently formed 11th (Service) Bn, the Royal Scots (Lothian Regt) as a second lieutenant in September 1914. He went to France on the 11th May 1915. He was Mentioned in Despatches in France in 1915. During the Battle of Loos, on the 25th September 1915, Morey was severely wounded in the shoulder and on 4 November 1915 he was awarded the Military Cross, *"for conspicuous gallantry and devotion during the fighting on September 25, 1915 at Loos, in France. He volunteered to cross the open space between the opposing lines to obtain information, and although he was wounded and therefore should have sent a written report, he went for some distance personally to report to the brigadier before his wound was dressed."* He spent a long period convalescing in England, at Chatsworth. Morey then joined the Royal Flying Corps; he learnt to fly on a Maurice Farnham Biplane at the Military School, Shoreham, and received his wings on the 29th April 1916. While undergoing subsequent training at Gosport, his machine collapsed in mid-air on 20 June 1916 and he fell 300-500 feet to the ground. He was severely injured and hospitalized. He was crippled so badly by the accident that he never walked again without the aid of two sticks. He was transferred to the general list of officers on 29 June 1916 and in August 1917 received compensation of £250 for his injuries. Nevertheless, once his rehabilitation was complete, he continued with his training, and on completion, volunteered to serve in France. He was posted to 60 Squadron RFC, on 5 December 1917. Morey and eleven other aircraft took off at 12.10 hours on the 24th January 1918 on an offensive patrol over Menin and Roulers, during which seven enemy two-seaters were sighted, engaged, and driven back eastwards. During the combat, at about 1250 hours, when the patrol was at a height of 8-12,000 feet to the south-west of Becelaere, an Albatros Scout dived down out of the sun on Lieutenant Clark's aircraft from behind and fired about ten rounds. Clark's combat report then reads: *"He then turned over my back towards the right. Lieutenant Morey, who was on my right, did a left-hand bank towards the Hun, and immediately collided with him. I saw Lieutenant Morey's wing come off and they both crashed".* Morey was due to be promoted from lieutenant to captain on the following day. Alan Wilson Morey was aged 24, and he was the only South Australian Rhodes Scholar to die in WW1. His death was confirmed on 25th March 1918, when the Germans dropped a message over the British lines. He has no known grave. His name is on the Arras Flying Service Memorial, the AWM aviation section and the Memorial Hall and the Memorial plaque in the entrance to the large quadrangle at St Peter's College.

Sources:

Courtesy of the *Slow Dusk* project, Magdalen College, Oxford, edited by Richard Sheppard, David Roberts, Roger Hutchins and Robin Darwall-Smith.

The Kadina and Wallaroo Times 13 December 1913.

The Register Adelaide 22nd June 1916

MORRIS Bedlington Howell
MB BS

1868 - 1936

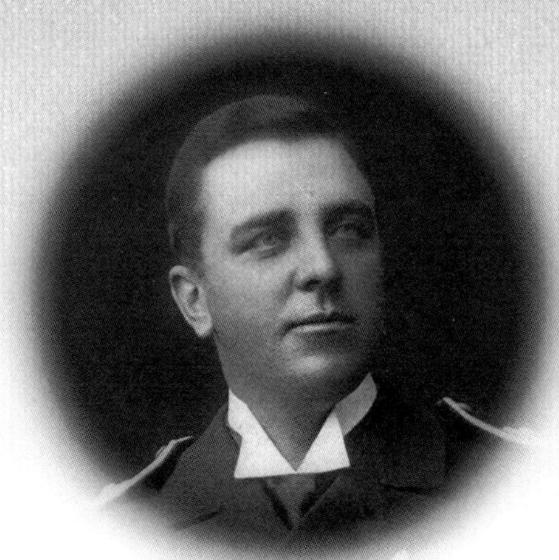

Bedlington Howell Morris was born on the Isle of Anglesey, North Wales on the 22nd April 1868. He was educated at St Thomas College and the Beaumaris School and then in 1893, MB BS with 1st Class Hons from Durham University, first prizeman in surgery, and obtained first-class honours in anatomy and surgery. He was the Goyder memorial scholar in clinical medicine and surgery and the Luke Armstrong scholar in 1893. He held several clinical appointments in England in Mental Disease and Tropical Diseases. He also spent a time as Transport Medical Officer in the Ocean Steamship Company on the Netherlands India Service in Java and Malaya. Morris previously was a resident medical officer in Denbigh Infirmary, and was in practice in Swansea when appointed to the Adelaide Hospital in 1896. Morris arrived at Largs Bay, Adelaide on 22nd December 1896 on the board the RMS *Oroya* from Plymouth. Morris was one of the "strike breaker" doctors brought to the Adelaide Hospital from the United Kingdom to replace doctors who had resigned in the 'Adelaide Hospital Row'. He joined the South Australian Public Service in 1896 and was appointed medical officer to the destitute poor and State Children's department in June 1899. He was granted leave of absence whilst he was engaged on naval duties and served with distinction as staff surgeon on the HMCS *Protector* in China from August 1900-January 1901. Morris married Ada Jessica Shearer on 11th August 1902 at St Luke's Church Adelaide. In 1913 Morris was appointed Inspector General of Hospitals. This important position required him to be responsible for the administration of the Mental Defectives Act, the inspection and supervision of all country hospitals and all the duties formerly held by the Colonial Surgeon. It also entailed being Chairman of the Mental Defectives Board, the Dental Association Board and the Medical Board.

Morris was keen to serve in WW1 as he had during the Boxer Rebellion but was not granted leave by the South Australian Government. He had to be content to remain as a Fleet Surgeon, Permanent Naval Force, at the Adelaide Port Depot assisting the District Naval Medical Officer.

After the war in 1920 to 1921 he with his many other board appointments became the Chairman of the newly formed Nurses Registration Board. He also had a long association with the Australian Red Cross Society. He commenced long service leave from the State Department on 1st March 1936 and was living at Pembroke Street, College Park. Bedlington Howell Morris died in Calvary Hospital Adelaide, aged 68, after a short illness on the 10th July 1936. He was survived by his widow and three sons, C H Morris of Union Bank, Warracknabeal, Victoria; C L Morris of Adelaide, Solicitor and H M Morris of the ES&A Bank, Applia Yarrowie, South Australia.

Sources:
Photo: AWM, B6401
Find my Past website
Register Adelaide 11 Jun 1899
Adelaide Advertiser 12 September 1922
The Mail Adelaide 4th September 1920

South Australia
From our Special Correspondent

We rather anticipated His Majesty's views on abstinence, as the following resolution will show:

That in view of the evidence frequently coming before us as medical men of the dangers to our troops from excessive alcoholism, and hoping to exert influence towards temperance among them, members of the Branch of the British Medical Association are of the opinion that in the present national emergency all medical men will do well to become and remain total abstainers during the continuance of the war.

BMJ, 3 July 1915, p. 32

MORRIS Edward Walter

MRCS (Eng) LRCP (Lond) LSA (Lond)

1863 - 1942

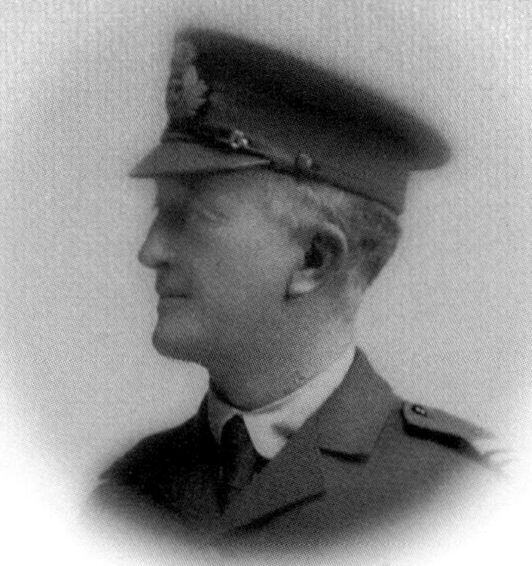

Edward Walter Morris was born at Reading, England on 25th December 1863. He was the son of Edward Morris, a draper, and his wife Kate. He had moved away from home and was a draper's apprentice, age 17 years living in Windsor, Berkshire in 1881. There is no confirmation as to when he and/or family moved to Adelaide but he did study medicine at St Thomas's Hospital, London with qualifications in 1888 and 1889. He married Dora Anne Jacobsen in 1889 at Semaphore, South Australia and is recorded as a medical practitioner in St Vincent's Street, Port Adelaide in 1893. He was appointed assistant health officer Port Pirie in 1901. He appears as lieutenant and staff surgeon in the lists of the CNF (Citizen Naval Force) South Australia and the RANR from 1907 as the District Naval Medical Officer with his superior being Fleet Surgeon Bedlington Howell Morris. Morris, was confirmed as a member of the South Australian Medical Board in March 1915.

Morris is unusual in that during WW1 he served in two arms of the Defence Force, the Navy and Army, two enlistments in the AIF and in three styles of deployment. He served as a staff surgeon on the little known Royal Australian Naval Bridging Train (RANBT) at Gallipoli from 26th April 1915. The RANBT was the most highly decorated Royal Australian Navy unit during WWI. The RANBT was formed in Melbourne on 28 February 1915 and was manned by Reservists. Three hundred Naval Reservists were selected for the RANBT and began training in horsemanship, engineering and pontoon bridging at the Domain in Melbourne. They left Melbourne on 4th June 1915; once deployed they acted as an engineering unit to support the British landings at Suvla Bay to the north of ANZAC Cove on the Gallipoli Peninsula. During this time they were to be under British command and control. Morris was transferred to the 5th Field Company Australian Engineers for 6 months from March 1916. He was struck off strength in November 1916. He returned to Australia. At the age of 54 years he was deemed "permanently unfit for Active Service" for dental fractures which were not service related in February 1917. Morris again applied for enlistment after 12 months and was accepted as captain in the AAMC for duty at the Mitcham Army Camp and the 7th AGH at Keswick. He was 5ft. 10ins, 178lbs, of fair complexion, grey eyes and red hair. His wife of Hall St, Semaphore was named as his next of kin care of Mrs Claridge of 97 Jeffcott St, North Adelaide He was promoted to major in July 1918 and was appointed to the 5th Sea Transport Section. Whilst in England from late 1919 he performed AIF duty at Australia House later posted as SMO at AIF HQ when ADMS Lieutenant Colonel Lewis Wibmer Jefferies returned to Australia. His AIF appointment was terminated in London on the 10th October 1921. He was issued with the 1914-15 Star, Victory Medal and the British War Medal

Morris was appointed chief medical officer Australia House, London from Sept 1921 until July 1926. In that period he remained on the navy list as Commander, RANR. On return to civilian life in Adelaide the Morris family was prominent in social life with children, reunions, weddings and Morris' appointment to executive positions with the Navy League 1930 to 1937 and the South Australian branch of the Royal British Nurses' Association. Edward Walter Morris of Grant Avenue Toorak died 17th May 1942. He was survived by his wife and two sons and a daughter.

Sources:
http://recordsearch.naa.gov.au/scripts/Imagine.asp?B=7981832,
Likeman R., Gallipoli Doctors, Slouch Hat Publications, 2010
Photo: SLSA: GRG26_5_4_0_2327
South Australian Register 15 March 1899
Adelaide Advertiser 17 May 1901
Adelaide Advertiser 18 May 1942

MUECKE Francis Frederick

CBE MB BS FRCS

1879 - 1945

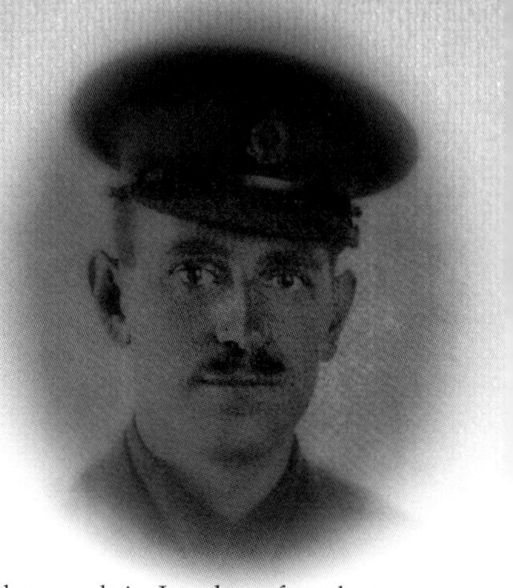

Francis Frederick Muecke was born in Adelaide on 6th December 1879. He was the son of the Honourable Hugo Carl Emil Muecke and Margaret Julia Elizabeth, nee Le Page. His father was a Member of Parliament and German Consul in South Australia. He was educated at the Queen's School and Prince Alfred College. He studied medicine at the University of Adelaide graduating in 1901. He spent a year at the Adelaide Hospital as a resident medical officer before moving to England and joining The London Hospital in 1903. Muecke, on 11th April 1905, married renowned singer Ada Jemima Crossley, who was born in Tarraville, Victoria. Ada Crossley had received wide acclaim in England and was commanded to sing for Queen Victoria five times in a two year period.

Muecke joined the RAMC in 1914 at the rank of lieutenant and was present at the Suvla landing and took part in the big offensives in France. He was promoted temporary captain in 1917. He was later transferred to the Royal Air Force, which was formed as a separate service on 1st April 1918, as a temporary lieutenant colonel in 1919. He was Mentioned in Despatches and appointed CBE for gallantry

Muecke continued to work in London after the war and rose to be one of the leading consultant ear, nose and throat specialists in England. Ada Crossley died on 17th October 1929 at Woodlands Park, Great Missenden, Buckinghamshire, England. He married Jean McMurtrie in 1930 of Cumnock, Ayrshire, Scotland and they visited Adelaide in 1935. Muecke and Ada had no children. Francis Frederick Muecke died on 14th April 1945 in The London Hospital, England. He was survived by his wife and his three brothers Edwin Charles, Alfred Eugene, Walter Le Page and sister Amelia Caroline.

It should be noted that some sources incorrectly report that Muecke had three sisters and a brother.

Sources:

The Adelaide Advertiser 18th September 1935, 16th April 1945
The Chronicle 20th May 1905
Obituaries Australia 1879-1945 National Centre of Biography, Australian National University.
http://oa.anu.edu.au/obituary/muecke-francis-frederick-16992
www.forceswarrecords.co.uk/ViewRecord/5390261?reference=arrowLinks
South Australian Indexes of Births Death and Marriages
Missen M., 'Crossley, Ada Jemima (1871–1929)', Australian Dictionary of Biography, National Centre of Biography, Australian National University, http://adb.anu.edu.au/biography/crossley-ada-jemima-5829/text9899.
Photo: PAC Collection

MUIRHEAD John Robb

DSO MB BS

1883 - 1932

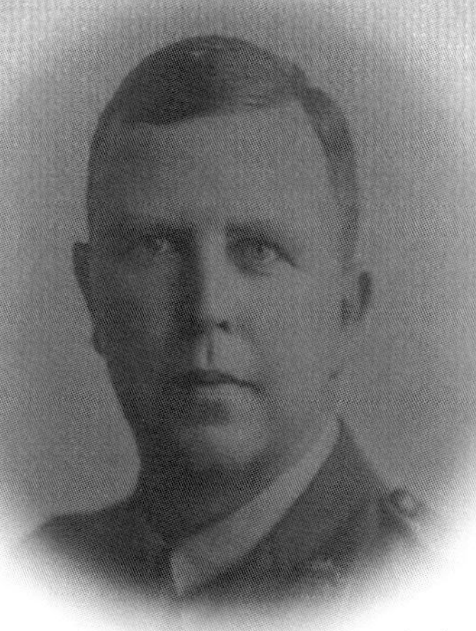

John Robb Muirhead was born at Glenelg on 28th December 1883. He was the eldest son of Charles Mortimer Muirhead, a barrister, and his wife Margaret Sarah nee Robb. Margaret's father, John Robb was an engineering contractor with extensive building projects in the eastern states and South Australia (including the railway from Kapunda to the river Murray and the Granite Island breakwater at Victor Harbour). Unfortunately his fortune turned and in 1894 he became bankrupt with debts over £680,000. Muirhead's father Charles was to engage in 1908 in extended litigation with his wife's family on his wife's behalf who was suing for a seventh of her father's estate. Charles' investments had taken a hit in the 1890s and as a result of this, and the unsuccessful internecine legal action, went bankrupt in 1909. Notwithstanding these family troubles Muirhead was educated at St Peter's College and studied medicine at the University of Adelaide where he graduated MB BS in 1908. After graduation he practised in Laura and Gilberton. He also served in the school cadets for 3 years prior to WW1.

Muirhead enlisted in the AIF in Adelaide on 23rd November 1914, he was single, 30 years old and living in Tyne Street, Gilberton. He was 5ft 8½ins tall and weighed 15 stone 3 pounds. He initially served at the Oakland's Camp. He was attached to the 2/3 reinforcements for 1 ASH and left Australia, from Sydney, on the *Hymettus* on 5th February 1915. He served in Egypt, on Lemnos and Gallipoli when 1 ASH moved there late in 1915. He proceeded to join the BEF on the 11th March 1916 and attached to 2nd Div Engineers and travelled with them to France. He remained with them until he was promoted major and posted as an RMO to 24 Bn in June 1917. He was wounded when blown up in Broodseinde in October 1917 and evacuated to England. He did not return to duty until April 1918 when he joined 1 AAH. He was posted, second in command, to 6 FdAmb in August 1918 and went with them to France. He was Mentioned in Despatches with 6 FdAmb and, for his courage and organisation during the October offensive, awarded the DSO. The citation reads: *As second in command of 6 Aus FdAmb served throughout the big advance from Villers-Brettoneaux until the capture of the Hindenburg line. In the attack on Montebrehain north east of St Quentin on 3rd and 4th October he was in full charge of the evacuation of divisional casualties to the Advanced Dressing Station and it was due to his energy and careful arrangements that this evacuation was one of the most expeditious on record and as the enemy shelling on the evacuation route was very intense this rapid evacuation was the means of saving many lives*". He was promoted temporary lieutenant colonel and returned to Australia in 1919 and his appointment terminated in February 1920. He was issued the 1914-15 Star, the British War Medal, and the Victory Medal with Oak leaves. His three younger brothers, Henry Mortimer Muirhead (b 1885) had served as a private with 10Bn, Francis Charles Muirhead as a gunner and Gordon McKinnon Muirhead (b 1895) a gunner-Lt with 6 Fd Art Brigade.

Muirhead married whilst in England. After the war he returned to medicine in Adelaide and in 1925 was noted to be practising as an opthamologist in Verco Buildings on North Terrace, Adelaide. Muirhead was a keen yachtsman and in 1925 in Sydney won the Australian Dinghy Championship in White Cloud. John Robb Muirhead died in North Adelaide at the young age of 48 on 17th November 1932, predeceasing his father. He was survived by his wife Kathleen.

Sources:

National Archives
http://recordsearch.naa.gov.au/NameSearch/Interface/ItemDetail.aspx?Barcode=7987481
Trove
http://trove.nla.gov.au/newspaper/result?q=Margaret+Sarah+Robb
Photo: from Family

MUIRHEAD Leonard Graham

MB BS

1887 - 1964

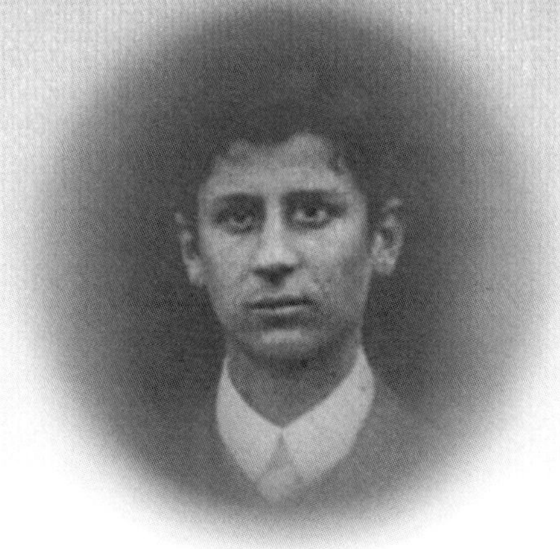

Leonard Graham Muirhead was born 19th April 1887, son of Graham David Muirhead and Eliza Helen nee Hogg. He attended Prince Alfred College (1903-1905) and then studied medicine at the University of Adelaide graduating MB BS in 1911. He was a house surgeon and physician at the Adelaide Hospital 1911 to 1912 and subsequently went into practice at Grange, South Australia. Muirhead began a Citizens Naval Forces posting as acting District Naval Medical Officer (DNMO) at Port Adelaide in July 1915. He was replacing Edward Walter Morris who was deployed on 27th April 1915 to Gallipoli and France. The role of the DNMO is similar to that of the MO of 4 MD. Muirhead was relieved of his duties as DNMO when Morris returned to the position by April 1917.

Muirhead applied for a commission in the AIF in April 1917. He was 30 years old, single 5ft 8ins tall, and weighed 10st 4lbs. He had slight knowledge of French, and noted his next of kin as Graham David Muirhead of Grange, Adelaide. He was recommended for general duties and embarked from Melbourne on *Ascanius* on 11th May 1917 to England and then to France on 15th October 1917 to the 1st Aust Tunnelling Company for a year then to No. 3 AAH. Muirhead returned to Australia in November 1918 with his appointment in the AIF terminated on 29th January 1919 owing to the cessation of hostilities. He was issued with the British War Medal and Victory Medal.

Muirhead became engaged to Freda Mary Chinner, daughter of Mr. and Mrs. Hubert Chinner, of Glenburnie, Upper Mitcham in October 1922. They married on 3rd March 1923. The couple lived at 1 Crosbie St, Brighton and 9 Sturt Place, Beaumont. Muirhead enlisted again in WW2 on 12th February 1942, and served at the Loveday Prisoner of War camp. Leonard Graham Muirhead died on 2nd January 1964 and is buried in Centennial Park. He was survived by his wife Freda who died in 1988 when she was 88 years old.

Sources:

http://recordsearch.naa.gov.au/scripts/Imagine.asp?B=987485
Adelaide Advertiser 22 December 1903
Photo: Adelaide University Archives; Medical Students 1906
Tunnellers Association http://www.google.com.au/url?sa=t&rct=j&q=&esrc=s&source=web&cd=1&ved=0CCkQFjAA&url=http%3A%2F%2Fwww.tunnellers.net%2Fprofiles___photos%2Fmuirhead_leonard_graeme_capt.doc&ei=Z8vIUt7fMs-2lQX_moHoDQ&usg=AFQjCNE-0PCw_biN5YXsykOiVkhPhDXRWA

Field Ambulance Work at ANZAC

By June 26th the operating tent was riddled with bullets and a number of the orderlies and patients had been hit, so we came to the conclusion that cases, and incidentally ourselves, ran so much risk of further injury that operative procedures in the tent were unjustifiable. We set to work to excavate a room underground, as timber was now available, and by the evening of June 26th had an operating room fitted up and lighted with acetylene gas.

BMJ, 4 December 1915, p. 806

MUNDAY Neill Horace

MB BS FRCS(Ed)

1894 - 1955

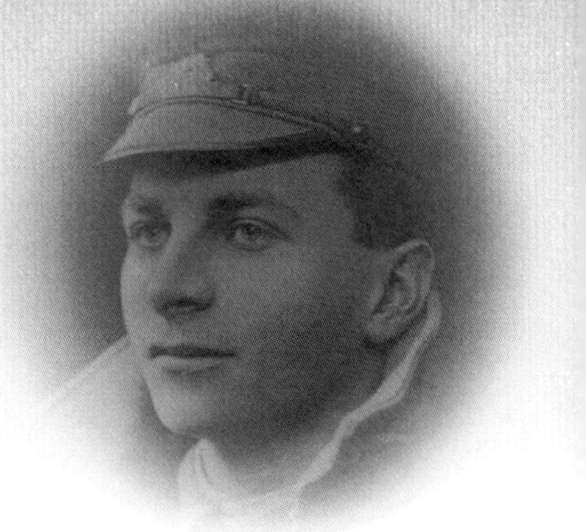

Horace Munday was born in 1894 in Marryatville, South Australia, the fifth child and fourth son of Fred and Elizabeth, nee O'Neill of County Clare, Ireland. He was educated at Marryatville High School and later Muirden College where he topped the commercial examinations at the age of 16 before enrolling in first year medicine at the University of Adelaide in 1916.

Munday enlisted in the AIF on the 30th May 1916 whilst he was still a medical student as a private soldier in the AAMC. He was 22 years old and still serving in the 19 AAMC CMF. He gave his mother of 121 King William Rd, Hyde Park as his next of kin. He was 5ft 6ins tall and 130lbs, (by 1918 he was 140lbs), of fresh complexion blue eyes and light brown hair. He was posted to No. 5 Section Sea Transport Nursing Staff from the 27th October 1916. He travelled back and forth between Australia and the United Kingdom, as a medical orderly/nurse, for the next three years on various P&O Liners converted into troop ships. These included *Borda, Beltana, Suevic* and *Gaika*. He was promoted to sergeant on the 1st January 1918. At the time of discharge he had served with 2 years 269 days total service with 2 years 46 days aboard. He was discharged to the 4th MD with the rank of sergeant medically unfit (suffering from influenza) on 22 February 1919. He was issued the British War Medal.

Munday resumed his medical studies at the University of Adelaide in 1919 and also added the name "Neill" (derived from his mother's maiden name) by deed poll and thus was known as Neill Munday for the rest of his life. He completed his medical course MB BS at the end of 1924. During his university years he played Intervarsity lacrosse in 1924 and was captain of the University B Cricket Team. After serving his internship at the Adelaide Hospital he entered general practice at Murray Bridge from 1926 until May 1935. He married Dorrie Eva Ellershaw in October 1925; they had two children Mary born in 1927 and Robert born in 1930. In order to further his studies in surgery, Munday took himself and his family to the United Kingdom in May 1935. After a short stay in London with his elder brother William, Munday decided to move to Edinburgh where he spent nine months studying in the Edinburgh Royal Infirmary under Professor John Fraser who was Regius Professor of Surgery at Edinburgh University at the time. He passed the Fellowship Examination in Surgery in July 1936. Munday and his family returned to Adelaide in 1937 to enter a general practice partnership in the Unley area of Adelaide with two brothers, Drs Herbert Henry Ernest Russell and Ernest Albert Harold Russell. Munday was the surgeon in the group. After several years with the Russell brothers Munday elected to enter private surgical practice with consulting rooms in the Bank of New South Wales. Munday was appointed honorary clinical assistant in 1939 at the Adelaide Hospital and on the 1st December 1942 he was promoted to the position of temporary honorary assistant surgeon to Sir Henry Newland and held this position until 3rd January 1946. He was also gazetted as a captain in the AAMC and was a recruiting medical officer during the early part of WW2. While operating at Memorial Hospital North Adelaide in October 1950, Munday suffered a major stroke and it was feared he would die shortly thereafter. However, showing great courage over the next six months, he recovered enough to walk with the aid of a stick but was never able to return to work. Neill Horace Munday died on the 19th October 1955, at the age of 61 after a long illness, survived by his wife and 2 children.

Sources:

http://recordsearch.naa.gov.au/scripts/Imagine.asp?B=7987679

Biography and photo from son, Dr Robert Munday, 2012.

NEWLAND Sir Henry Simpson

CBE DSO MS FRCS FRACS LRCP

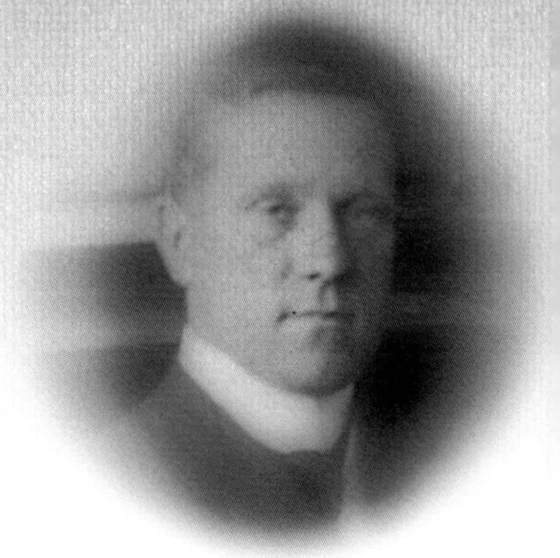

1873 - 1969

Henry Simpson Newland was born in Adelaide on 24th November 1873. He was the eldest son of Simpson Newland and Jane Isabella, nee Layton. His father was the author of "Paving the Way", a wealthy property owner and Member of the SA Legislative Assembly. His grandfather had migrated to Encounter Bay in South Australia in 1839. Newland was educated at St Peter's College and studied medicine at the University of Adelaide where he graduated top of his class in 1896. Newland travelled to London in 1898 where he used his prowess as an oarsman in The London Hospital eight to impress Sir Frederick Treves who gave him an appointment as house surgeon at The London. This appointment required Newland obtaining a medical degree registrable in England so he took the conjoint exam passing MRCS LRCP. He subsequently had appointments at The London and The Hospital for Sick Children in Great Ormond Street before returning to Adelaide with his FRCS. He obtained the first MS (Adel) in 1902 and commenced private practice in Adelaide. Subsequently he held surgical appointments at The Adelaide Children's Hospital and at the Adelaide Hospital (initially as an honorary radiographer).

Newland joined the AIF on 14th November 1914 at the rank of major. He was 41 years old, 5ft 9ins tall and weighed 11 stone. He had married Ellen Mary Lindon in 1910; she was the daughter of his classics master at Saints. He was posted to 1 Australian Stationary Hospital and travelled to Egypt on the *Kyarra*. 1 ASH landed in Alexandria and were established in the Cairo suburb of Maadi in January 1915. Newland was deployed with Henry Arthur Powell and Joseph Stanley Verco to Ismailia for the first Turkish attack on the Suez Canal. Subsequently 1 ASH moved to Mudros on Lemnos to support the Gallipoli campaign where Newland saw service on Lemnos, on Hospital ships and at Gallipoli. Sir Frederick Treves visited 1 ASH on Lemnos in May. Newland was described by his CO, Lieutenant Colonel HW Bryant, as one of *'the best officers any commanding officer could wish to have under him'*. He transferred to 1 ACCS in January 1916 and promoted to lieutenant colonel to 3 AGH in November. He was posted to 1 AAH Harefield in January 1917 and served in France with 3 ACCS from March 1917. Later in 1917 he served at Queen Mary Hospital, Sidcup where he headed the Australian Facio-Maxillary Section. The Australians with their Commonwealth colleagues pioneered the art of plastic surgery in the management of the most horrific traumatic injuries at this hospital. He was Mentioned in Despatches and decorated with a DSO on 1st January 1918 and the CBE on 3rd June 1919.

Newland returned to Australia in 1919 and resumed surgical practice in Adelaide. His interests were principally plastic surgery with additional interests in neurosurgery and thoracic surgery. He was knighted in 1928. Newland was a founder and founding Fellow of the Royal Australasian College of Surgeons (RACS) and President of the College from 1929-1935. He was President of the South Australian branch of the BMA 1919 to 1921 and President of the Federal Council of the Australian branch of the BMA from 1932 to 1949 and a Vice President of the BMA from 1932 to 1965. He was the Acting Dean of the Adelaide University Medical School during WW2. He was awarded the gold medal of the BMA and subsequently that of the AMA. He was a founder of St Mark's College in Adelaide and chaired the council from 1927 to 1954. He was president of the Adelaide Club. Sir Henry Simpson Newland died on 13th November 1969 and was survived by his wife and two children.

Sources:
Photo: The ACH Cup Book.
http://recordsearch.naa.gov.au/scripts/Imagine.asp?B=7994923
Hicks N., Leopold E., 'Newland, Sir Henry Simpson (1873–1969)', Australian Dictionary of Biography, National Centre of Biography, Australian National University.

NOTT Harry Carew

MB BS FRCRA DMRE (Cantab)

1888 - 1973

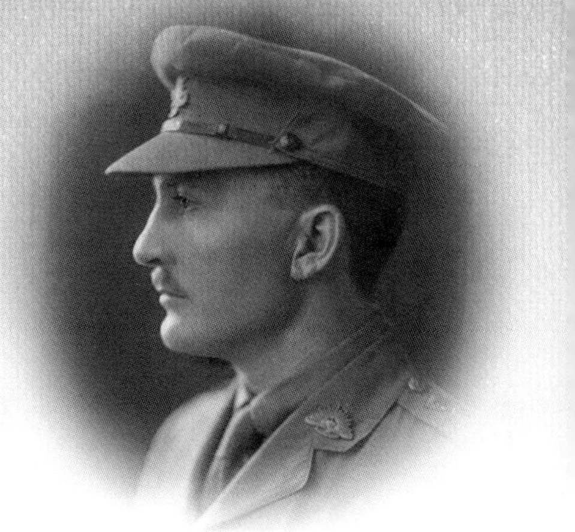

Harry Carew Nott was born on the 1st August 1888 at Walkerville SA, the only child of Albert Edward Nott, the manager of the South Australian Brewing Company, and Harriett Augusta, nee Taylor. He was educated at St Peter's College where he was a senior lieutenant in the cadets. He studied medicine at the University of Adelaide, excelling in cricket, tennis and lacrosse and graduating in 1913.

Nott enlisted in the AIF on 4th August 1914, the day that war was declared. He was described as 26 years of age, single, and 5ft 10ins tall and weighed 158lbs. He had normal vision and was commissioned as captain in August 1914, and posted as RMO of 10 Bn at Morphetville South Australia. His father was named as his next of kin and they lived at St. Georges, Lower Mitcham SA. Nott left for Egypt on the *Ascanius* on 2nd November 1914 which was the first troop ship to leave from Adelaide for the war. Nott later landed at Gallipoli on 25th April 1915. Nott lost touch with his Bn on the beach through stopping to dress the wounded. He recalled, *"All my knowledge of medical arrangements came out of the RAMC Training Manual. This looked easy enough on paper, but I soon found out in the landing that in practice it wasn't so simple'.* The Bn moved up to Victoria Gully in May then White Gully, close to Capt Goldsmith's 12 Bn RAP. Here they withstood the fierce Turkish attack of 19th May. This was followed on 24th May by an armistice to collect the dead and wounded. *'It was a gruesome sight, as the bodies were all blown up and swarming with maggots; and the stench was horrible. We moved the bodies by rolling them on stretchers with the aid of shovels'.* By June dysentery had taken hold of the Australians and Harry Nott was involved in the reserve sanitary squad. Sanitary conditions were very poor and dysentery was a major problem; about 45% were affected in varying degrees, and they were being admitted to hospital at the rate of 10 per day. Nott was re-infected, and transferred to 1 ASH Lemnos then Alexandria then back to Australia for three months. Whilst back in Australia he married Marjorie Lowe on the 22nd February 1916 before being sent to England. He was attached to 3 Trg Bn, and promoted major in November. He was posted to 2 FdAmb in January 1917, He remained with the FdAmb until July 1918, During the summer he was attached to 10 Bn and to 1 ACCS then to 2 FdAmb,. In July 1918 he was promoted temporary lieutenant colonel and posted to 1 AGH at Rouen. Nott was then posted SMO of the Australian Base at Le Havre. He remained there until June 1919. Nott applied for discharge in England to further his studies in radiology at Kings College Hospital in London. He returned to Australia in 1920 and appointment in the AIF was terminated on18th December 1920. He remained in the CMF until 1925. He was issued with the 1914-15 Star, the British War Medal and the Victory Medal.

He was an early full time radiologist in Adelaide and conducted a private practice from his home in Hutt St, (now the Naval, Military and Air Force Club) and in 1921 he was appointed as Honorary Radiologist at the Adelaide Hospital and later at the Repatriation Hospital. He was Radiologist with 2/2 AGH in WW2. In 1941 he was also appointed consultant radiologist to the AIF. Nott was discharged in January 1946. He was a more than competent golfer, won trophies at the Royal Adelaide Golf Club and on one occasion qualified and played in the British Open. He married twice and lived in Palm Beach, NSW with his second wife and, about 1969, returned to Adelaide. Harry Carew Nott died on the 3rd January 1973. He was survived by his second wife, two daughters from the first marriage and a son from the second.

Sources:

Likeman R., Gallipoli Doctors, Slouch Hat Publications 2010.
MJA April 4th 1973 p 773.
Letter to University of Adelaide undated 1916
http://recordsearch.naa.gov.au/NameSearch/Interface/ItemDetail.aspx?Barcode=7999716
Photo: SLSA GRG26_5_4_0_76

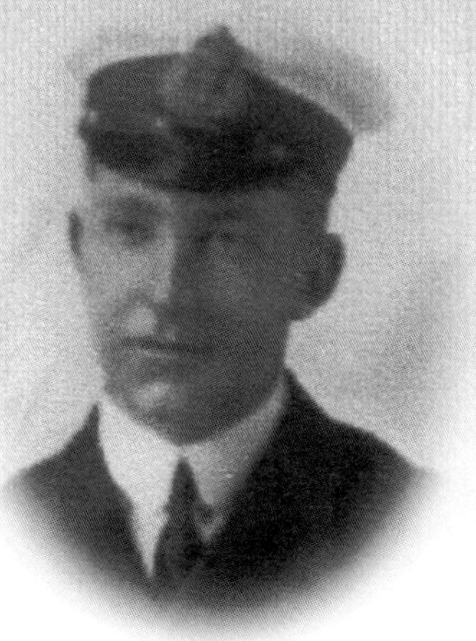

O'NEILL Sydney

MB BS FRCS

1895 - 1961

Sydney O'Neill was born in Richmond, Victoria on the 25th January 1895, son of Arthur O'Neill and Maud Evelyn nee Williams. He was educated at the Adelaide High School and qualified for a Government Bursary to study medicine at the University of Adelaide with his best friend John Besley Gillen. O'Neill graduated in July 1917 and lived at Palmerston Rd, North Unley.

O'Neill joined the naval cadets prior to WW1; the University of Adelaide archives record that he served in the RAN. The RAN service card is the only record of his service during WW1 as a temporary surgeon PNF (S) with his appointment from the 6th August 1917 until demobilisation on 1st December 1919.

O'Neill completed his FRCS in London after the war and returned to Australia where he established a practice in Sydney, NSW. He married Grace Mary Smith, daughter of Mrs Theresa Smith and the late Charles Smith of "Fairholme", Guildford, Western Australia on 7th February 1924. The couple left for Sydney on the overland express train on the evening of the wedding. However, by March 1925, he was living in Western Australia and had commenced a practice at 1290 Hay St, Perth. Whilst attending a function at Government House ballroom in Perth, on 26th August 1925, he unfortunately witnessed the shooting of a man close to him and was a witness in the subsequent court case. O'Neill moved back to NSW in the 1940s, and was embroiled in a legal case in 1943 when the house he owned at 13 Carr St, Coogee, was rented out and used as a convalescent and rest home for aged people. O'Neill required the home to be vacated for his wife and two children. He won the case and the house was vacated. He continued to practice in NSW. Sydney O'Neill died on 14th November 1961 in NSW and was survived by his wife and his son and his daughter.

Sources:

Personal Interview and Photo Bob Gillen.
The Register Adelaide 16th December 1911
The Register Adelaide 23rd November 1912
The Register Adelaide 10th July 1917
Sunday Times Perth 17th February 1924
Daily News Perth 21 March 1925
Daily News Perth 8th October 1925.
The West Australian 2nd March 1943
Ancestry .com

Proposed Mobile Operating Theatre

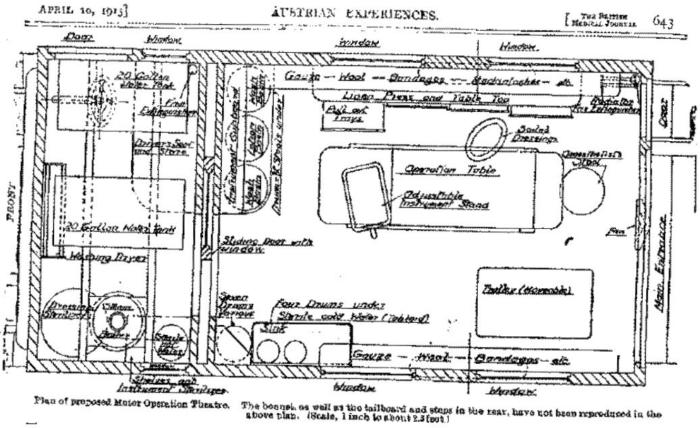

PARKHOUSE Devon

MB BS

1883 - 1973

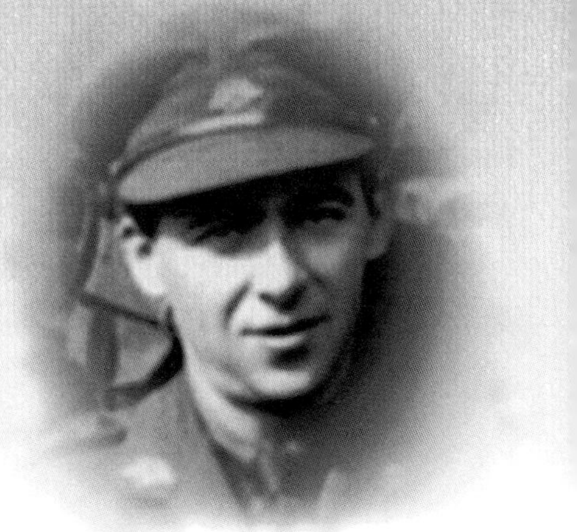

Devon Parkhouse was born at Henley Beach, South Australia, in 1883. He was son of Thomas Anstey Parkhouse and his wife Elizabeth Sarah Harper, nee Beck. He was educated at the Grange School and studied medicine at the University of Adelaide. He received the Dr Davies Thomas scholarship 1905 when he was in third year and graduated in 1907. He completed his residency at the Adelaide Hospital in 1908-09. He entered general practice in Woodville SA in 1912 with Christopher Bollen. He visited England and the USA in 1914; this included a visit to Belgium before the German invasion. He returned to Australia in December 1914.

Parkhouse volunteered for the AIF in March 1917 as a single 33 year old Medical Practitioner of Woodville. His father of Belmore Terrace, Woodville was nominated as his next of kin. He embarked from Melbourne on the *Ascanius* in May 1917, and landed at Devonport in July and was attached to the AAMC Trg Depot at Parkhouse for a month before being sent to France. He was first attached to 3 AGH at Abbeville and then in September posted to 4 FdAmb at the height of the Third Battle of Ypres. He was detached for short periods to 16 Bn and to 4 FdAmb Bn. He was transferred to 2 AGH at Wimereux in May 1918, and served there until March 1919 when he was briefly attached to 3 AGH once again. He returned to England in May 1919 and sailed for Australia the same month. His appointment was terminated on the 29th July 1919 and he was issued with the British War Medal and the Victory Medal.

He returned to his practice in Woodville, but withdrew from his partnership in 1920 due to ill health. He later settled at 12 Gloucester Street, Prospect South Australia. Devon Parkhouse died in 1973.

Sources:

Photo; Adelaide University Archives Group photo of Medical Students 1906

Advertiser Adelaide 16 December 1907.

http://encore.slsa.sa.gov.au/iii/encore/record/C__Rb2186689__SPhysicians%20--%20South%20Australia%20--%20Diaries__P0%2C1__Orightresult__X3?lang=eng&suite=cobalt

http://recordsearch.naa.gov.au/NameSearch/Interface/ItemDetail.aspx?Barcode=8007280

Grousing

The main duties of the regimental medical officer when his regiment is actually fighting are to see that the first dressing is properly applied so as to arrest haemorrhage and mitigate as far as possible the risk of infection, to put up fractured limbs so that the man may be carried away or walk away with minimum of suffering; to diagnose conditions such as wounds of the head which may seem trifling but which are really serious; and to treat men suffering from the shock of chest and abdominal wounds while dispatching them as quickly as possible with a note of the gravity of their condition to the nearest casualty station.

BMJ, 9 October 1915, p. 541

PELLEW Leonard James

CBE MB BS

1880 - 1957

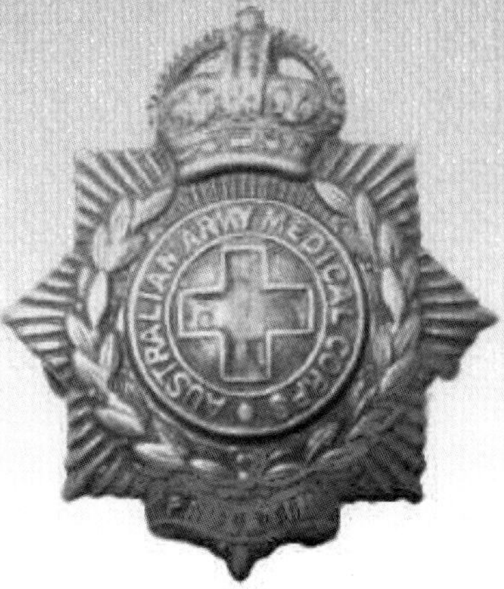

Leonard James Pellew was born on 21st April 1880 in North Adelaide, the son of James and Mary Jane Pellew, nee Beatty. He had one brother and two sisters. He was educated at Prince Alfred College and studied medicine at the University of Adelaide where he graduated in 1906. He clearly enjoyed his university life as it was widely reported throughout Australia in 1904 that he was fined five shillings for disturbing the peace in Adelaide with a fellow university student. Pellew entered general practice in Balaklava in 1913 and he moved to Port Augusta at the time the transcontinental railway was being built. His additional duties included practice at the government hospital where he was instrumental in having the hospital accredited as a training school for nurses. He devoted himself enthusiastically to his demanding job taking particular interest in general surgery; he was able to develop sound surgical techniques. He married Hirell Alice Ternouth daughter of Alfred H Ternouth on 17th December 1906 at Balaklava; they had two sons and a daughter.

Pellew applied for a commission in the RAMC at the outbreak of war hoping to move overseas without delay. He left for England with his wife and family in May 1915. He joined the RAMC and was posted to the 21st Casualty Clearing Station in France and achieved his desire to practice war surgery. His diagnostic acumen was of a high order and he became recognized as a capable surgeon. He was Mentioned in Despatches.

Pellew returned to Australia in 1917 and, at that time, still had responsibility for the Port Augusta practice. However he decided to dispose of it before attempting to enlist in the AAMC. The irritating delay in the sale of his practice prevented him joining the AAMC in time for overseas service. Pellew took over the practice of Dr Charles Todd, a prominent Adelaide surgeon with rooms fronting on to Victoria Square, Adelaide in 1918. His busy surgical practice and numerous duties with public bodies and charitable institutions left him little free time. He spent a year in postgraduate studies in the USA and UK in 1926 and made short visits to Japan and other countries in South East Asia. Pellew was the official surgeon to the South Australian Fire Brigade Board and President of the South Australian Football League. He made the study of history a special hobby and his general knowledge was extensive. This and his facility for expression made him greatly in demand as a lecturer by many organisations in South Australia. He sought re-enlistment to serve in WW2 in 1939 but then was deemed too old for service. Pellew was widely reported in the newspapers throughout Australia when he refused to pay a £1 parking fine and faced 6 days in gaol in 1948. He had many offers to serve his sentence by well-meaning friends. A friend paid the fine despite Pellew's wishes. It was while leaving the official box at the Adelaide Oval in June 1957 that he slipped and fractured his femur; he endured the long months of enforced rest with reasonable equanimity. Leonard James Pellew was just returning to work after this accident and died 3rd November 1957. He is buried with so many of his family in the Norton Summit Cemetery. He was survived by his wife and children; Jane Pellew BDS, LJT Pellew FRCS and RAA Pellew FRACP MRCP.

Sources:
MJA 1958 45(4) 127-8
The Daily News Perth 31 March 1904
Sunday Times Perth 12 September 1948
The New Adelaide 11th September 1948
Ancestry.com

The Need for Motor Ambulances

Sir Frederick Treves

From the point of view of the wounded, the motor ambulance is a very urgent need... Rapid transport is everything.

BMJ, 10 October 1914, p. 641-642

PENNY Harold John

MB BS

1888 - 1968

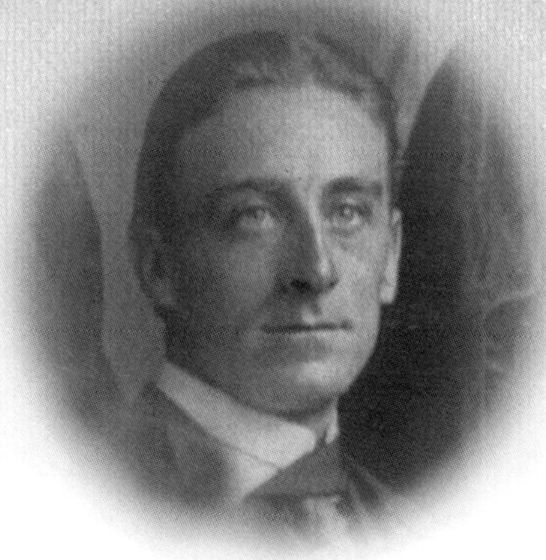

Harold John Penny, always known as 'Hockett', was the youngest son of Charles James and Emma Stephens Penny of Semaphore in SA, and was educated at St Peter's College and the University of Adelaide where he graduated MB BS in 1913. He was a talented sportsman and played interstate tennis and cricket. He rowed (No 4) in the Adelaide eight: Adelaide University came third in the 1911 and 1912 intervarsity eights boat races. He was a resident medical officer at the Adelaide Hospital in 1915 and Adelaide Children's Hospital in 1915. He treated at least three gunshot injuries during this time: one where the master of the four masted barque *Hougemont* shot at an inebriated sailor, one of self inflicted gunshot wounds resulting in death and a woman with three gunshot injuries.

Penny travelled, on the *Mongolia*, to the UK in March 1915 to join the RAMC as one of 'Kitchener's 100'. He was given the rank of temporary lieutenant on 26th March 1915 and registered on 3rd May 1915. He married Winifred Annie Lake of Bristol shortly after arriving in England. His mother described her son as having met with an accident after undergoing his training which prevented him from being fit for active service for a long time. He was appointed surgeon at the De Walden Court Hospital, Eastbourne, where he remained until early 1916. Promoted to captain in April 1916 and now fit for active service he went to France on 6 November 1916.

Penny returned to Australia and is recorded as being in practice in Hackney, South Australia. He returned to England with his wife whom he subsequently divorced (1925) for her adultery with a dentist. Later that year he married a vicar's daughter, Mary Violet Risdale, from Harrow-on-the-Hill; it is believed that they travelled to South Australia and Harold joined a practice in Nailsworth. They indicated their intention to move to Western Australia in 1928; whatever became of these plans they had returned to England in 1938, initially to Stoke-on Trent and finally to Tunstall in Staffordshire. Penny was a world class croquet player, amongst the best in Britain, winning at least two gold medals in the sport. He seemed to be the bete noir of a number of members of the Mills family against whom he played many tournaments. During his 1948 visit to Adelaide, his first for 18 years, it was noted that he had three sons, one on the land and two still at school, and a daughter studying medicine. Harold John Penny died in Bournemouth in 1968.

Sources:

Emma Penny, 7th December 1916, Letter to the Registrar, University of Adelaide, University of Adelaide Archives
The Advertiser, Friday 16January 1948
The Mail, Saturday 17January 1948
"Who is George Mills?" Posted by Sam (also known as Harry) 5th JULY 2011
Photo: Adelaide University Archives; Medical Graduates 1913.
Medical Directory 1919

The End of the War

The capitulation of Bulgaria, Turkey, Austria-Hungary and of Germany to the allied Powers after four and a quarter years of the most destructive war the world has ever seen, marks an epoch for every class of the population and for every interest of mankind. This medical profession has perhaps more reason for rejoicing than any other section of the community...The Pride of belonging to an Empire that always wins its way through to victory...is tempered by the knowledge that British medicine has triumphed on account of its human character, its high ideals and its scientific practicability...Today we dare to forget everything else than the fact of victory, and the fact that no further sacrifices are needed to safeguard the whole world.

MJA, 23 November 1918, p. 411

PHILLIPS William James Ellery

MC MB BS

1891 - 1952

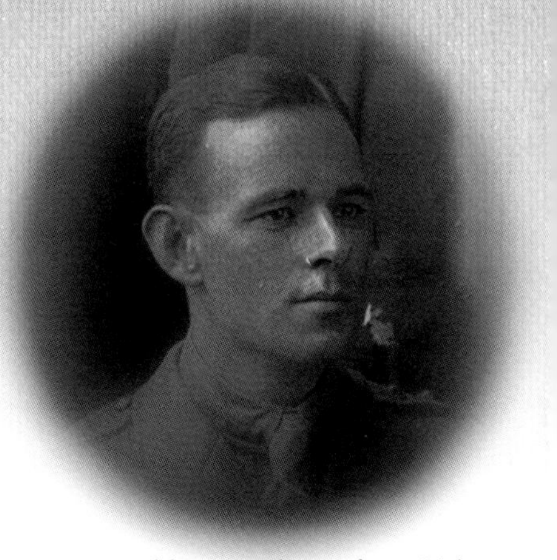

William James Ellery Phillips was born in Adelaide on 18th September 1891, the second of nine children. His father was James Henry Phillips, a compositor, and mother was Esther Jane, nee Ellery of 107 Mitchell Street, Hyde Park. He was educated privately and at Goodwood School where he was awarded a bursary in 1904 for Prince Alfred College. He was awarded a university scholarship in 1911 and studied medicine at the University of Adelaide. He was named the St Alban's scholar for 1913 and graduated MB BS in 1915. Prior to WW1 he had served in the school cadets.

Phillips enlisted on 30th November 1914 at Oakland's Camp, South Australia. He was a single, fifth year medical student. On the order of the PMO he was discharged on 26th February 1915 to complete his medical degree. He re-joined on 23rd September 1915 having completed his degree and 3 weeks of practice at the Adelaide Hospital. He was 5ft 8½ins, weighed 133lbs, of dark complexion with grey eyes and light brown hair. His father was named as his next of kin. Phillips was allotted to the 3rd Reinforcements for 1 ASH. He embarked from Sydney on the *Kanowna* on 22nd December 1915. He was appointed RMO to the 13 Bn and on 20th August 1916 he was transferred to the 4 FdAmb and later still to the 2 AGH. He was sick on two occasions; the first saw him admitted to 3rd London General Hospital and he was admitted again to 20th General Hospital on 15th February with bronchitis. He was transferred to the 1 FdAmb on 17th May 1917. He was severely gassed and admitted to the 5th British Red Cross Hospital on 8th March 1918 and transferred to 3rd London General Hospital on 13th March 1918. He was promoted major on 10th September 1918. He was awarded the Military Cross *"for conspicuous gallantry and devotion to duty on 6th-7th September 1918. During an advance on Roisel. He worked continuously for 48 hours in charge of the evacuation of the wounded from the forward aid posts. Although the area was heavily shelled, he got his ambulance cars right up and cleared the wounded with great rapidity. His energy and perseverance set a splendid example to those working with him."* He was granted leave with pay from 24th June 1919 to 24th December 1919 and leave without pay from 25th December 1919 to 30th June 1920. He returned to Australia with his wife accompanying him on the *Narkunda* disembarking in 4 MD on 19th August 1920. His appointment was terminated in 4MD on 19th October 1920. He was issued the British War Medal and Victory Medal.

Phillips moved to England and was a ship's doctor after the war; he was a senior medical officer in Palestine from 1937 to 1945 and had served in the British and American sectors of UNRRA. He had retired by the time he was 45 years of age and in a report of him pleading guilty for stealing chairs from a sports club he said he had not been well. At the time of the court case he was resident in Blackheath, England. William James Ellery Phillips died on the 25th December 1952, when he was living at Chateau de la Freyere La Bocca, Cannes, Alpes Maritimes in France.

Sources:
National Archives of Australia
http://recordsearch.naa.gov.au/NameSearch/Interface/ItemDetail.aspx?Barcode=1991514
South Australian Bibliographical Index 1836-1885
Morning Bulletin Rockhampton Queensland 6th September 1946
Chronicle 14th August 1920
Photo: Adelaide University Archives Medical Graduates 1915
Prince Alfred College archives.

The Germans
Medical Profession in War Times

Germany is suffering from a severe dearth of medical men many thousands of whom have joined the colours

BMJ, 24 October 1914, p. 726

PITCHER Cyril Frederick

MB BS

1887 - 1955

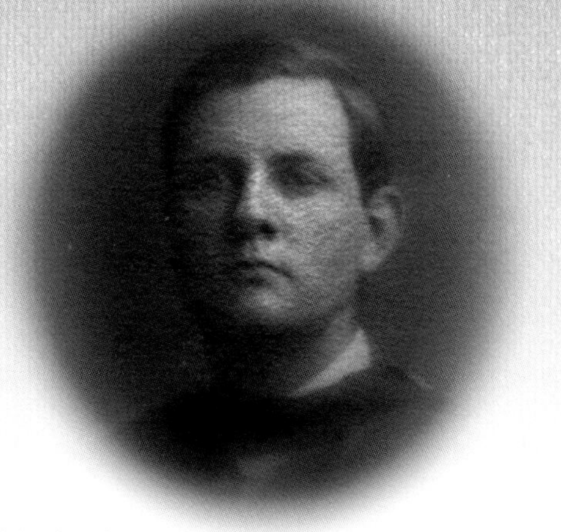

Cyril Frederick Pitcher was born at Medindie, South Australia on the 14th June 1887, the third son of Rev John Garlick Pitcher J.P. and Mary, nee Butler. She was the sister of a Premier of South Australia Sir Richard Butler and the aunt of Sir Richard Layton Butler who also became Premier of South Australia. Pitcher was educated at St Peter's College and graduated in Medicine from the University of Adelaide in 1911. He served in the militia as a captain in the Light Horse Field Ambulance in 1912 and the Reserve in 1913. At the time of his enlistment in the AIF he was a medical practitioner at Victor Harbor.

He applied for a commission in the AIF on the 19th October 1914, a 27 year old single graduate living at 23 Erskine St, Goodwood Park. He stood 6ft 1ins tall, and weighed 14st. His brother Ronald Owen Pitcher was his next of kin, later Mrs. Isabel Warren Elizabeth Pitcher, his wife, c/- W Gilchrist Esq, "Marindalk", Mulders Vlei, Cape Colony, South Africa. He embarked from Brisbane with 2 LHFdAmb in December 1914. He did not go to Gallipoli with 2 LHFdAmb when it first landed in May, but remained at Mudros. He went with the second landing on the 3rd Aug 1915, but was immediately detached to 3 Bn for three weeks and then to 5 LHR for 10 days. Pitcher was evacuated to Egypt in September 1915 with sciatica, a condition with which he had suffered prior to enlistment. This was followed by jaundice. He was declared unfit for general duties for six months, and served with 1 ASH from March to August 1916. He was promoted major on 14th November 1916 and posted to 2 ACCS at Trois Arbres, France. Soon after the Battle of Messines, Pitcher developed renal disease, and was sent back to England. He rejoined his unit in August, but soon became ill again and was sent back to Australia in September 1917. He returned to England on the *Borda* in January 1918, but disembarked in Cape Town to spend 2 months with his older brother Richard Charles Pitcher who had enlisted in the South African medical corps as a private soldier. His brother had been in the 4 FdAmb with a short active service from February 1916 until he was diagnosed with carcinoma of the tongue from which he died on the 18th May 1919. Pitcher reached London in April and, in October 1918, was posted to 3 AAH. He returned to France and joined 7 FdAmb. All five Australian divisions were then in the Fourth Army rest area around Abbeville, and in the first week of November moved up towards the front line again. They were spared further combat by the Armistice. Pitcher returned to London in January 1919, and sailed for Australia in February with his AIF appointment terminated on the 16th June 1919. Pitcher was issued with the 1914-15 Star, The British War Medal, and the Victory Medal.

Pitcher set up practice at Hindmarsh, South Australia on his return. He was appointed as Hon Medical Officer to the Mareeba Babies' Hospital, with Drs Helen Mayo and Frederick Neill Le Messurier in 1923 and they made a lifelong association. They contributed to important advances in the care of sick and particularly premature babies. He subsequently became Chairman of the Board of the Babies Hospital. He lived at Dutton Terrace, Medindie, South Australia. Cyril Frederick Pitcher died in 12th May 1955 in Adelaide.

Sources:
http://recordsearch.naa.gov.au/scripts/Imagine.asp?B=8017770
Likeman R., "Gallipoli Doctors", Slouch Hat Publications 2010
Letter to the University of Adelaide 1916Photo: Adelaide University Archives Graduate 1911
Adelaide Advertiser 5th January 1903
Adelaide Advertiser 14th December 1911
The Register Adelaide 15 March 1923

POMROY Harry Roy

MB BS FRCS

1895 - 1943

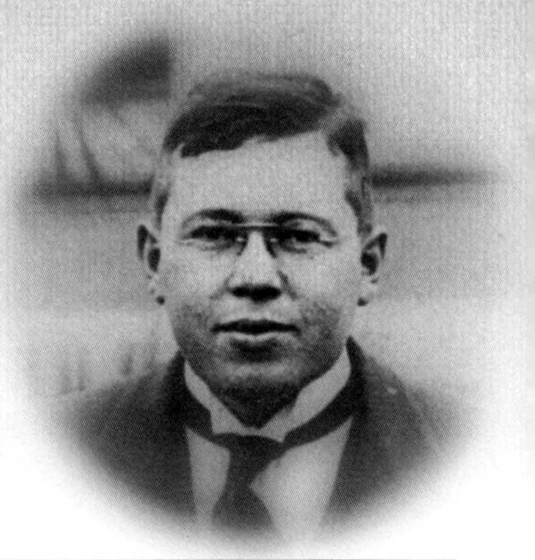

Harry Roy Pomroy was born in Moonta on 3rd March 1895. He was the son of Mr H Pomroy of Wallaroo Mines, South Australia. He was educated at Wallaroo Mines District High School and gained a scholarship to Adelaide High School in 1910. He was seventh in the Higher Public Examination in 1912 thereby gaining a bursary for the university which included a £40 per annum maintenance allowance. He studied medicine at the University of Adelaide graduating MB BS in 1918.

Pomroy enlisted in the AIF on 26th November 1918 in Adelaide and proceeded to 5MD. He had influenza in the Western Australia quarantine station in December 1918. He returned to 4MD on the *Marathon* on 24th December 1919. His appointment in the AIF was terminated on 17th January 1920.

His post-war address was given as Cowell, South Australia. He later spent three years in England to gain his FRCS which he achieved in 1925. He was appointed assistant honorary surgeon and, after the retirement of Henry Simpson Newland, honorary surgeon at the Adelaide Hospital. He enlisted again in WW2 at Wayville, South Australia rising to the rank of lieutenant colonel. Harry Roy Pomroy died in 105 Military Hospital Adelaide on 10th March 1943 aged 48 years. He was survived by his wife Elisabeth and son Andrew.

Sources:
National Archives of Australia
http://recordsearch.naa.gov.au/NameSearch/Interface/ItemDetail.aspx?Barcode=8017949
Kadina and Wallaroo Times 24th December 1912
The Register 11th August 1928
The Advertiser 11th March 1943
Photo: Adelaide University Archives; Medical Graduates 1918.

Call for Civilian Medical Practitioners

The war Office notifies as follows:

Civilian medical practitioners desiring to serve at home or abroad as surgeons with the army should communicate with the Secretary, War Office London SW.

Gentlemen accepted for such service will be granted the temporary rank of lieutenant in the army and must fulfil the following conditions:

1. They must be registered practitioners
2. They must engage for a period of twelve calendar months or until their services are no long required, whichever shall first happen.
3. Their pay to be 24s a day, inclusive of all money allowances except travelling allowances and expenses when travelling on duty.
4. They will be granted free passages to and from any country abroad to which they may be sent.
5. They must devote their whole time to military service.
6. They will receive a gratuity of £60 at the termination of their engagement if they have rendered satisfactory service.
7. They should not exceed 35 years of age, but in exceptional circumstances gentlemen between 35 and 40 may be accepted.
8. They must furnish:
   (a) A medical certificate showing that they are in good health, of sound constitution, and fit for hard physical work.
   (b) A statement of any previous service with the army.
   (c) A recommendation as to character from a person of position and responsibility.
   (d) A certificate as to age.

BMJ, 8 August 1914, p. 318

POWELL Henry Arthur

CMG VD MB BS FRACS

1868 - 1944

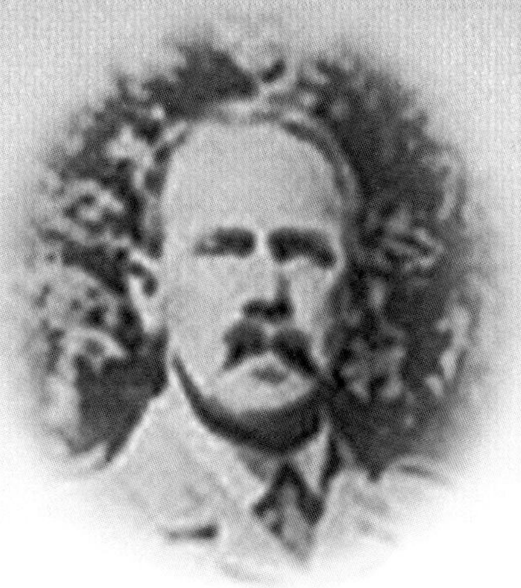

Henry Arthur Powell was born on the 31st January 1868 in Kadina, SA, the son of Charles Bendin Powell and his wife Mary Ann nee Ward. He was educated at Glenelg Grammar School and the University of Adelaide where he graduated MB BS in 1891. He first practised in Angaston and subsequently established a surgical practice in Kadina for 18 years where he was Mayor in 1902 to 1904. He was commissioned as a lieutenant in 1900, promoted captain in 1905 and he was advanced to the rank of major in 1913 and posted as RMO of 23rd (Barossa) LH. He married Katie Frances Smith of Yalumba in the Barossa Valley.

Powell joined the AIF in October 1914 as second in command of 1 ASH. Aged 46 years he was 5ft11ins tall and weighed 12st 12lbs. He travelled to Egypt on the *Kyarra* and, shortly after arrival in Cairo on 27th January 1915, took half the unit which included Henry Newland and Stanley Verco to Ismailia in support of the Australian Light Horse defending the Suez Canal. Captain Charles Bean, writing for the The Press describes; *The personnel of the 1st [Australian] Stationary Hospital also took a route march through the desert on the other side of the canal which was suspiciously like a picnic.* Their first patient was a Dutch woman who gave birth in the hospital. The officers observed the Turkish attack on the canal on 3rd February 1915 before returning to the Cairo suburb of Maadi. He served on Lemnos where 1ASH was the first medical unit on the island, at sea during the early part of the Gallipoli campaign, before the threat of enemy submarines sent the unit back to Lemnos and, when Lieutenant Colonel Bryant was evacuated, was promoted to command the unit in December 1915 and established the unit at North Beach, Anzac. Bryant described Powell as "a most capable and efficient officer, and his executive ability was of great value". He was Mentioned in Despatches by General Sir Ian Hamilton for his work at Gallipoli. He was promoted lieutenant colonel in January 1916, and took the unit to Ismailia until September, and then to Dartford in England, where it became 3 AAH. In October 1916 Colonel Neville Howse VC wrote of him, *"He is one of the best officers in the AAMC, and his work at Lemnos, Anzac, and Ismailia was of the highest order".* He was appointed CMG in May 1916 for good and hard work with the Australian Hospitals established in England. Powell worked at 3 AAH until June 1917 when he was posted to 2 AGH at Wimereux as CO. He was made temporary colonel in July, and in August he was brought to notice. He commanded the hospital for 16 months, and was given substantive rank in May 1918. He relinquished command in November, a few days after the Armistice and was returned to Australia. His AIF appointment terminated on the 8th March 1919. Powell transferred to the Reserve at the end of the war, and retired from the Army in 1926. He was issued 1914-15 Star, the British War Medal and the Victory Medal with Oak Leaves. He received the VD in 1920.

Powell resumed his practice at Norwood; with his appointments to the Adelaide Hospital, where he was honorary assistant gynaecologist; on the consulting staff at the Queen's Home, and with rooms at Brougham Place, North Adelaide. He succeeded Dr Alfred Austin Lendon as president of the District Trained Nursing Society in 1929. His family interests included Arbor Day and the success of the Kiosk at the Adelaide Hospital. The Director General Medical Services, Lewis Wibmer Jefferies described his valuable and important work as Controller of Medical Equipment in the Medical Coordination Committee in the early part of WW2. Henry Arthur Powell died on 7th June 1944 at home, at Le Fevre Terrace, North Adelaide.

Sources:

The Advertiser, Adelaide, 8th June 1944

Bryant HW LTCOL (1916) "Some notes taken whilst on Active Service with the No1 Australian Stationary Hospital" Medical Journal of Australia, 13 257-265

Bean Charles (1915) "Close to Battle" The Press 25March 1915 Volume L 1 issue 15236 p8

POWELL Harold

MC MB BS

1886 - 1963

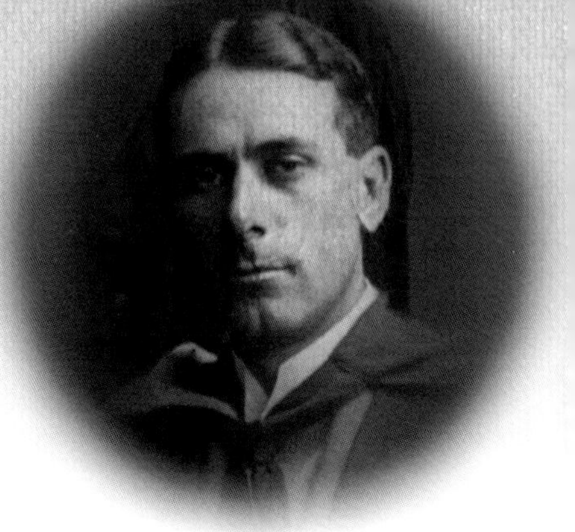

Harold Powell was born on 29th September 1886 at Wilpena near Hawker South Australia, son of Charles Bendin Powell and his wife Mary Ann nee Ward, and grandson of Charles Powell who had landed at Kangaroo Island South Australia in 1836. He was educated at St Peter's College and studied medicine at the University of Adelaide and graduated in 1913. He married Mary Elizabeth Milne on 8th October 1914.

Powell enlisted in Adelaide on the 8th November 1915 when he was 29 years, 5ft 10ins tall, weighing 10st 11lbs, of dark complexion with grey eyes and dark brown hair. He nominated his wife of 57 Cheltenham St, Malvern South Australia as next of kin. He was commissioned in December 1915 and posted to 4 FdAmb and sailed for Egypt on the *Kanowna* in December 1915. He joined the unit in Egypt in February 1916, and went with it to France in June. The 4 Div did not take part in the Battle of Fromelles, but moved to the Somme in August 1916 to relieve 1 Div. where their objective was to capture Mouquet Farm; after six successive night attacks they failed to take the Farm. Their losses were 4649 men, and the FdAmb was swamped with casualties. Powell was transferred to 50 Bn as RMO in December 1916. He remained with the Bn until October 1917 and was awarded the Military Cross in August 1917. The citation refers to *'his complete disregard for his personal safety working under heavy fire and the most adverse conditions'*, but it does not identify a particular action in which he showed his *'conspicuous gallantry and devotion to duty'*. He suffered concussion from a shell burst in September 1917, and was evacuated to England. After recovering he was posted to 3 AGH at Abbeville with the temporary rank of major. He was admitted to hospital with pleurisy in January 1918, and again evacuated to England, where he was admitted to 3 LGH. He returned to Australia in March 1918 with his appointment terminated on the 26th October 1918. Harold Powell was issued with the British War Medal and the Victory Medal.

Powell settled in Largs Bay, and in 1920 was commissioned as a surgeon lieutenant in the RAN Brigade (SA). He was appointed MO to St Margaret's Convalescent Hospital in, Semaphore in 1933. Harold Powell died on 9th July 1963. Both of Harold Powell's brothers and one of his sisters served in WW1. Henry Arthur Powell served at Gallipoli, and in France as CO of 2 AGH. Charles Baxter Powell served as a trooper in 9 LHR and was killed in action at Bir el Abd in August 1916. He is buried in the Kantara War Memorial Cemetery. Edith Mabel Powell served as a Nursing Sister on the *Karoola* and at Auxiliary Hospitals in London. She returned to Australia in March 1919.

Sources:

http://recordsearch.naa.gov.au/scripts/Imagine.asp?B=8019785
Photo; Adelaide University Archives 1913 Graduates
Likeman R., 'No time for Regrets: Doctors of the Western Front', in Press, Rosenberg Press, 2013.
The Register 22 Dec 1903
The Register Adelaide 12 June 1918
The Chronicle Adelaide 13 September 1934
Barrier Miner Broken Hill 18 May 1920
Ancestry.com

PREST Henry Gordon

KCStJ MB BS

1899 - 1989

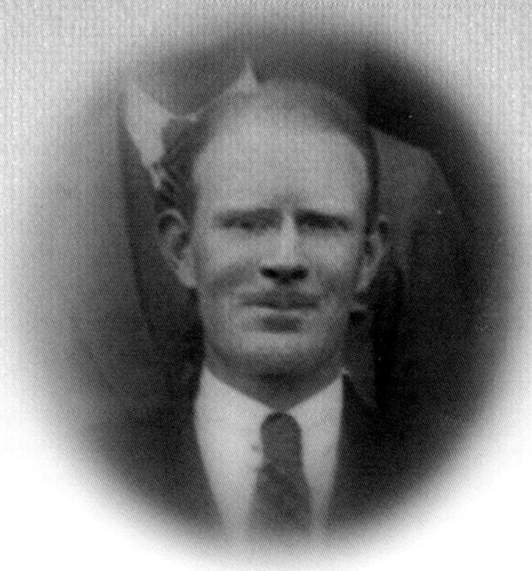

Henry Gordon Prest was born in Port Pirie, South Australia on 10th January 1899 to Henry Prest and Eleanor, nee Clark. His father was a highly regarded businessman in Port Pirie until his death in 1903. Prest was educated at Kyre College and Prince Alfred College. He was captain of the school at Princes. He studied medicine at the University of Adelaide graduating in 1925. He captained the University A Grade cricket, football and lacrosse teams and was awarded University Blues for cricket and football.

Prest enlisted in the AIF on 7th May 1918 in Adelaide, South Australia. He was single and a medical student and had 4 years previous cadet experience. His mother, Eleanor, at the time of his enlistment was living at 9 George Street, Unley Park, South Australia and was given as his next of kin. He was recorded as 5ft 6ins tall, and weighed 139lbs, of fair complexion with blue eyes and fair hair. He embarked on the *Marathon* in Melbourne on 23rd July 1918. Prest disembarked in London on 24th September 1918 and posted to 10 Bn but subsequently transferred to the artillery as a gunner on 8th December 1918. He was transferred to France on 14th December 1918. He left France for England on 30th January 1919 and embarked on the *Anchises* for Australia on 28th February 1919. Prest arrived in Port Adelaide on 13th April 1919. He was discharged on 27th April 1919. He was issued with the British War Medal. He later applied for the Victory Medal but as he had not been in a war zone was deemed ineligible.

He married Ethel Irene Hunwick on 9th September 1926 in Kent Town Methodist Church. Ethel was born on 18th March 1904 in Semaphore, South Australia. Her father was Henry Charles Moore Hunwick and her mother Fanny Louise, nee Crawley. Prest was registered to practice in South Australia in 1926. After registration, Prest, with his wife, went to England where he worked at The London Hospital. During this time Ethel gave birth to a daughter. They returned to South Australia in 1928 and he had a practice in Jamestown. He then moved to a medical practice in Wakefield Street, Adelaide, where he remained for 20 years. This practice, which included his residence, was later demolished to build the Wakefield Street Private Hospital, which still exists today. Prest and his family moved across the road from the hospital. Finally they moved to Unley Road, Malvern, where his continued his practice. He was restored in rank as an honorary captain from November 1939 in WW2. Prest was an honorary anaesthetist at the Adelaide hospital for 25 years and co-founder and foundation member of the Australian Society of Anaesthetists. He was an active member of St John's Ambulance as a medical officer for 21 years, and continued his association with the organisation for 33 years. Later in his life he worked with the School Health Service screening primary school children both in city and country areas. He was involved in medical politics holding executive positions with the BMA and the SA Medical Defence Association. Prest also had a long association with the Order of St John of Jerusalem. He became vice-president on the Council of the Order, representing them on several boards, including the SA Red Cross Society, Royal Doctor Flying Service and the Asthma Association. For his devotion to the Order he was invested as a Commander of the Order of St John of Jerusalem in 1965. Henry Gordon Prest died on 17th October 1989; he was living in Rutland Avenue, Unley Park, South Australia. He was 90 years old. His daughter and grandson both graduated in medicine from the University of Adelaide. His daughter, Elisabeth, served as a medical officer in 9RAANC in 1954 and 1955.

Sources:
National Archives of Australia
http://recordsearch.naa.gov.au/NameSearch/Interface/ItemDetail.aspx?Barcode=8018665
South Australian Indexes of Births Deaths and Marriages
The Register Adelaide 2nd December 1924
The Register Adelaide 18th January 1926
The News Adelaide 6th November 1939
http://www.findagrave.com/cgi-bin/fg.cgi?page=gr&GRid=102087944
Photo: Adelaide University Archives Medical Graduates 1925
Elizabeth Puddy, Family records

PROCTOR John Smith

LRCPI LRCSI LMI

1869 - 1941

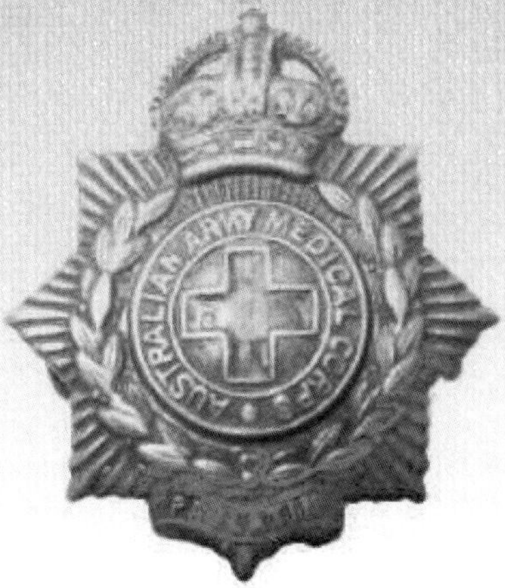

John Smith Proctor was born in Ballina, County Mayo, Ireland on 23rd September 1869. He immigrated to South Australia and was married to Marion Louise Crampton on 5th February 1898 at St Matthews Church, Kensington, South Australia. They were living at St Anne's, Norwood, South Australia. He graduated LRCP, LRCS, LM (Ireland) in 1891. He was appointed a Public Vaccinator on 21st May 1896. He also was practising in Mount Pleasant, South Australia. He was appointed to attend the destitute poor and Aborigines in the Tungkillo district of South Australia in 1911. Later he gave his postal address as the Adelaide Club, Adelaide and his wife's postal address as the Queen Adelaide Club.

Prior to enlistment in the AIF he was an honorary captain in the AAMC Reserve. He enlisted in the AIF on 22nd March 1918 at Keswick Barracks. He was 48 years and 6 months old, 5ft 10ins tall, weighed 192lbs, of dark complexion with brown eyes and black hair. His wife was named as his next of kin. He entrained for the 2 MD on 15th July 1918 for embarkation on *Borda* on 17th July 1918. He disembarked in London on the 27th September 1918 and was admitted on arrival to Fort Pitt Military Hospital, Chatham with an abscess on his right buttock. He was discharged fit for duty on the 23rd of October 1918. He was attached to the 3 AAH at Dartford on 27th November. He proceeded to France via Folkstone on 24th January 1919 and was posted to 2 AGH. He was then attached to 3 AGH from March until the following May. After leave in Paris from 11th May to 3rd of June 1919 he re-joined his unit before returning to London. There he had leave for medical education purposes from the 7th August to the 31st October 1919 while staying at the Royal Automobile Club in Pall Mall. He embarked for Australia on 20th December 1919 on the *Runic* as the ship's senior medical officer. He became unwell with rheumatic pain and jaundice on 8th January 1920. The *Runic* arrived in Australia on 3rd February 1920. He was apparently accompanied by his wife. His appointment in the AIF was terminated on the 3rd April 1920. He was issued with the British War Medal and the Victory Medal.

After the war he had a practice on North Terrace, Adelaide, remaining there for many years. Proctor and his wife were known for entertaining guests on the Floating Palais and also at their home in Wakefield Street, Adelaide. His wife died on 8th February 1934. He was fined four pounds with ten shillings costs for speeding with a pillion passenger on a motorbike in 1939. John Smith Proctor died at Glenelg Private Hospital, South Australia on 19th February 1941. He was survived by his son Basil St John Guy Proctor who served in WW2 and who died on 2nd June 1958.

Sources:

National Archives Australia
http://recordsearch.naa.gov.au/NameSearch/Interface/ItemDetail.aspx?Barcode=8021792
The Adelaide Advertiser 22 May 1896
The Adelaide Advertiser 8th December 1925
The Adelaide Advertiser 9th February 1934
The Adelaide Advertiser 19th December 1939
The Adelaide Advertiser 20th February 1941
Indexes Birth, Deaths and Marriages

Uniforms and Outfits

As things are he can within limits, decide for himself what sort of outfit he will take abroad. If he is a wise man he will decide to bring out as little as possible, and certainly to regard as superfluous many other the things likely to be pressed upon his notice by outfitters at home. Among positive superfluities may be written down revolvers, swords, and whistles, and many changes of garment.

BMJ, 2 January 1915, p. 31

PRYOR William Arthur

MB BS

1895 - 1981

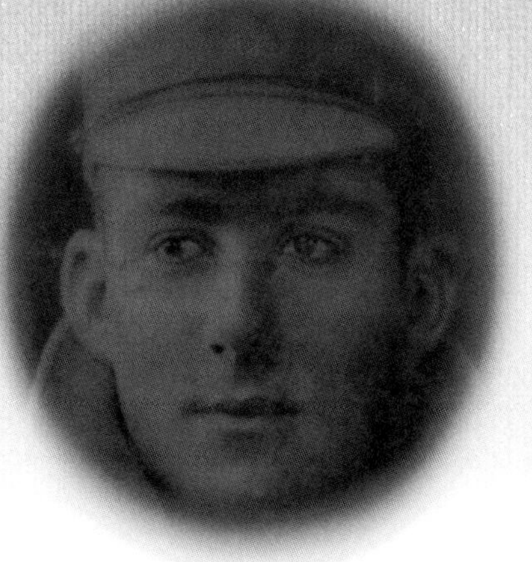

William Arthur Pryor (affectionately known as Woppy) was born on 16th October 1895 to William George Pryor and Mary Mowbray nee Richardson in Mundulla, near Port Augusta, South Australia. He was educated privately, at Adelaide High School and St Peter's College. He studied medicine at the University of Adelaide and graduated in 1919. During his school years he served in the Cadets and Senior Cadets.

Pryor joined the AIF on 25th August 1915 whilst he was still a medical student and required his mother's approval to enlist. He was 19 years old, 5ft 9ins tall and weighed 153lbs of fair complexion with hazel eyes and dark brown hair. He had a vaccination scar on his left upper arm. He was initially posted in the reinforcements for 3 FdAmb as a private soldier. He remained at the Mitcham camp until his embarkation on the *Borda* in the Outer Harbour on 11th January 1916. He was transferred on the 9th March 1916 to the 7 FdAmb in Egypt and was transferred to France departing on 12th March 1916 arriving in Marseilles on 19th March. He was detached from that unit on 21st Jun 1916 and was attached to administrative HQ in London whilst waiting for his return to Australia to resume his medical studies. He embarked on the *Karmala* for Australia on 21st July 1916. He was discharged in 4 MD on the 18th September 1916. He was issued with the British War Medal and Victory Medal.

Pryor resumed his medical studies at the University of Adelaide and graduated in 1919. He married Phyllis Angela Field on 22nd September 1921; they divorced in 1936 when they were living in Brighton, South Australia. They had three children William John Pryor, Colin Huston Pryor and Nancy Mowbray Pryor. He moved to Ballarat, Victoria after his divorce where he remarried and became a much respected anaesthetist. He served as a reservist during WW2. He had a farm at Millbrook south east of Ballarat and retired at the age of 75 years. William Arthur Pryor died in Ballarat Victoria in 1981.

Sources:
National Archives of Australia
http://recordsearch.naa.gov.au/NameSearch/Interface/ItemDetail.aspx?Barcode=8023487
The Adelaide Advertiser 14th February 1895
The Adelaide Advertiser 28th November 1919
The Adelaide Advertiser 17th April 1936
Indexes of Birth, Deaths and Marriages
Colleague's personal recollections.
Ancestry.com

Remarks on the Mechanical treatment of compound and suppurating fractures occurring at the seat of war.

I have been asked to offer some suggestions as to a suitable way of treating certain fractures of the upper and lower limbs as they occur at the seat of war. We realize that wounds as met with during the Boer and Russo-Japanese campaigns were very different in character from those occurring on the richly manured fields in Flanders where suppuration so commonly follows. The point therefore, is to decide upon the best way of immobilizing compound fractures in the presence of pus. The method employed must be both efficient and simple; it must allow easy and painless access to the wound, and protect the limb from harm during transport. From experiences gained by a short visit to the front, and from conversations with many surgeons at home and abroad, I feel strongly that surgeons should abandon all operative methods designed to immobilize the fractured ends. They are fraught with danger, and have no place in this campaign.

BMJ, 16 January 1916, p. 101

RAMSAY SMITH William

FRS(Ed) DSc MD

1859 - 1937

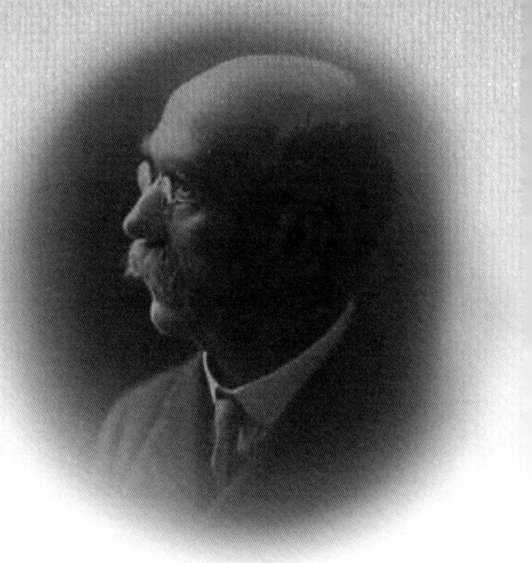

William Ramsay Smith was born in King Edward, Aberdeenshire, Scotland on 27th November 1859 the son of William Smith, a farm servant and later stationmaster, and Mary, nee MacDonald. Educated at Cairnbanno Madras Public School he became a pupil teacher and studied Arts at Edinburgh University. At the age of 20 years he was appointed a school headmaster at Invergordon Public School. He graduated with a BSc in 1888 he was appointed assistant professor of natural history. He graduated MB ChM in 1892 and MD in 1913. For two years he was an examiner for the Royal College of Physicians. He married Margaret MacKenzie, headmistress and linguist, daughter of James MacKenzie, on 1st June 1889 in Scotland. He was brought to Australia by the South Australian Government in 1896 to work at the Adelaide Hospital after the resignation of the consultant staff; as a consequence the SA Branch of the BMA expelled him for life in 1897. He was the subject of a government inquiry into his competence and exonerated by a Government Tribunal in 1899. He was appointed as city Coroner and permanent Head of Public Health. He was dismissed from coronial duties in 1903 because of misuse of human remains. He later was reinstated and continued to collect human remains. He resigned from the Adelaide Hospital because of "conflict of interest". He completed his DSc at the University of Adelaide in 1904.

Ramsey Smith had previous military service in the Boer War as surgeon captain. He was awarded the Queen's Medal with two clasps. Prior to enlisting in the AIF Ramsay Smith was a major in the AAMC Reserve. He was promoted to the rank of lieutenant colonel on enlistment and appointed CO of 1 AGH on 2nd October 1914. He was described as 5ft 9ins and weighed 11st 5lbs. His wife was named as next of kin and was recorded as living at Belair, South Australia. He embarked with his unit on the *Kyarra* on 24th October 1914 which disembarked in Heliopolis, Egypt. He was replaced by Colonel J. W. Barrett as Commanding Officer of the unit by February 1915 and returned to Australia on the *Kytell.* There had been a management problem with Matron Bell over the control of the nurses of 1AGH. She also returned to Australia. Colonel Barrett also resigned and transferred to the RAMC. Smith's appointment to the AIF was terminated on 5th October 1915 by order of the Governor-General on the advice of Executive Council. He was issued with the 1914-15 Star, British War Medal and Victory Medal.

Ramsey Smith continued to publish after WWI; in the main concerning the indigenous population and Coroner's duties. Some works were said to be plagiarised including that of David Unapion regarding aboriginal customs. He continued to collect and experiment on human remains and was responsible for Edinburgh University's collection of 500-600 individual skeletons. After his death in 1937 more than 100 skulls were found in his house. He was awarded a Fellowship of the Royal Society of Edinburgh, Honorary Fellowship of the Royal Anthropological Institute and Honorary Membership of the Association of Military Surgeons of the United States amongst others. William Ramsay Smith died at Belair on the 28th September 1937. His wife Margaret predeceased him on 13th April 1936. They had four daughters and a son who survived them.

Sources:

Tyquin M., "Neville Howes" Oxford University press 1999
Elmslie R. Nance S., Australian Dictionary of Biography, Vol 11 (MUP) 1988.
http://adb.anu.edu.au/biography/smith-william-ramsay-8493
http://recordsearch.naa.gov.au/NameSearch/Interface/ItemDetail.aspx?Barcode=1793501
Photo SLSA B7479

RAYNER Howard Luscombe

MB BCh (Oxon)

1896 - 1975

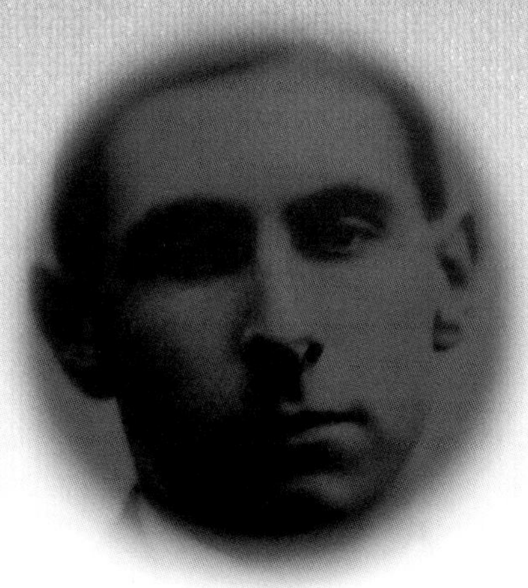

Howard Luscombe Rayner was born on the 12th March 1896 at Glenelg, South Australia the son of Rev George Rayner of the Glenelg Congregational Church, and a missionary in the Fiji Islands. He was educated at Prince Alfred College where he was an outstanding student and athlete. He represented Sturt in the final against Port Adelaide. He gained a government bursary and an Elder Scholarship and began his medical degree at the University of Adelaide until, at the age of 21 years, he was awarded a Rhodes scholarship in 1916 and continued his studies at Oxford. After the announcement of the Rhodes scholarship in December 1915 he went to England and enlisted for active service and subsequently, in 1918, to Balliol College, Oxford to study medicine. He was also awarded the Burney Yeo Scholarship to King's College Hospital, London in 1918. He was reported to be a fine cricketer and the most consistent batsman in the Varsity combination.

During the war he served in the Royal Navy, and, after the Armistice, returned to Balliol and Kings College Hospital, London graduating in 1921 and subsequently entered general practice in 1923 at Twickenham. He took a great interest in sport including cricket, tennis and rugby and later golf. He was too old to enlist in WW2 but took over the International Rugby Ground at Twickenham and turned it into a first-aid post. After WW2 he was appointed doctor to the Twickenham Rugby Club. He was interested in anaesthetics and continued with anaesthetics from 1938 until 2 years after his retirement in 1965. He was an active member of the BMA and chairman of his local division. Howard Luscombe Rayner died on the 13th June 1975 aged 78 years and was survived by his wife.

Sources:

BMJ 19th July 1975 p 164
The Adelaide Advertiser 23 December 1914
The Adelaide Advertiser 9th December 1915
Photo: PAC Collection

Extracts from the Gallipoli Landing by Harry Carew Nott

...On Thursday morning (29-4-15) we marched down to the beach and round to the right, and bivouacked in a small gully just off the beach on our right flank (subsequently know as Shell Green)... Most of us went for a swim but the Turks began shelling the beach, and stopped our ablutions. 15-5-15 moved our HQ into White's Gully and the regimental pioneers dug some good dugouts, and covered them with timber...24-5-15 armistice arranged from 7.30 am to 4pm to bury the dead between the trenches...It was a gruesome sight as the bodies were all blown up and swarming with maggots: the stench was horrible. We moved the bodies by rolling them on to stretchers with the aid of shovels...carried across to a neutral zone where they were handed over to some Turks who buried them, after taking any equipment off that was useful – boots were especially rushed!!

...The flies, which became a plague after a few weeks, no doubt spread infection very considerably among men who were already in a poor state of health. Disease was also spread by the water, which was obtained almost universally from a contaminated source... for the first few days on the Peninsula, all the rules of sanitation were disregarded. It was the usual thing for men to use the nearest bush or gully for a latrine, without even troubling to dig a hole or cover up the deposit. So that from the start, all the gullies, from which water could be obtained, were grossly contaminated with faeces and urine....There are many lessons to be learned from the early days of the AIF and I think they have been learned and acted upon: but it is just as well to keep the original faults in mind to prevent their occurrence.

Source: AWM

RENNIE Henry Charles Cadell

MB BS MRCS (Eng) LRCP (Lond)

1891 - 1925

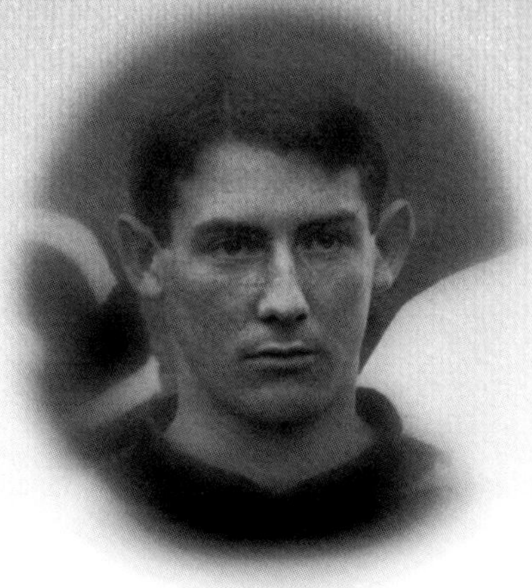

Henry Charles Cadell Rennie was born in Adelaide on 10th April 1891 the youngest child of Professor Edward Henry Rennie, the Angas Professor of Chemistry at the University of Adelaide, and his wife, Agnes Alison, nee Cadell. Rennie was educated at the Queen's School in North Adelaide and studied medicine at the University of Adelaide where he was the Everard scholar of 1912. He was a house surgeon at the Adelaide Hospital in 1913 followed by some time at the Broken Hill Hospital where he was assistant to Dr Birks. After returning to Adelaide he decided to travel to England for post-graduate experience and took his MRCS LRCP about the time of the declaration of war.

Rennie joined the RAMC as a lieutenant and served with the 52 FdAmb in France. His time in the trenches resulted in him developing the 'malady' that was to later take his life. While never specified, it is presumed he developed tuberculosis at this time. He was invalided back to Australia in 1916. He was given the rank of honorary captain on 15th May 1918.

He was appointed Medical Superintendent of the Bedford Park Sanatorium in June 1917 and later undertook private work at the Nunyara Sanatorium at Belair. His health began to fail and he returned to the Bedford Park Sanatorium until ill health forced him to relinquish this appointment. He was untiring in his efforts for the 'inmates' of the Bedford Park Sanatorium and Myrtle Bank Institution which gained him the love and esteem of all who knew of the skill and sympathy in his ministrations. To the Tubercular Soldiers Association and the Tubercular Soldiers Aid Society he was a valuable helper having given great assistance in framing appeal cases for the Repatriation Department. Indeed, he lobbied forcefully on behalf of those with tuberculosis: he reported 123 beds for tuberculosis sufferers in South Australia of which only 64 were available to the public when there were 500-600 new cases each year. He wrote "The neglect of the State and medical profession to make an organised effort to cope with the spread of tuberculosis has prompted me to draw attention to the existing provision for sufferers from this disease and what seems to me its inadequacy".... as a State we are grossly neglecting our duty". He is described as a man with a loveable character, a clear, original and deep thinker who kept himself abreast of the most recent treatment of tuberculosis. He enrolled for the Doctor of Medicine (MD) at University of Adelaide in 1923. He was a keen student of animal husbandry and bred cocker spaniels and Jersey cattle; he exhibited successfully in a variety of shows and was successful in obtaining prizes. Henry Charles Cadell Rennie died, aged 34, on 2nd September 1925 at Victor Harbour having moved there 12 months earlier. Doubtless his health precluded completion of his doctorate. His father, Professor Edward Henry Rennie, died 13 months later on 8th January 1927.

Sources:

Photo: Adelaide University Archives; 1910 Lacrosse Intervarsity Team.

The Adelaide Register, 3rd Sep25

Rennie HCC (1919) "The problem of Tuberculosis in the State of South Australia" Medical Journal of Australia 17 347-8

The London Gazette 14th May 1918 p. 5715

REYNELL Walter Rupert

DM MA FRCP MRCS

1885 - 1948

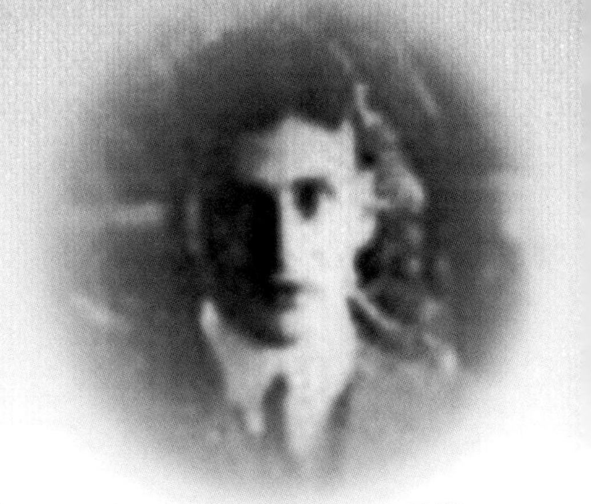

Walter Rupert Reynell was born at Payneham, South Australia on 5th July 1885. He was the son of noted South Australian wine grower and pastoralist Walter Reynell, who died in 1919, and his wife Emily nee Bakewell. He was educated at Queens's College where he won 17 prizes for his academic ability and was dux of the school before going to St Peter's College where he excelled at cricket. He was the South Australian Rhodes Scholar for 1906. He studied medicine at Balliol College, Oxford, and Guy's Hospital graduating in 1913. Walter married Una Mary Shaw-Stewart the daughter of Reverend Charles Robert Shaw-Stewart and Ida Fannie Caroline, nee Afken on the 5th June 1916. Their children were Peter Carew Reynell (1917), Joan Katherine Reynell (1918), Anne Lenore Reynell (1923) and Anthony Charles Reynell (1930)

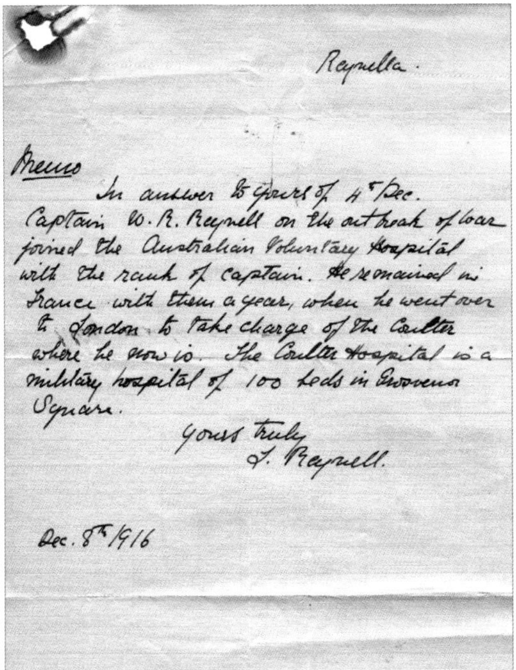

Reynella.

Memo

In answer to yours of 4th Dec.
Captain W. R. Reynell on the outbreak of war joined the Australian Voluntary Hospital with the rank of captain. He remained in France with them a year, when he went over to London to take charge of the Coulter where he now is. The Coulter Hospital is a military hospital of 100 beds in Grosvenor Square.

Yours truly
J. Reynell.

Dec. 8th/16

Reynell was appointed as a captain in the RAMC on the 2nd September 1914 whilst he was serving with an Australian Medical Unit and was posted to the Australian Voluntary Hospital. When the Hospital closed, he was transferred to the Seale Hayne Hospital at Newton Abbot, Devon, which was pioneering the treatment of shell-shock. His time at Seale Hayne stimulated Reynell's interest in neurological diseases, and led him to pursue a career in that field.

Reynell gained his MRCP in 1918 and his DM in 1919. He went on to become the Senior Physician at the West End Hospital for Nervous Diseases, London, and kept rooms in Harley Street. Walter Rupert Reynell died in London on 21st March 1948. Reynell's older brother Lieutenant Colonel Carew Reynell commanded 9 LHR for a short time at Gallipoli and was killed in August 1915 during the attacks on Hill 60.

Sources:

http://www.onkaparingacity.com/libraries/localstudies/view_photo_enlarged.asp?RefID=2182
The Register Adelaide 2n March 1902
The Adelaide Advertiser 23 December 1902
The Register Adelaide 9th April 1919
Photo: cropped from the University of Adelaide Archives, 1906 medical students group photo
Response to the University of Adelaide's request about Reynell's war service.

RICE Patrick William

MB BS DRCOG

1889 - 1952

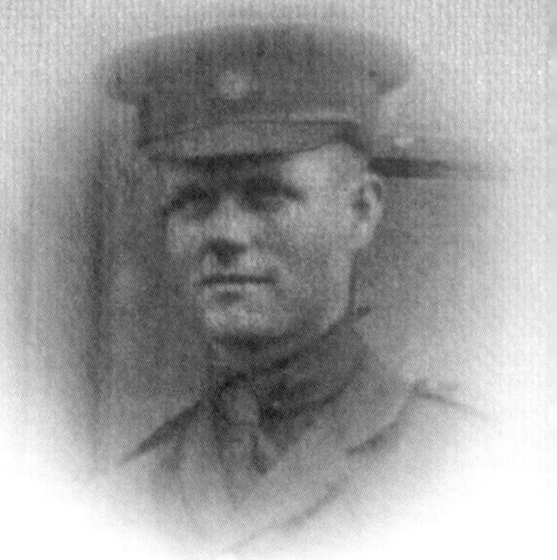

Patrick William Rice was born in Morgan, SA on the 18th May 1889, third son of Mr. and Mrs. J. J. Rice of Cockburn. He was educated at the Moonta Public School and the Christian Brothers College, Adelaide. He completed an apprenticeship in pharmacy at Main and Sons Dispensary and while doing this decided to enroll in medicine which initiated a brilliant academic career at the University of Adelaide, during which he topped every year of his course and obtained the Elder Prize, Dr. Davies Thomas Scholarship (twice) and the Everard Scholarship graduating in 1915. After graduating he worked for the next three years on the staff of 7 AGH (Keswick), first as pathologist and bacteriologist, and then in the orthopaedics and x-ray departments. He married Ruby Dunleavey Hill, youngest daughter of Mr. and Mrs. T. W. Hill, of Parkside, in September 1916.

Rice was commissioned in the AAMC in August 1918 and joined the ANMEF. He was 29 years, 5ft 6ins tall, and weighed 147lbs, of fair complexion, blue eyes and brown hair. His wife was named as his next of kin care of J J Rice of Mills Terrace, North Adelaide or his permanent address of 12 Victoria Avenue, Hyde Park South Australia. Rice sailed for Rabaul in October and in December he was posted to Kavieng in New Ireland. He was declared medically unfit in May 1919, and returned to Australia to the 2 MD on the 14th June 1919 and then to the 4 MD Adelaide, with his appointment terminated on the 1st September 1919. He was issued with the British War Medal and the Victory Medal.

After the war Rice entered general practice at Torrensville, but soon established a reputation as a gynaecologist. He went to England in 1935 and sat for and topped the examination for the Diploma of the Royal College of Obstetricians and Gynecologists. He acquired a large practice which he carried on until his death. Rice and his wife were prominent at Rostrevor and Loreto College's functions as committee and in executive positions. He lived on Portrush Road, Tusmore. Rice was a well-known figure in the sporting world; he was surgeon to the SA Trotting Club for many years. As a joint organiser each year of the Anzac trotting meeting, he was largely responsible for raising large sums of money for the Soldiers' Distress Fund. Patrick William Rice died at Calvary Hospital, on the 7th March 1952. He was survived by his daughter Therese and son, Dr Laurence Rice.

Sources:

http://recordsearch.naa.gov.au/scripts/Imagine.asp?B=8031333;
MJA 12th July 1952 p75, NLA Trove.
Photo; SLSA B26285-127.
The Adelaide Advertiser 13th December 1905
Daily Herald Adelaide4 October 1915
The Chronicle Adelaide 13 March 1952.

ROGERS Richard Sanders

DSc MD (Edin) MA FRACP FRS (SA)

1861 - 1942

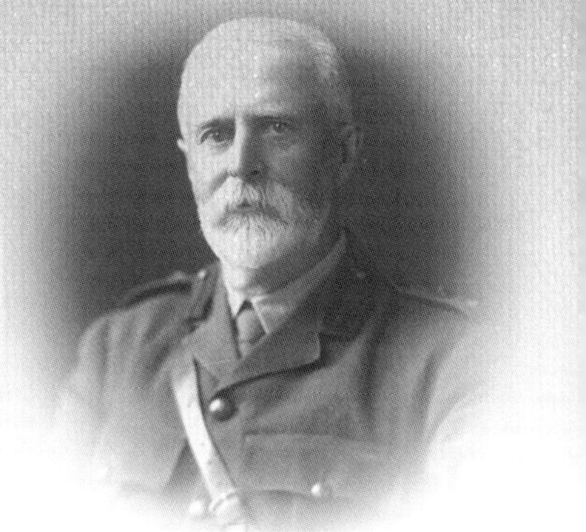

Richard Sanders Rogers was born on the 2nd December 1861. He was the son of Joseph Rogers and Ann Childers Williams. Joseph was a contractor/mason from Lyndoch South Australia. Rogers was educated at the Pulteney Street School in 1879. He became the first public school boy to matriculate, with Greek as a supplementary subject, which earned him a scholarship to the University of Adelaide to study a Bachelor of Arts graduating with 1st class honours in 1882. He then undertook teaching at Prince Alfred College before travelling to the University of Edinburgh to study medicine graduating MB ChM in 1887. On August 3rd 1887 he married Jane Scott Paterson. In 1893 he also gained his MD at Edinburgh University. He returned to Australia with his wife to commence general practice in Adelaide. Their home, with surgery attached, was located in Flinders Street, East Adelaide, within easy reach of the Adelaide Hospital. He undertook further study at the University of Adelaide gaining a MD and MA in 1897. He was appointed as an Honorary Physician to the Adelaide Hospital in 1897 and served as a member of the hospital Board from 1896-1922. In 1893, Rogers' became interested in hypnosis and used it as an adjunct to his methods of treatment. His private practice flourished and he was a notable exponent of mesmeric art from 1894. Furthermore, in 1895, The Advertiser reported that Dr Rogers *"successfully removed a cyst from the breast of a young woman while acting as both a surgeon and hypnotist while she was awake and talking to assistants and witnesses standing nearby"*.

Rogers had brief military service in South Africa in 1901. In 1914 he was appointed as the Medical Superintendent, 7th Australian Base Hospital at Keswick Barracks, South Australia with the rank of Lieutenant Colonel. He served in this position until the end of the war.

After the war Rogers became Superintendent and visiting Psychiatrist to Enfield Receiving House, Northfield Mental Hospital. He was also Consulting Psychiatrist to all Mental Institutions from 1929 until 1942. He recommenced study at the University of Adelaide and gained a DSc in 1936. He was a member and President of the state Medical Board and a lecturer in Forensic Science to medical students. He occupied positions on numerous public institutions including the Museum, the Public Library, and the Art Gallery of South Australia. Rogers was a Foundation Fellow of the Royal Australasian College of Physicians. Rogers was also interested in native orchids. He wrote papers on orchids and published in the Transactions of the Royal Society of South Australia. He was credited with the discovery of 85 new species of Australian native orchids. His wife accompanied him in searching for orchids in Australia, New Zealand and New Guinea. He was elected a Fellow of the Royal Society of SA, he served as its President from 1920-1922. In 1924 Rogers was elected Fellow of the Linnean Society of London for the many contributions he made on orchids and their taxonomy. Richard Sanders Rogers died on 28th March 1942. He was survived by his wife, his son and his daughter whom he disowned because of her secret marriage. He bequeathed his research and material on orchids to the University of Adelaide and the rest of his collection is at the Adelaide Herbarium.

Sources:

Gibberd J, 'Rogers, Richard Sanders (1861–1942)', Australian Dictionary of Biography, National Centre of Biography, Australian National University, http://adb.anu.edu.au/biography/rogers-richard-sanders-8259/text14465.

Presentation to the SAMHS by Dr W. S. Lawson March 2012.

The Adelaide Advertiser 7th November 1896

Transactions of the Royal Society of South Australia, Vol 30, and page 225.

RUSSELL Ernest Albert Harold

OBE VD KStJ MB BS

1885 - 1969

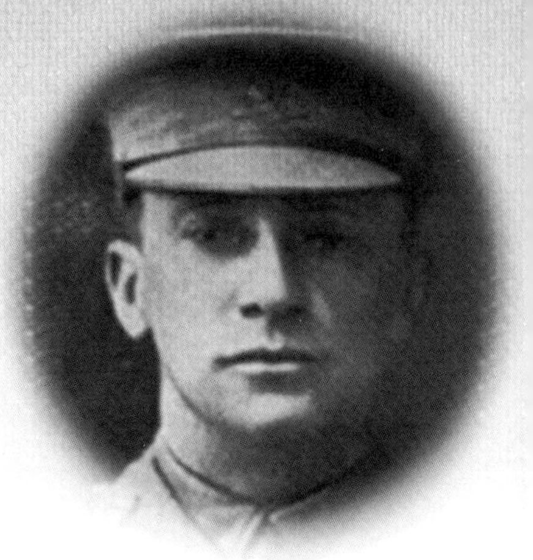

Ernest Albert Harold Russell was born on the 28th August 1885 at Unley, South Australia. He was the third son of James Thomas Russell and his wife Susanne Charlotte, nee Bird. He was educated at Prince Alfred College and studied medicine at the University of Adelaide graduating in 1911. At University he was Captain of the successful Inter Varsity Lacrosse team. He completed his residency at the Adelaide Hospital, and was commissioned as a Captain in 1911 in the AAMC reserve. He was posted first to 31 LHFA, and then to 19 FdAmb. He set up practice at Unley and Westbourne Park with his older brother Herbert Henry Ernest Russell.

Russell enlisted in the AIF in May 1915; his father, of St. Raymond's, Unley Rd Unley was nominated as his next of kin. His service records contain no details of a physical examination on enlistment. He was subsequently posted to 3 AGH. He travelled with the unit to England and on to Lemnos, and remained there throughout the Mediterranean campaign. He was promoted major in January 1916, and posted to 6 FdAmb. He remained with 2 Div but served at various times with both 7 and 8 FdAmb through the Somme battles of 1916 and for much of 1917. He contracted trench fever in November 1916, and the fever returned twice in 1918. Russell had had a lung abscess as a child, and his oldest brother had died of tuberculosis. He was therefore carefully watched by successive medical boards. No firm diagnosis was made apart from fibrosis of the lung. He was posted to 1 Sanitary Section in September 1917 (which by an anomaly was part of 2 Div), and in October promoted lieutenant colonel and posted back to 3 AGH. One year later he was reviewed, and found unfit for another winter in the field, and invalided back to Australia. He was allowed to proceed via Canada at his own expense, and was discharged from the AIF in February 1919. Russell was issued with the 1914-15 Star, The British War Medal and the Victory Medal.

Russell married Janet Manson Ward of West Payneham on 17th December 1921. They had a daughter and a son. He remained in the CMF and was CO of 3 FdAmb from 1921-26. He set up practice at "Corowa", Napier Terrace, Westbourne Park, and from 1920-23 was an honorary obstetrician at the Queen's Home, and afterwards a consultant. He was an ardent supporter of St John's Ambulance and the Australian Red Cross Society, and was President of the SA Branch of the BMA in 1943-44. He loved yachting and was a member of the Royal SA Yacht Squadron. He was appointed OBE in 1949 and a Knight of St John in 1953 for services to the Queen Victoria Hospital. In 1967 his address was 401 The Parade, Kensington Gardens, SA. He died on the 19th May 1969.

Sources:

Photo: SLSA; B26285_5

http://recordsearch.naa.gov.au/scripts/Imagine.asp?B=8071627

Likeman R., "Gallipoli Doctors" Slouch Hat Publications, 2010

The Register Adelaide 15 December 1911

The Chronicle Adelaide 6th January 1949

The News Adelaide 23 December 1953

Off to the War

Extract from Claude Morlet's diary written on a troop ship

10th December [1914]

Today it is delightfully milder and the sea is calm and slightly misty...From then till lunch listened to the gramophone belonging to the Adelaide Stationary Hospital of which Le Messurier and Verco are the captains. Both, especially the former, are bonzer chaps.

Morlet G, Eyes Right: the life of Claude Morlet, DSO, Eye Surgeon and Soldier, 2007, Lythrum Press, Adelaide Australia, p. 34

RUSSELL Herbert Henry Ernest

OBE VD KStJ MD

1875 - 1951

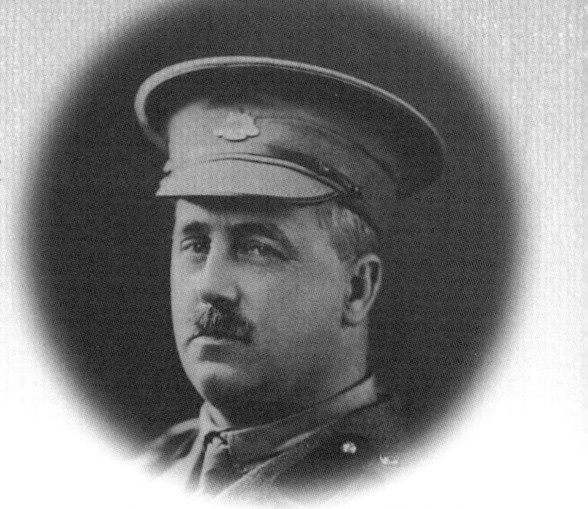

Herbert Henry Ernest Russell was born on 28th October 1875. He was the second son of James Thomas Russell, inspector of the Adelaide Milling Company, and his wife Susanne Charlotte, nee Bird. He had three brothers and five sisters. He was educated at Prince Alfred College. He started to study medicine at the University of Adelaide but continued at Melbourne University because of the 'Adelaide Hospital Row', graduating MB ChB in 1899 and at the University of Adelaide, MD, in 1905. He became a lieutenant in the AAMC militia in 1906.

At the outbreak of WW1 Russell wanted to enlist in the AIF but was told that his services as a PMO were needed at home. He was compulsorily retained in Australia at the rank of lieutenant colonel. Russell proved to have exceptional administrative qualities and management and supervision of the medical services of 4 MD received high commendation from distinguished officials and other sources, including the Royal Commission on Navy and Defence Administration, the Board of Business Administration, and the Commission of Enquiry into the Home Service Personnel. Many of the methods of control and procedure in the 4 MD were adopted by other military districts in the Commonwealth. This led to Russell going to Melbourne to report on the system in operation at the Curative Workshops in that district.

Russell returned to his general practice in Unley after the war. He was appointed OBE in 1920. He was made a member of the Nurses Board in 1933. In 1938 he gave evidence in the Royal Commission into the remuneration of doctors under the national insurance scheme. He remained in general practice at Unley for 50 years and was the Unley Health Officer for 45 years. Herbert Henry Ernest Russell died on the 10th July 1951. He never married.

Sources:

News Adelaide 11th July 1951
The Adelaide Advertiser 25 November 1905
The Adelaide Advertiser 30 January 1906
The Mail, Saturday 13th December 1919
The Adelaide Advertiser 16 October 1920
The Chronicle Adelaide 2 March 1929
The Adelaide Advertiser 15 October 1938
http://www.ww1sa.gravesecrets.net/ru---ry.html

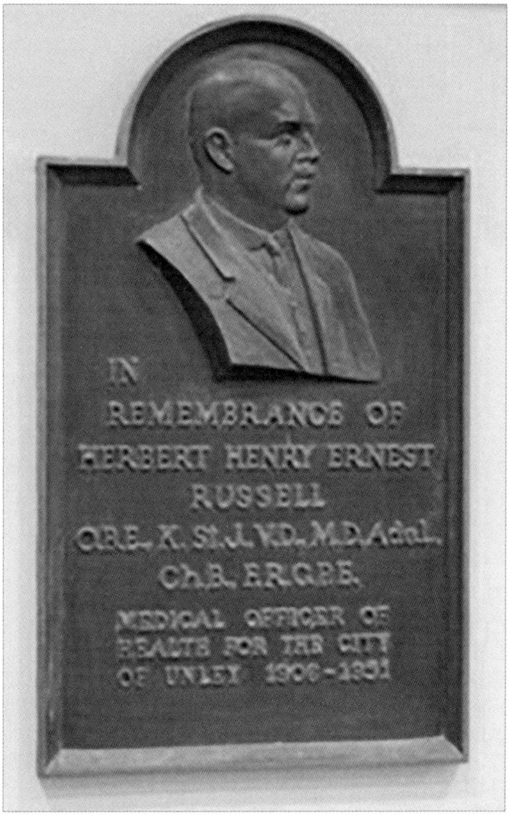

SCOTT Malcolm Leslie

MS MB FRCS FRACS

1882 - 1931

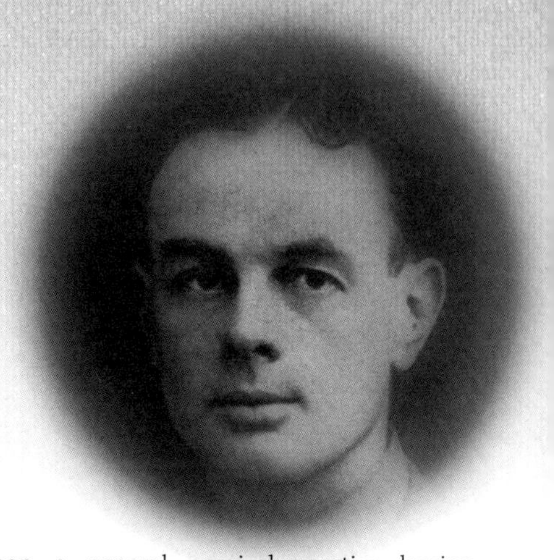

Malcolm Leslie Scott was born at College Park on the 25th June 1882, the son of Paul and Clara Scott, nee Waterhouse. He attended Prince Alfred College and studied medicine at the University of Adelaide graduating MB BS in 1904. He was appointed to the Adelaide Hospital in 1905 and then spent 2 years as assistant to Dr Henry Arthur Powell at Kadina followed by 2 years in post graduate surgical training obtaining the FRCS in 1909 in England. Following his return home he was in general practice in Mt Barker 1910-1916; he married Irene Gertrude Hunter at the Methodist Church, Kent Town on 4th August 1910. He had a love of golf and was President and Captain of the Mount Barker Golf Club in 1914. He was medical officer to the West Adelaide Military Training Area in 1911.

Although it was reported that he first attempted to enlist in July 1915 he did not enlist at this time. It was also reported in the Adelaide Register in August 1915 that he had been the recipient of a "white feather". Despite this Scott enlisted in the AIF in May 1916. He was 33 years old and his wife was nominated as his next of kin. He was 5ft 9ins tall, 154lbs, of medium complexion with brown eyes and hair. He could ride and had a slight knowledge of German. Scott embarked from Adelaide on the 13th July 1916. He was appointed to the permanent surgical staff of 1 AGH at Rouen in early 1917, detached to a British CCS at Passchendaele, later in 1917 to the 5th British General Hospital. As a temporary major he was posted to the 3 FdAmb with 10 Bn in September 1918 and finally in December back to the 1 AGH at Rouen in Command of the Surgical Division. Scott maintained that the war experience enhanced his surgical knowledge, especially the drainage and treatment of infected joints particularly the knee joint. He returned to Australia on 24th December 1918 having served in many British and Australian General Hospitals and with FdAmb in France with his only sick leave being Influenza and an inflamed face. His appointment was terminated from the AIF on the 11th May 1919. Scott was issued with the British War Medal and the Victory Medal.

Scott began a general surgical practice having gained his MS on returning to Adelaide in 1919 He was appointed an honorary surgeon at the Adelaide Children's Hospital and in 1927 an honorary surgeon to the Adelaide Hospital. Scott was a foundation fellow of the RACS. He was also involved on the as a demonstrator, lecturer and examiner at the Medical School of the University of Adelaide from 1919 to 1927. Scott's commitment to education was also demonstrated by his Committee and Council memberships of Scotch College and Presbyterian Ladies College and to the profession by membership and 2 years on the Council of the SA Branch of the British Medical Association. Malcolm Leslie Scott died on the 3rd November 1931. He was survived by his wife and six children.

Sources:
http://recordsearch.naa.gov.au/scripts/Imagine.asp?B=3003472
MJA: p 64, January 9th 1932
The Register Adelaide 13th August 1910
The Register Adelaide 8th August 1915
The Adelaide Advertiser 4th November 1931

South Australia
From our Special Correspondent

The War

Our thoughts are all of the war; we have no time for anything else. Every entertainment almost that is given is either for our patriotic fund or for the relief of the Belgians, or for the British Red Cross Society, or for supplying comforts to troop horses, or for nurses going with the hospital. Ever the cinema show seeks patronage by advertising "war prices" not, as one might expect, increased prices of admission, but reduced. Some drugs, especially morphine, have increased in price; at one time we were told there would be a famine of anaesthetics.

BMJ, 16 January 1915, p. 137

SHEPHERD Arthur Edmund

CBE DSO VD L&LM RCP&S (Edin) LFPS (Glas)

1867 - 1942

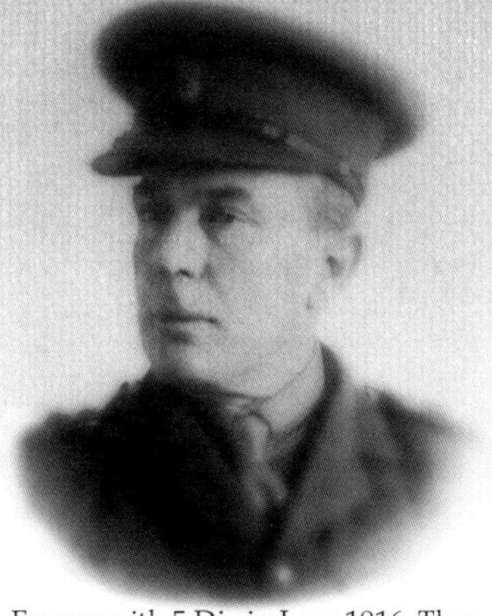

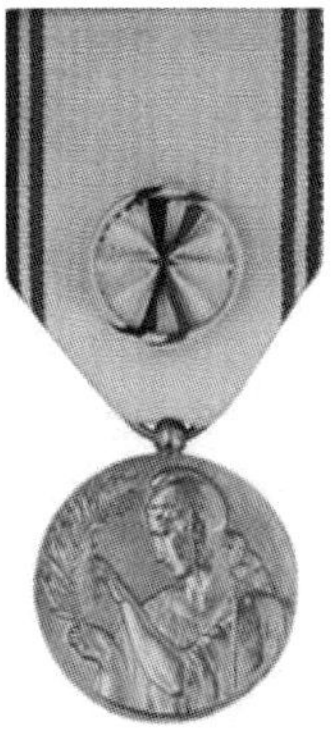

Arthur Edmund Shepherd was born at Norwood South Australia on 21st October 1867, the son of Richard Webb and Susan, nee Bennetts. Richard Webb died in 1870, and in 1872 Susan married Emmanuel Shepherd, a Yorkshire-born land-broker. Emmanuel Shepherd adopted Arthur when he was 5 years old and his surname changed to Shepherd. The family home still stands at 205 Magill Road, Maylands, and is heritage listed. Shepherd was educated at Norwood Grammar School and Prince Alfred College. He studied medicine in Edinburgh. He returned to Australia in 1891 and set up a practice in Norwood. He married his father's niece, Emma Tarrant Amanda Shepherd in 1895. When the Adelaide Hospital Row led to the resignation of the honorary medical staff in 1895, Shepherd obtained an appointment to the staff as a surgeon, and in 1903 as a gynaecologist. Shepherd also was club doctor and Vice President of the Norwood Football Club. He was the first medical health officer for East Torrens. Shepherd was commissioned as a lieutenant in 1900 in the Volunteer Medical Corps, and in 1903 when this was incorporated into the AAMC he was promoted to captain. He was promoted to major in 1910, and in 1912 promoted lieutenant colonel as CO of 19 FdAmb.

Shepherd enlisted in the AIF when he was 47 years old. He had been acting PMO of 4 MD until he was given command of 8 FdAmb on the 16th August 1915. His wife, of Molesworth Street, North Adelaide, was named as next of kin. He was described as of slight build and medium height. His departure for Egypt was delayed by his temporary appointment as DDGMS while Surgeon General Richard Herbert Joseph Fetherston was visiting Egypt and England. Shepherd finally sailed for Egypt in December 1915. The unit went to France with 5 Div in June 1916. They took part in the Battles of Fromelles, the Somme, and Ypres. Shepherd was appointed ADMS of 2 Div in November 1917, and promoted colonel in April 1918. He was awarded the DSO in June for his services rendered in France. He continued to play a key role in casualty evacuation in the fighting at Peronne and Mont St Quentin, and the advance to the Hindenburg Line. He was appointed DDMS of 1 Aust Corps in April 1919. He was mentioned in Despatches three times. His AIF appointment was terminated in November 1919 and he was issued with the 1914-15 Star, British War Medal and the Victory Medal with Oak Leaves. He was also awarded the Medaille de la Reconnaissance Francaise.

On the 15th September 1919 he was appointed CBE. Shepherd was invited to become the Principal Medical Officer of the South Australian branch of the Repatriation Department on his return to Australia. He held this position from 1920 to 1932, while continuing his appointment at the Adelaide Hospital and his private practice. Two of his four sons served as privates in 3 LHR in the Middle East. Shepherd died in Adelaide in 1942, survived by his wife and six children.

Sources:
http://recordsearch.naa.gov.au/scripts/Imagine.asp?B=8081685
Photo, PAC Collection
Refshauge W. D., 'Shepherd, Arthur Edmund (1867–1942)', Australian Dictionary of Biography, National Centre of Biography, Australian National University, http://adb.anu.edu.au/biography/shepherd-arthur-edmund-8412/text14775,
The Register Adelaide 4 June 1918

The Médaille de la Reconnaissance française (French Medal of Recognition) is a French honor medal created 13 July 1917 and awarded solely to civilians.
"gratitude extended to all individuals or communities, who have arisen in France, with the Allies and the whole world, to help the wounded, the sick, families of soldiers killed in combat, the maimed, disabled, blind, orphans and people whose lives were destroyed by the invasion

† SHIERLAW Norman Craig
MC FRCS(Ed) LRCP

1883 - 1917

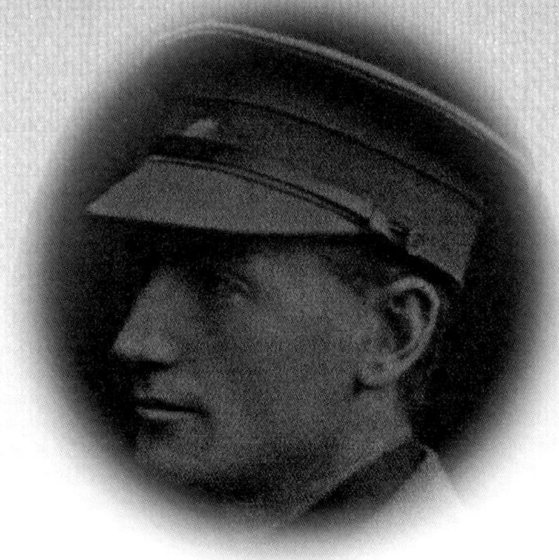

Norman Craig Shierlaw was born on the 23rd August 1883 in Adelaide son of Joseph Craig Shierlaw and Emma née Baldwinson, brother of Howard 1879, Allan 1881 and Edith 1886. His father owned 'Sheirlaw and Co.' which was a Tailors, Clothiers, Outfitters and Hatters business in Hindley Street Adelaide. He was educated at Prince Alfred College, the University of Adelaide and Edinburgh University. The Prince Alfred College Chronicle reported that *"He was much interested in social problems in civil life before he went to the war".*

Sheirlaw joined the AIF in June 1915 at the age of 31 years and applied for a Commission in the AAMC. He was single and his father of 52 Eaton St, Malvern, SA was named as his next of kin. He was posted to a Convalescent Depot, in England. He embarked from Melbourne on the 17th July 1915. He was attached as MO to the 1st Anzac entrenching Bn at Etaples on the 11th June 1916 and remained with them until a posting to the Australian 4 FdAmb and then to the 13 Bn as RMO in August 1916. He died of wounds received in action on the 11th April 1916 and was buried in the Australian Dressing Station Cemetery. He was re-interned to the British Cemetery in 1929, ½ mile SW of the Vaulx-Vraucourt Corps British Cemetery, France Plot 2, Row B, Grave 13 , 3 miles NE of Bapaume. He was awarded the Military Cross posthumously on 22nd February 1917 for; *"conspicuous gallantry in action and devotion to duty. He continually attended to the wounded for two days and nights under heavy fire. He has on many occasions done fine work".* Correspondence between his father and the AIF for the receipt of the MC and the details of his son's death took more than a year for a satisfactory response. His family received his 1914-15 Star, the British War Medal and the Victory Medal, and the Memorial Scroll and Kings Message in 1921 and the Memorial Plaque in 1922.

Sources:
http://recordsearch.naa.gov.au/scripts/Imagine.asp?B=083156
Photo; PAC collection
Cemetery or memorial details: Vraucourt Copse Cemetery, Vaulx-Vraucourt, France
AWM145 Roll of Honour cards, 1914-1918 War, Army
PAC Chronicle No. 119 of August 1917

During the late South African war, when medical men for the moment began to think of military medical affairs, one not infrequently heard of schemes by which civil effort would provide for the supply of personnel, and of even complete hospitals in war, such hospitals to be affiliated to, or exist as, offshoots from the great civil institutions. The idea was undoubtedly a good one, but as the years have passed the zeal and enthusiasm has lessened.

BMJ, 17 February 1906, p. 362

SHIPWAY Graham Stuart

MB BS

1889 - 1956

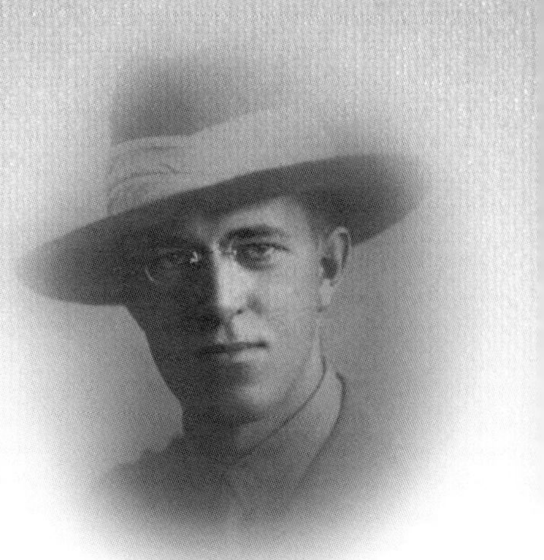

Graham Stuart Shipway was born on the 26th February 1889 at Victor Harbor, South Australia. He was the son of postmaster Cornelius John Shipway, of Meningie and later Victor Harbor and his wife Agnes Ann, nee Graham of "Glenwreath" Long Valley, Strathalbyn. He had a brother John and sister Margaret. He was educated at Prince Alfred College and studied medicine at the University of Adelaide graduating in 1916.

Shipway joined the AAMC in July 1916 and enlisted in the AIF on 5th February 1917 after completing his residency. He was 26 years old, single, and his father was named as his next of kin. He was 5ft 9ins tall, and weighed 11st, of dark complexion, green eyes and dark hair. He could ride and had a fair proficiency in German. He was posted to the Australian Camel Brigade Field Ambulance (ACBFA) and embarked on the *'Itria'* from Sydney for the Middle East in May. He was appointed adjutant of the unit in September 1917 and one story of his escapades said; *"he infiltrated enemy lines on his camel in the dead of night to steal drugs for the patients he was looking after, as supplies had failed to arrive."* Shipway was detached to 4 Bn ICC as RMO from October 1917 until January 1918. He transferred to 5 LHFA when the ACBFA was disbanded in August 1918. When the FdAmb reached Damascus in October 1918, Shipway fell victim to malaria, and was admitted to the English Hospital in Damascus. He was promoted temporary major in May 1919, and left Egypt for England with a group of casualties. He was granted study leave in England, and used the time to work at the Bristol Royal Infirmary. There he met one of the first two female medical graduates of Bristol University, Hilda Elizabeth Reynolds. Shipway returned to Australia in April 1920 with his appointment terminated on the 8th August 1920. On discharge Shipway was granted the honorary rank of major. He had served for 1494 days with 1142 overseas. Shipway was issued with the British War Medal and the Victory Medal.

He set up practice in Victor Harbor. Hilda followed and the couple were married in 1922 at Unley and had four children, Mary, Phyllis, Gerald, and Margaret. He became a prominent member of the community, was a trustee of the newly built Victor Harbor and South Coast District Hospital in 1925, and was President of the Sub Branch of the RSL for 15 years. He is noted, with Dr W A Verco, as a prominent exhibitor at the Inman Valley Flower Show in 1935, and a member of the Council of the Victor Harbor High School. He was a visiting MO at the South Coast Hospital, and in 1938 was President of the Recruiting Committee for the CMF. The Victor Harbor Rifle Club had a competition for the Dr G S Shipway Trophy. Hilda helped in the Red Cross and also helped him in his practice; they were both well-known and much loved in Victor Harbor. Graham Stuart Shipway died in 1956 and is buried at Victor Harbor.

Sources:
http://recordsearch.naa.gov.au/NameSearch/Interface/ItemDetail.aspx?Barcode=8082691
The Advertiser 27th July 1916
The News Adelaide 6th November 1939
Encounter Bay Family History Group.

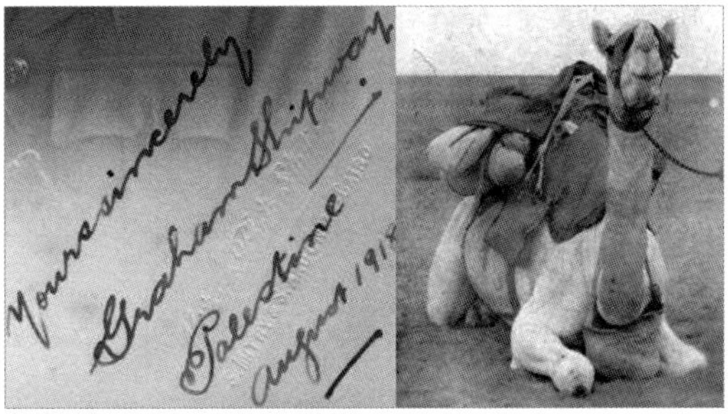

SINCLAIR William Malcolm

MB BS

1882 - 1942

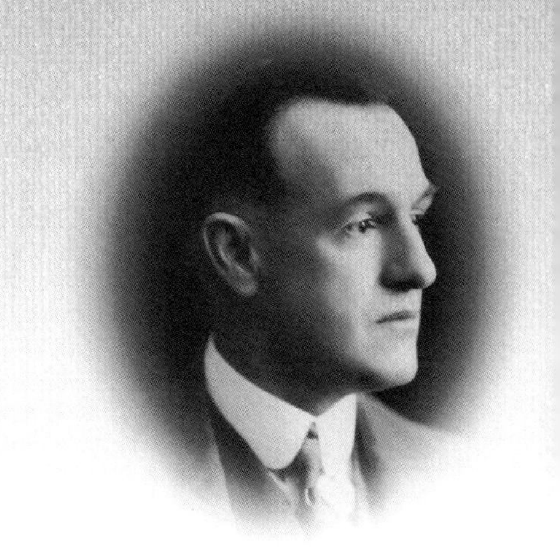

William Malcolm Sinclair was born on the 18th April 1882 at Rocky River in the Clare district, South Australia. He was son of John Sinclair and Agnes, nee Miller, youngest daughter of Mr John Miller, of Stonehenge Farm near Athelstone and one of seven children. Sinclair's grandparents John William and Christina Sinclair were early colonists of South Australia arriving in 1839 in the ship *Palmyra*. Sinclair's family settled on a property called Sunny Brae, on the Rocky River near Crystal Brook, where they lived for forty-five years. Sinclair's father was a leading breeder of exhibition and high class Lincoln sheep and Hereford cattle. Sinclair was educated at Prince Alfred College and studied medicine at the University of Adelaide graduating in 1911. After graduation he practiced at Gladstone, and later at Crystal Brook. Sinclair married Pearl Edith Elizabeth McLean (1891-1963) of "Sunny Bank" Mt Pleasant, South Australia in the Presbyterian Church Goodwood on the 15th April 1913.

Sinclair enlisted in the AIF on the 24th April 1915 at the age of 33 years; he had no previous military experience. He was 6ft 3ins tall, and weighed 12st. His wife of "Farina" Crystal Brook was nominated as his next of kin. He was allotted to 1 AGH in Egypt with reinforcements. He arrived in Egypt in July and in August was posted to 3 AGH on Lemnos. A month later he was in hospital with amoebic dysentery. He was sent back to 17 General Hospital in Alexandria, and from there to 1 AGH at Heliopolis, for ten days to the Al Hayat Convalescent Depot at Helouan, and finally to 2 AGH at the Ghezireh Palace. There he was seen by Colonels Ryan and Manifold, who agreed that he should be returned to Australia as permanently unfit. He was transferred to the *Karoola* at Suez, and transported back to Australia. He was issued with the 1914-15 Star, the British War Medal and the Victory Medal.

Sinclair returned from the war and continued to practise in Crystal Brook working in conjunction with his sister, Florence May Orr, a nursing sister who owned the local hospital until 1926. During the 1920s Sinclair became interested in producing motor fuel from prickly pears. He went to Brisbane in 1925 to demonstrate a model for doing this. He then moved to Toowoomba Queensland and had a general practice. He had a disagreement with the Toowoomba Hospital Board over his appointment as a full honorary medical officer on the hospital staff in 1932. The issue was settled out of court. He retired in 1938. William Malcolm Sinclair died at Ashfield NSW on 23rd April 1942. He was survived by his wife and four children, one of whom, Bruce Alexander Sinclair was also a doctor. His wife died in August 1963 at Inverell NSW.

Sources:
http://recordsearch.naa.gov.au/scripts/Imagine.asp?B=8085469;
Sinclair History and photo by Heather Klose
The Adelaide Advertiser 4th June 1913
The World News Sydney 7th March 1925
Queensland Times 28 July 1932
The Adelaide Advertiser 1st June 1942

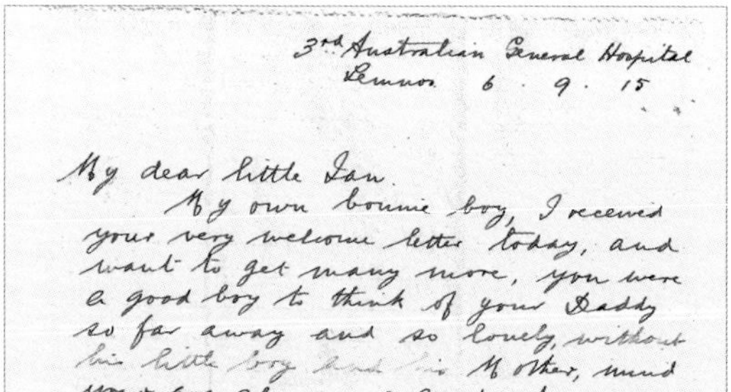

3rd Australian General Hospital
Lemnos 6 . 9 . 15

My dear little Ian.
My own bonnie boy, I received your very welcome letter today, and want to get many more, you were a good boy to think of your Daddy so far away and so lonely, without his little boy and his Mother, mind you are always a good chap, and make Mummy happy because she has so much to worry her.
I was afraid to send you a present from Egypt for your birthday as you have not been vaccinated, and Egypt is such a dirty place. But Daddy sent you many happy returns of the day a long while ago. Give Mummy many kisses for me, and look after her every day until I come back, and then we will have some fine old times, with much love from your far away Daddy.

Letter to Sinclair's son.

SMEATON Bronte

MB BS FRACS MRCS (Eng) LRCP (Lond)

1873 - 1956

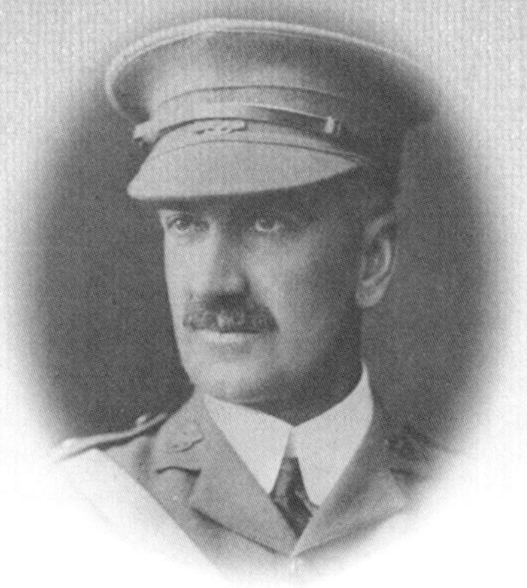

Bronte Smeaton was born on the 6th October 1873 at Menindie, South Australia. He was the second son of an English engineer Thomas Drury Smeaton and his second wife Selena, nee Witt. Thomas Smeaton was a manager of the Bank of South Australia. Smeaton was educated at Prince Alfred College and studied medicine at the University of Adelaide where he shared the Everard Scholarship with Henry Newland. He graduated in 1896 which coincided with the 'Adelaide Hospital Row' and therefore completed his residency in country hospitals at Port Augusta, and Wilgena South Australia. Smeaton went to London, and took up house appointments at The London Hospital, St Mark's and St Peter's Hospitals. He returned to Australia in 1899 and went into general practice at Murray Bridge. He was appointed Medical Superintendent of the Adelaide Hospital in 1901 and remained there until 1904. He moved to Mount Barker until he was given a position on the staff of the Adelaide Hospital as an assistant surgeon in 1910 and moved to Tynte St, later Barton Terrace and finally to Palmer Place, North Adelaide. Smeaton married twice, Elizabeth Florence Moule in 16th June 1900 at the St Peters College but she died on the 10th October 1900. He married again to Josephine Lucy Cordelia Wigley on 18th May 1904 in Glenelg and they had four children; Patricia Constance, Joan Mary, Bronte Creagh and John Anthony.

Smeaton volunteered for the AIF and was commissioned as a major in 1915. He was 41 years old, 5ft 11ins, and weighed 12st 6lbs. He sailed from Sydney in June 1915 on the *Orsova*, and joined the *Karoola* in Alexandria. His appointment was to the 1 Hospital Ship. He served on the voyage from there to England and back to Australia in 1915, and on the ship's next round trip to England. Smeaton was discharged in March 1916. Smeaton re-joined the AIF in June 1918, he was 44 years old and embarked for England in August. He arrived in October and was posted to 3 AGH at Abbeville. In May 1919 he was briefly transferred to 1 ADH at Bulford, and then just before the cessation of hostilities he returned to Australia as his eldest son, Bronte Creagh, had been in an accident. His appointment terminated on the 30th July 1919. He was issued with the 1914-15 Star, the British War Medal and the Victory Medal

Smeaton was President of the SA Branch of the BMA in 1921. After some years as an assistant surgeon, he was finally appointed an honorary surgeon at Adelaide Hospital in 1925 on Sir Arthur Cudmore's retirement and at the Repatriation General Hospital, Keswick. He became a Foundation Fellow of the RACS even though he did not possess a senior surgical qualification; *"he was a sound and practical surgeon"*. He retired in 1933. He was described as *"a man of striking appearance who possessed a ready and trenchant wit."* In his professional life it is said that *"he did not suffer fools gladly......... he did not suffer them at all"* an *"excellent raconteur"* and *"he knew how to handle troublesome neurotics with firmness and dignity without the slightest display of rudeness"*. Bronte Smeaton died 20th December 1956 survived by his wife and two of his children. His son Dr Bronte Creagh Smeaton, radiologist and surgeon, predeceased him in 1950.

Sources:

NAA: B2455, Item barcode 8086621

Lendon G. A., MJA 20th March 1957 p444

Escourt Hughes J.J., A History of the Royal Hospital. 1967.

http://recordsearch.naa.gov.au/scripts/Imagine.asp?B=8086621

Ancestry.com

German Doctors tried for looting

Even doctors belonging to the best families in Germany...They have not refrained from plundering works of art, silver plate jewels, money...

BMJ, 13 March 1915, p. 478

SMITH Walter Leonard

MC MB BS

1890 - 1971

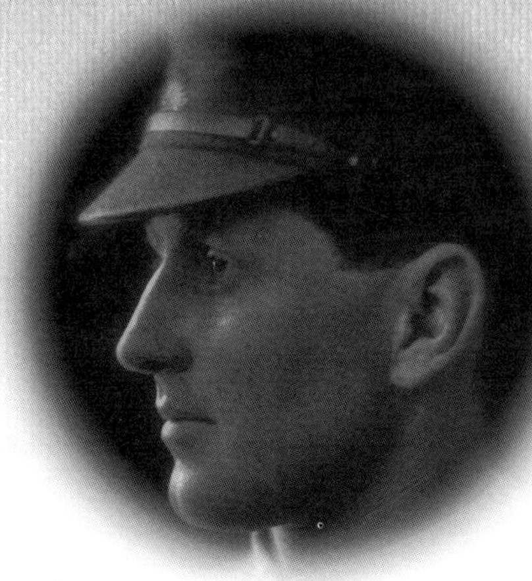

Walter Leonard (Len) Smith was born on 3rd January 1890 in Broken Hill, New South Wales. He was the son of Mr Arthur Smith, a surgeon dentist. His family moved to "Martindale" in Gawler, South Australia. He was educated at St Peter's College and studied medicine at the University of Adelaide and graduated in 1914. He then became a house surgeon at the Adelaide Hospital in February 1915.

Smith enlisted into the AAMC on 17th September 1915 with the rank of captain. He was described as being 5 feet 10 inches tall, weighed 10st 7lbs with blue eyes and black hair. Smith embarked on the *Kanowna,* although one record suggests the *Kyarra,* on 22nd December 1915. He was admitted to hospital with measles on 15th July 1916 later re-joining his unit. He was re-hospitalised in March 1917. He was attached to 13 Field Artillery Brigade as Medical Officer on 3rd February 1917 subsequently returning to his unit, 13 FdAmb, on 18th April 1917. On several occasions he was detached from FdAmb to 60 Bn Division Base Depot and other Field Ambulances. He was awarded the Military Cross in February 1918. His citation read: *"For conspicuous gallantry and devotion to duty while in charge of stretcher bearers and posts. He did significant work in attending to the wounded and organising their removal, and by his fearlessness and determination set a splendid example to the stretcher bearers."* Smith was transferred to 1 Convalescent Depot as MO on 30th August 1918. He was promoted major on 10th September 1918. He returned to Australia on the *Ceramic* disembarking in Australia on 24th September 1919. His appointment to the AIF was terminated on 16th November 1919. He was issued with the British War Medal and Victory Medal.

He married Isabel McPherson and they lived at The Parade, Norwood, South Australia, where he continued in general practice. He came under criticism from the coroner for failing to appreciate the seriousness of bed sores which contributed to the death of an elderly nursing home patient in 1947. Walter Leonard Smith died at Daw Park on 13th April 1971 aged 81 years.

Sources:

Biographical Index of South Australia 1836-1885
Resources of South Australian Genealogy and Heraldry Society Inc.
http://recordsearch.naa.gov.au/NameSearch/Interface/ItemDetail.aspx?Barcode=1790629
The Bunyip Gawler 1st December 1911
The Register Adelaide 19th December 1917
The Adelaide Advertiser 1st February 1947
Photo: CCI05092012

† SOUTER John Francis

ChM MB

1866 - 1916

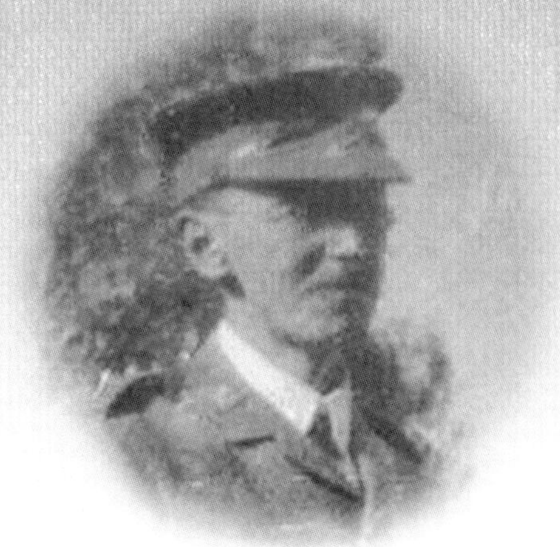

John Francis Souter was born 11th September 1866 in Aberdeen, Scotland. He was the son of John Clement Souter, general practitioner, and his wife Helen, nee Coutts. Souter an accomplished pencil and watercolour artist, collected 'rare classical books, old English china and coins'. He graduated from Aberdeen University MB ChM. Souter moved to Nottingham, England, and in 1872 to Upper Holloway, London by this time he was married with a family. Souter, with his family, immigrated to Sydney in March 1879; on the advice of Archbishop Vaughan they settled inland at Coonabarabran. They moved to Adelaide in 1896 where he became a public vaccinator.

Souter applied for a Commission in the AAMC at the age of 48 years on the 17th August 1915. He had no previous military experience but had past experience as a MO at the Hilston Hospital in NSW. He was 5ft 5ins tall and weighed 8st. His wife Agnes Emma Souter of Uraidla, South Australia was named as his next of kin. He could ride and spoke moderate French. He was accepted for one voyage in the Transport Service. Souter embarked at Adelaide on the *Star of England* on the 21st September 1915 for Egypt. He arrived in Egypt in good health but shortly after arrival he contracted dysentery and Nile fever. He recovered from the immediate effects of these illnesses and returned on the *Star of England* on Transport Service on the 27th November 1915; he did not report any illness and was discharged as he had completed his one voyage. He was admitted to a private Hospital with his present condition as "grave". He had surgery in December which disclosed a pneumococcal empyaema with a discharging sinus in the chest. The Medical Military Board concluded the cause was the abrupt climate change and ordinary military service. He died of tetanus and liver failure in a North Adelaide Hospital on the 26th February 1916. A Memorial Scroll was received by his wife Agnes Emma Souter in Oct 1921 and later a Memorial Plaque in February 1923. She was also issued with his British War Medal.

He was survived by his wife and 5 children. The following children Hugh Godfrey, Madeline Theckla, Agnes Helen, Dorothy Phyllis and his wife received War Pensions. Two other sons served in WW1. Francis Henry Souter enlisted on the 24th August 1915 and serviced in the 10, 27 and 48 Bn and was killed in action on 12th October 1917. John Herbert Ignatius Souter an 18 year old student, served as a private soldier in the 6 FdAmb. He had joined the AIF on the 10th January 1917.

Sources:
http://adb.anu.edu.au/biography/souter-charles-henry-8588/text14995
The Adelaide Advertiser 12 June 1896
Sydney Morning Herald 18th January 1890
The Adelaide Advertiser 28 February 1916
http://recordsearch.naa.gov.au/NameSearch/Interface/ItemDetail.aspx?Barcode=8087803

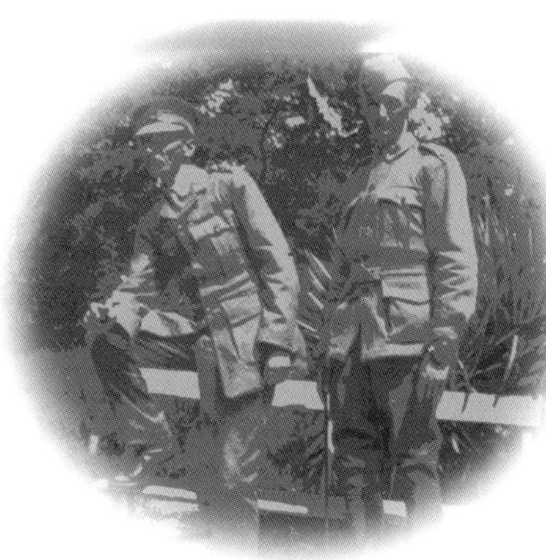

Father and Son WW1

SOUTHWOOD Albert Ray

CMG ED MS FRACP MRCP

1894 - 1973

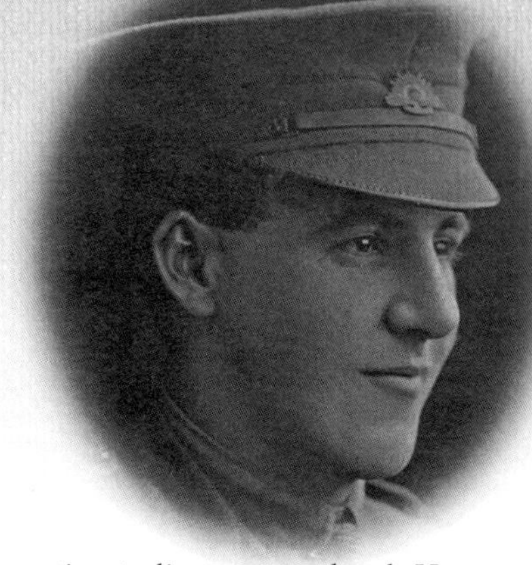

Albert Ray Southwood was born on the 15th June 1894 at Katoomba, NSW. He was the son of John Albert Southwood and Elizabeth Jane, nee Walters; his parents were married in Sydney in 1889. His father was the proprietor of the Kadina newspaper *The Plain Dealer.* John Albert Southwood had strong political views which were based on the philosophy of the Labour and Union movements surrounding the print trade. Southwood was educated at the Wallaroo Mines School where he was awarded a scholarship to Prince Alfred College. His family moved to St Peters, South Australia for the children's education. He studied medicine at the University of Adelaide and graduated in 1916.

Southwood had attempted to enlist in the AIF at the outbreak of WW1 but was advised to complete his medical training. He eventually enlisted in the AIF on the 10th October 1916 as a captain in the AAMC. He was single, aged 22 years, his mother of Fourth Avenue, St Peters South Australia was his next of kin. He had previous military experience as a lieutenant in the school cadets 1912-1916; he could not ride and spoke moderate German. He was 5ft 10ins tall, and weighed 11st in weight, of dark complexion, brown eyes and black hair. He was posted for general duty to the 1 HS *Karoola* and embarked from Melbourne on the 9th December 1916. He completed two voyages with the ships in December 1916 and January 1918. His period of service was from September 1916 to March 1919. He disembarked from *Karoola* to the 4 MD on the 13th February 1919 with his appointment terminated on the 23rd April 1919 owing to "cessation of hostilities". He was issued with the British War Medal and the Victory Medal. Southwood remained in the CMF after the war; he was CO of 8 Field Hygiene Section in 1932, and CO of 3 FdAmb from 1933 with promotion to lieutenant colonel. He was awarded the ED in 1937, and appointed CMG in 1947. During WW2 he was DDMS for 4 MD from 1940-43 with the temporary rank of colonel.

After WW1 Southwood completed his residency at Broken Hill, and then spent five years in general practice in Grote St, Adelaide from 1920-25. During this time he married Elva May Dillon at the Methodist Church Kent Town. He moved to South Terrace, Adelaide, before embarking on a career in public health. Later, in 1931, the family lived at 5 Wootoona Terrace, St Georges, next door to Malcolm Leslie Scott. Both doctors were members of the Council of the nearby Seymour College. He became Chairman of the Central Board of Health in South Australia in 1931 to 1959 and also appointed Head of the State Health Department, and ultimately Director General of Health for South Australia. He held these positions during the time TB, polio, mosquito and fly borne disease were public health issues. At the same time he was an honorary physician at Adelaide Hospital. Southwood was a devoted father, a prodigious reader with a large library and author of many articles on Public Health. Like his father he was very conscious of and compassionate for the common man. Albert Ray Southwood died in 2nd January 1973 survived by two sons and two daughters.

Sources:

http://recordsearch.naa.gov.au/scripts/Imagine.asp?B=8086882
Photo and personal history from daughter Audrey Lord and her Daughter Felicity and son Richard Southwood
Letter to the University of Adelaide dated 13th December 1916
http://www.racp.edu.au/page/library/college-roll/college-roll-detail&id=703 author R. Hecker
Chronicle Adelaide 2nd January 1947

STEELE David MacDonald

MC and Bar MB BS

1886 - 1964

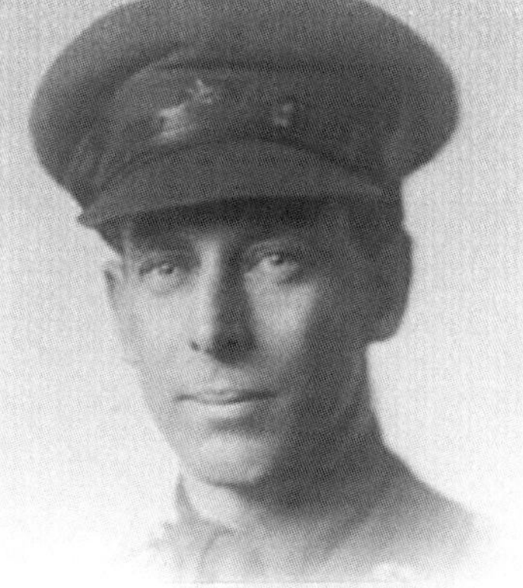

David MacDonald Steele was born on the 9th January 1886, son of Robert Moore Steele and Theresa, nee O'Leary of Jeffcott St, North Adelaide. He was educated at Prince Alfred College and studied medicine at the University of Adelaide graduating in 1909. He was a house surgeon at Brisbane General Hospital returning to South Australia where, on the 21st May 1911, he took over the practice of Alexander Ruan Caw in Burra.

Steele applied for a Commission in the AIF on the 5th October 1915 at 4 MD, Adelaide. Adelaide with his postal address, Kooringa, SA, aged 29 years, 5ft 6ins tall, and weighed 9st 2lbs. He nominated his father of Jeffcott Street, North Adelaide as his next of kin. He was posted captain to 1 AGH, Heliopolis, Egypt. He embarked from Melbourne on the 11th October 1915 arriving in England on the 5th November 1915. During his service with the AIF overseas he spent 3 months at 1 AGH in Egypt followed by 13 months as a RMO with the 16 Bn until March 1917. It was during this period that on the 25th October 1916, he was awarded the Military Cross for *conspicuous gallantry and devotion to duty when in charge of the evacuation of the wounded from a whole divisional front during thirteen days operations. On several occasions when it was impossible to bring casualties through by the existing route he personally inspected the new line of evacuation on each occasion and made admirable arrangement for getting them clear and avoiding further casualties.* His next postings were RMO to the 52 Bn for 2 months and other short postings during 1917 to 49 Bn and 52 Bn and finally 13 FdAmb. During this time, on 15th December 1917, he was awarded Bar to his Military Cross whilst attached to 49 Bn. He was promoted major in July 1918 and Mentioned in Despatches in Sir Douglas Haig's despatch of 8th November 1918. He returned to Australia in April 1919 with his service terminated on the 23rd June 1919. Steele was issued with the 1914-15 Star, the British War Medal and the Victory Medal with Oak Leaves.

Steele returned to Burra after the war and remained in practice there for over thirty years, resigning in 1946. He was the first president of the Burra High School Council and retained this post for 26 years. Steele House won the High School Swimming Carnival just prior to his death and a minutes silence was observed. He showed a keen interest in education and encouraged *"give boys and girls every chance, this was a duty parents owed the child and the nation"* He was interested in golf, tennis and bowls in Burra and his Koo-owie Merino Stud which he relinquished in 1963 to Barton Hill Proprietors. David MacDonald Steele died on the 25th February 1964, aged 78 years, at Tusmore, South Australia. He was survived by his wife, two sons Dr D M Steele of Strathalbyn and Mr J R Steele and a daughter Mrs George Mollard-Humphrys. His brothers Dr Kenneth Nugent Steele and Dr Donald MacDonald Steele also served in WW1.

Sources:

http://recordsearch.naa.gov.au/scripts/Imagine.asp?B=8093787
Burra History Group
Burra Record 2nd October 1918
Burra Record 15th October 1946
Burra Record 3rd March 1964
Photo: PAC Collection, Steele in his car

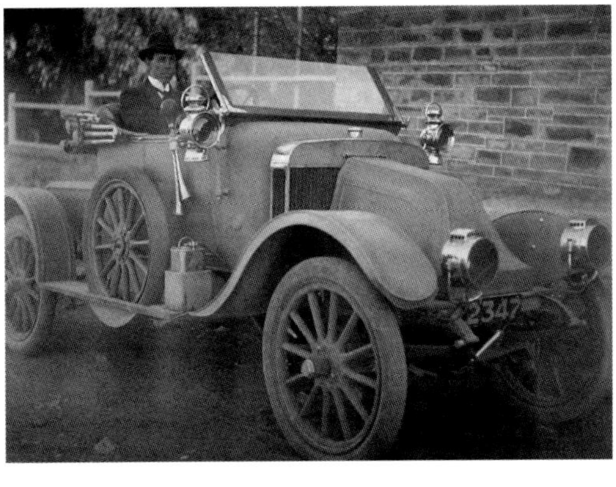

STEELE Donald MacDonald

MB BS

1893 - 1962

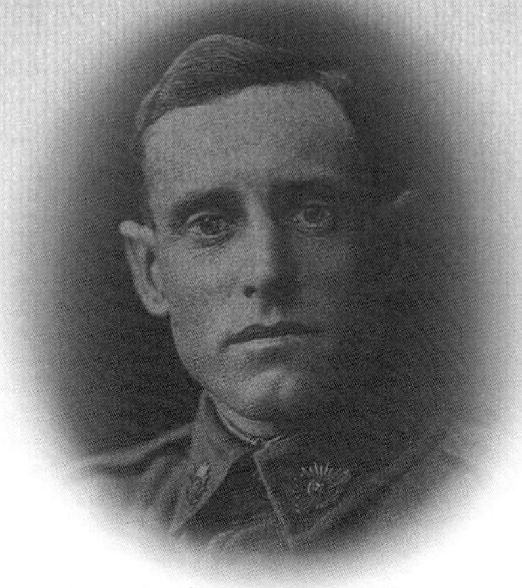

Donald MacDonald Steele was born in Adelaide on the 17th August 1892, son of Robert Moore Steele and his wife Theresa, nee O'Leary, of Jeffcott St, North Adelaide. His brothers were David McDonald Steele and Kenneth Nugent Steele. His parents had married at Norwood in 1875. His father was with the Liverpool, London Globe Insurance Company in the city and was also the Consul for Portugal. Steele was educated at Prince Alfred College and had some private tuition in his Science subjects for the March 1914 University entrance Examinations. He was the school captain in 1911 and an excellent athlete especially as captain of cricket, tennis and football for several years. He represented the State in cricket as a school boy under the mentoring of Clem Hill then the state captain. He studied medicine at the University of Adelaide where he acquired a Sports Blue in cricket and football.

Steele enlisted in the AIF on the 19th June 1918 at Adelaide as a 4th Year medical student, single, aged 24 years with his father as nominated as his next of kin. He was 5ft 5ins tall, 125lbs, of medium complexion, blue eyes and brown hair with normal vision. He had two years' experience in the sea cadets. He was not called up for duty and discharged as a private, B Coy, Mitcham AIF, on 18th November 1918 due to the cessation of hostilities.

Steele continued with his studies and graduated in 1919 after his discharge. He became the captain of the South Australian Cricket team in 1921 and on the 23rd November 1921 he married Winifred Ringwood at Christchurch, North Adelaide, and moved to Port Lincoln to join in a general practice with Dr Reg Goode. He was a keen gardener and played consistently at a high standard in golf and lawn bowls. He lived in Glenelg, South Australia from 1937. Donald MacDonald Steele died on the 16th July 1962 and was survived by his wife Winifred and children Ian, a doctor, and Janet.

Sources:

http://recordsearch.naa.gov.au/scripts/Imagine.asp?B=8093787
Personal information from son Dr Ian Steele,
Photo: Family collection taken after enlistment 1918.
The Register Adelaide 20 December 1921

The Duty of the Profession to the Army

In the first place we have no hesitation in advising that for medical men who have no urgent domesticities, and are not yet established in practice, especially, that is to say, for young men, the duty is clear. They should put their names on the waiting list kept by the Director-General Army Medical Services, at the War Office... The Director-General's list at present contains about 1,000 names of men deemed fit to undertake the arduous work of service in the field. This number, we learn on high authority, is not enough; the list is constantly being depleted, not only by men who are called up by the War Office, but by men who, getting impatient, go to France to help the French.

BMJ, 21 November 1914, p. 884

STEELE Kenneth Nugent

MB BS

1889 - 1956

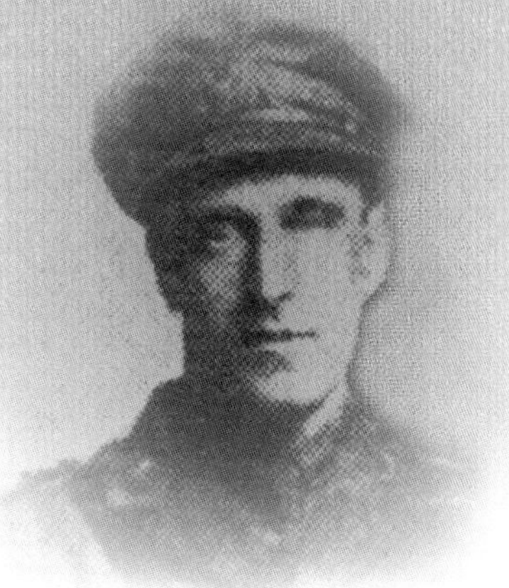

Kenneth Nugent Steele was born in Adelaide South Australia, on the 17th December 1889 son of Robert Moore Steele and his wife Theresa, nee O'Leary. His brothers were David Macdonald Steele and Donald Macdonald Steele. He was educated at Prince Alfred College and studied medicine at the University of Adelaide graduating in 1914. He then completed his residency at the Adelaide Hospital.

He enlisted in the AIF and was commissioned 19th May 1915. He was 5ft 9ins, and weighed 10st 10lbs. He had served as a lieutenant in the Cadet Corps whilst at school. His father was named as his next of kin. This later changed to his wife care of the Commonwealth Bank, London. He was sent to Egy.pt with reinforcements for 1 AGH. He embarked on the *Georgian* as SMO in August 1915 which was detailed to evacuate casualties from Gallipoli to Malta. Steele reported the very poor conditions suffered on this voyage when he arrived in Malta and the *Georgian* was withdrawn from service. On his return to Mudros in late September he was detached to the British 29 (Lowland) CCS which set up a convalescent depot for 1000 cases. Steele was posted to 3 AGH in November and remained on the strength of this unit for the next year, leaving it only as it was about to deploy to Abbeville from Brighton in March 1917. Whilst in England on 6th April 1917 Steele married Norah Elizabeth Taylor at St Peter's Church in Brighton. At that time he was posted to 3 AAH at Dartford, where he remained for another 12 months. He was promoted to major in June 1917. He was sent to France to join 8 FdAmb 5 Div in March 1918, then at Corbie, close to the confluence of the Rivers Somme and Ancre. A month later, and the day after the Australian success at Villers-Bretonneux, he was detached to 56 Bn (14 Bde). Within a few days he was gassed, and evacuated to 8 GH at Rouen, and from there to 3 LGH. He spent three months in hospital before being invalided back to Australia in July. Back home he was admitted to 4 AGH at Randwick, and then 5 AGH at St Kilda, and finally discharged in November 1918. He was issued with the 1914-15 Star, The British War Medal and the Victory Medal

Steele returned to his practice at Glenelg, in spite of his injury. In 1947 he was still living in Moseley Street, Glenelg and had his car drugs and instruments stolen. Kenneth Nugent Steele died in Glenelg on 19th December 1956. He and his wife Norah are buried together in the Mitcham Church of England Cemetery.

Sources:

http://recordsearch.naa.gov.au/scripts/Imagine.asp?B=8089321graduated

Likeman R.,"Gallipoli Doctors" Slouch Hat Publications, 2010.

Photo: Prince Alfred College

The Adelaide Advertiser 15th June 1917

The Mail Adelaide 10th August 1946

Ancestry.com

STEELE SCOTT Frederick

MB BCh BAO (RUI)

1873 - 1931

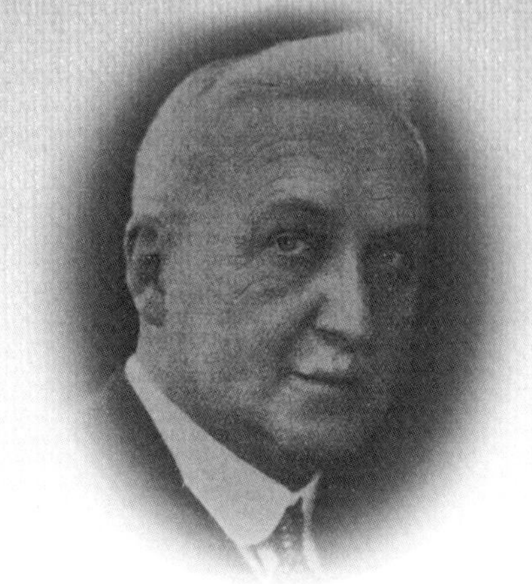

Frederick Steele Scott was born in Drumclamph, County Tyrone, Ireland on 13th September 1873. He was educated at the Royal University of Ireland and, after graduation, spent a period in England and as a ship's doctor and came to South Australia. He worked in the practice of his brother-in-law, Dr Arthur Kyle Gault in 1900 whilst Gault took his wife and 3 children to England for 12 months. He married Florence Love on the 13th September 1906 and from 1913 to 1916 he was an assistant surgeon at the Adelaide Hospital.

Steele Scott enlisted on the 1st November 1916; he was living in Unley Rd, Malvern. He was allotted to the 5 Sea Transport Section of the AAMC at the rank of major. He was aged 43 years, 5ft 11ins, and weighed 182lbs. He had been an honorary captain and area officer for 5 years. He could ride, speak French and his speciality was surgery. His first voyage was from Sydney on 25th November 1916 on the *Beltana* bound for Davenport, England and then from Adelaide on 23rd June 1917 to Plymouth disembarking 25th August 1917. Whilst overseas he was posted to Training Depot Parkhouse and 2 AAH between voyages. He appeared to do most of his sea time on board *Beltana*. His appointment was terminated at his request on 23rd July 1918 and he was issued the British War Medal.

After the war Steele Scott took a keen interest in the SA state branch of the BMA both as a member, on the Council and as President. He was on the Board of Health of the Unley Council. He was also involved with The Royal British Nurses Association (RBNA) (Australian Branch) and several Community based committees including that of surgeon to three local Racing Clubs. His patients regarded him as a friend as well as a medical advisor and he won and preserved the confidence of a wide circle of acquaintances. For many years he practiced in Unley and later in North Terrace, Adelaide. He had a love of floriculture, tennis and cricket. He returned to England to further his study in skin diseases in 1925 and during that time he also established his elder son, John, at Cambridge. Frederick Steele Scott died on the 6th June 1931; he lived at Gilberton and was survived by his wife and two sons.

Sources:

http://recordsearch.naa.gov.au/scripts/Imagine.asp?B=3002964;

Russell H H E, Obituary Frederick Steele Scott MJA, p117, July 25th 1931.

Photo: Ramsey Amy J., "One Hundred Years of Medical Practice The story of Ardmeen at 146 Belair Road Hawthorn" 1966.

The Advertiser 9th June 1931 p8.03

STOKES Alfred Francis

MB BS

1881 - 1943

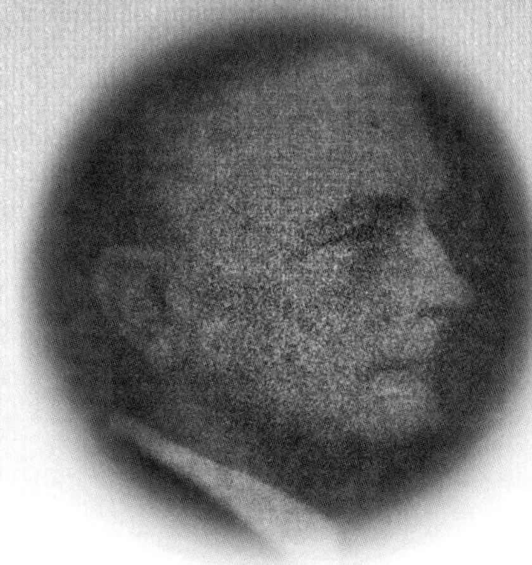

Alfred Francis Stokes was born on the 3rd July 1881, at Port Augusta the second son of the Rev Francis Herbert Stokes and Florence, nee Giles. He was educated at St Peter's College and graduated from Adelaide University with MB BS in 1904. He spent one year at the Adelaide Hospital as a house surgeon, then undertook some locums in South Australia. He proceeded to England and spent a year at the Hospital for Sick Children, Great Ormond St, London and as a Clinical Assistant at the Chelsea Hospital, London, and, later, in Vienna during 1907-1908. Stokes married Barbara Jessop of Barton Terrace, North Adelaide at St Magdalene Church on the 5th June 1912; the Rev Canon Hornabrook, the bride's uncle, officiated and Rupert Eric Magarey was his best man.

Stokes enlisted on the 12th July 1915 for one year to expire on the 26th August 1916. He was 34 years old, 5ft 11ins, weighed 12st 8lbs, and could ride. His wife of 24 Moseley St, Glenelg was nominated as his next of kin. He had been active in the AAMC Reserve from 1911 to 1914. He was appointed captain on the 26th August 1915 and posted to 1 AGH at Heliopolis, Egypt. He then went to the 7th F Amb then to the 6th on the 23rd Feb 1916 and on the 19th May detailed as the 6th Bde gas officer. He had two casualty episodes: in Nov 1915 to 3 Aux Con Depot with diarrhoea and on the 28th July 1916 invalided to England for one month with gastritis and was transferred to 1st AAH on the 24th August. He was discharged from the London General Hospital on 31 October 1916 after a week in hospital with gastritis. Stokes requested to the DMS whilst in France with the 6 FdAmb for a return to Australia before January 1917. His locum had applied for active service and he was needed both for financial reasons and for the family. If he did not return there would be only one doctor in the district. His request was accepted. Nigel Basil Gresley Abbott was posted in lieu on his departure. His appointment was terminated in Australia on the 22nd December 1916. He was issued with the 1914-15 Star, the British War Medal and the Victory Medal. Stokes youngest brother, Francis Herbert Stokes, was killed at the landing at Gallipoli in 1915.

After his discharge he was of indifferent health until his death at the age of 62 from a heart attack. Despite persistent heart pain as his age progressed, he was very active in the BMA, and became President of the SA Branch of the BMA in 1936. He was also on the Federal Council of the BMA. Stokes was involved with The Royal Flying Doctor Service and the St John's Ambulance Brigade. The Federal Council said of Stokes that *"he was a clear and logical thinker, always courteous in debate, his politeness to others never led to the deviation from a course he believed to be right"* Alfred Francis Stokes died on the 1st July 1943 at Glenelg, South Australia. He was survived by his wife and two sons who both served in WW2, Dr John Lewis Stokes as a Captain in the famous Z Special Unit, and Robert Francis Stokes as a Captain in 27 Bn.

Sources:
http://recordsearch.naa.gov.au/scripts/Imagine.asp?B=8095027
Likeman R., 2014, "No time for Regrets: Australian Doctors of the Western Front", Rosenberg Press.
MJA 14th August 1943 p 138, by Henry Newland,
The Adelaide Advertiser 2nd July 1943.
The Chronicle Adelaide 17th December 1898

STRACHAN James Charles Power

MB BS

1889 - 1959

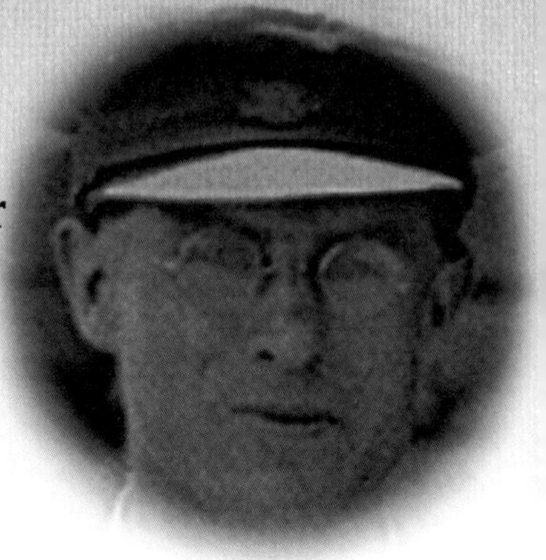

James Charles Power Strachan was born on 10th November 1889 in North Adelaide, the second son of a merchant, Roland Strachan, and his wife Edith Maud, nee Tuckett. He was educated at St Peter's College and served in the school cadets from 1906 to 1908, rising to the rank of 2nd lieutenant, before entering the University of Adelaide where he studied medicine. He graduated in 1914.

Strachan applied for a commission in the AIF on the 3rd March 1915. He was 25 years, single, 6ft tall, weighed 160lbs, and his father, of 172 Childers St, North Adelaide, was his next of kin. Strachan was sent to Egypt with reinforcements for 1 AGH, but immediately on arrival transferred to B Section of 7 FdAmb. He went to Gallipoli in September, where his unit relieved 4 FdAmb at Walden Grove. He spent some weeks detached to 1 LHFA. He was evacuated to Egypt in November with influenza but rejoined 7 FdAmb at the beginning of December. After several brief attachments to infantry Bns, he went to France with 7 FdAmb in March 1916. During the early stages of the Somme offensive, Strachan was briefly attached to 3 ACCS, but in August he was posted as RMO of 26 Bn. He was with the Bn through the series of unsuccessful attacks on Mouquet Farm. A month later he was evacuated with trench fever. He returned to the Bn in October as it moved back to the Somme from Ypres, and in time for the Battle of Flers and the attack on The Maze in November. Strachan again fell ill in Jan 1917, this time with mumps. After a variety of short term postings in the rear echelons, he was promoted major and posted to 16 FdAmb in 6 Div. After the losses of Bullecourt and Messines, the formation of 6 Div was abandoned, and Strachan was sent to 14 FdAmb which had lost three officers during the attacks on Polygon Wood. He remained with the unit until after the successful capture of Villers-Bretonneux on April 25th 1918. He was then recalled to England and posted to 1 ADH at Bulford on the Salisbury Plain, where he married Eleanor Marjory Isabel Tapp from Bath, Somerset in June 1918. Strachan obtained leave to attend a course at the Rotunda Hospital in Dublin after the Armistice. His appointment in the AIF was terminated at the 4th MD on the 13th February 1920. He was issued with the 1914-15 Star, the British War Medal and the Victory Medal. Strachan's older brother Captain William Leighton Strachan (6 Bn), aged 27 years, was killed on Bolton's Ridge on the 25th April 1915, a short time after the landing at Anzac Cove.

Strachan returned to Australia in October 1919 with his wife and first child, David Edgar who had been born in Salisbury in June. The family moved to Creswick, Victoria in 1920, where he set up practice. Strachan and his wife featured many times in the social pages of the newspaper. James Charles Power Strachan died in Creswick in 1959. He was survived by his wife and son. Strachan's son David Strachan, a celebrated Australian painter, was killed in a car accident in 1970.

Sources:

http://recordsearch.naa.gov.au/scripts/Imagine.asp?B=8092689
Likeman R., "Gallipoli Doctors" Slouch Hat Publications, 2010.
The Adelaide Advertiser 12 October 1904
The Adelaide Advertiser 16 March 1909
The Register Adelaide 12 February 1915
The Advertiser Adelaide 5 December 1934
Ancestry.com

The Effect of the War on the Price of Drugs

The scarcity of some of the more important drugs since the commencement of the war, on account of our dependence upon Germany for the production of many of them, has resulted in a very considerable inconvenience and in the establishment of fabulously high prices.

MJA, 17 June 1916, p. 489

STRANGMAN Cecil Lucius

LRCP LRCS(Dublin) DTM&H

1867 - 1942

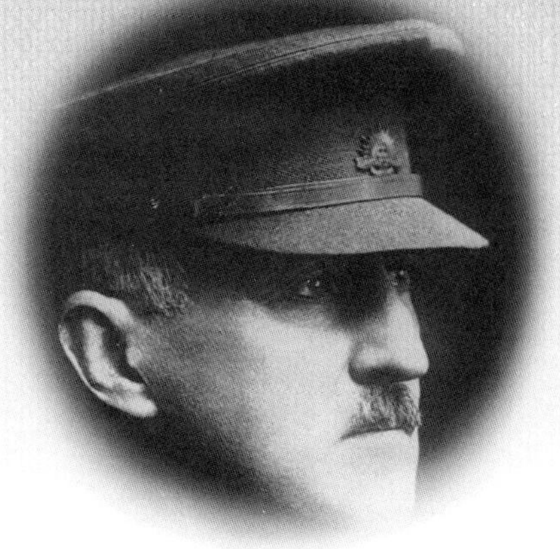

Cecil Lucius Strangman was born on the 1st August 1867 at Lissclan, near Tranmere, County Waterford, Ireland. He was the fourth son of the nine children of Thomas Strangman and wife Sarah White, nee Hawkes. Strangman graduated in medicine and surgery in Dublin in 1888; a brother and two sisters also became doctors. He began his career as a ship's surgeon which brought him to Port Adelaide in South Australia on the *SS State of Georgia*. He was registered as a medical practitioner in South Australia on the 7th August 1890. Here he worked at Port Lincoln, Carrieton, and Orroroo. Strangman met and married Edith Adelaide Moody in Orroroo in 1894 and stayed there for 16 years, then moved on to Port Darwin in 1907 as Medical Officer for the Northern Territory and the Protector of Aborigines. He attended post graduate study in London in 1909 and 1912 and obtained the Diploma in Tropical Medicine and Hygiene. He returned to Darwin, but by 1914, disagreed with the policies of the Administrator of the Northern Territory who abolished the Central Board of Health. Strangman resigned from his position. He had shown great empathy with the Chinese community whilst in Darwin and when he left, they presented him with a testimonial banner which was in the possession of the District Council of Waikerie, South Australia. He and his family returned to Cheltenham St, Malvern, South Australia in September 1913.

Strangman enlisted as a major in the AAMC on 22nd October 1914 as he had previous military experience with the SA Mounted Rifles, the 17 LH and 4 FdAmb. He was 47 years old, 5ft 10ins, and weighed 13st. In view of his expertise in tropical medicine, he was transferred to the AN&MEF which occupied the German Territories in the Pacific. He arrived in Rabaul in December 1914 during the wet season and malaria spread rapidly. He was made PMO and promoted to brevet colonel. His expertise in tropical medicine was invaluable and he remained in Rabaul until he took leave to return to Australia in 1917. He was returning from Sydney in the Burns Philp, *Matunga*, when, on the 6th August 1917, she was captured by the German raider *Wolf*. Nothing was known of the ship, its passengers or crew for five months as the *Wolf* roamed and caused havoc in the Indo-Pacific and Atlantic oceans with up to 200 prisoners on board. Also on board was John Wellesley Flood. Later, some prisoners, including Strangman and Flood, were transferred to another ship, a captured Spanish collier, which, whilst travelling north to Germany, on the 23rd February 1918, ran aground on the Danish coast near Skegen. The Danish authorities insisted on the release of the prisoners who reached London via Norway and the Shetland Islands on 10th March 1918. After release Strangman was in poor health and spent some time in the 3rd London General Hospital while his family resided in Ireland. He returned to Australia in December 1918 with his Service terminated in February 1919. He was issued with the British War Medal.

Strangman, using his newly acquired knowledge from courses in London, during recuperation from captivity, undertook the management of shell shocked soldiers by psychotherapy in major Australian Military Hospitals for the next 2 years. He settled in Glenelg in medical practice later retiring to the Adelaide Hills. Cecil Lucius Strangman died at Stirling West on 21st April 1942 and was cremated. He was survived by his wife and son John Handcock Strangman.

Sources:

http://recordsearch.naa.gov.au/scripts/Imagine.asp?B=8094484

NT Index of Biography. Written by daughter and son in law.

Guilliatt R., Hohnen P., "The Wolf"

Photo: SLSA, B26285_214

http://www.territorystories.nt.gov.au/handle/10070/226507

STUCKEY Edward Joseph

OBE MB BS BSc

1875 - 1952

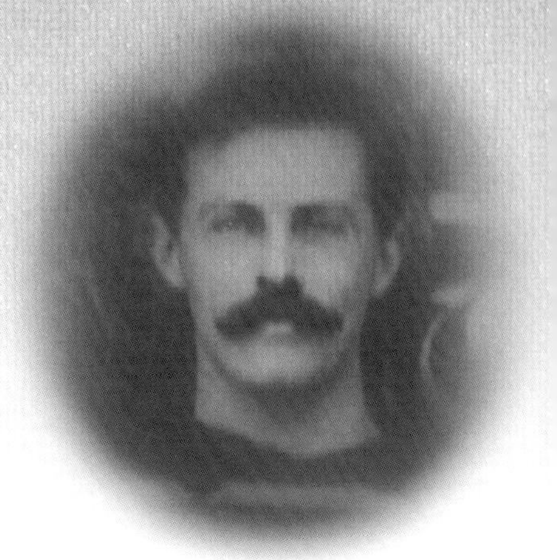

Edward Joseph Stuckey was born in Adelaide in 1875. He was the eldest of the ten children of Joseph James Stuckey, a solicitor, and Alice, nee Mann. He, along with Oliver Leitch, were appointed University Scholars in 1893 as they completed the first year of a BSc degree. He commenced his medical degree in 1899 graduating in 1904. He then worked as a house officer in the Adelaide Hospital for one year until the 31st January 1905. He married Frances Helen Campbell, the third daughter of J. M. Campbell of Kew in the Presbyterian Church, Kew, Victoria, on 12th July 1905. He was accepted by the London Missionary Society and proceeded to China in 1905. Four years later he was appointed to the Union Medical College in Peking. He continued his missionary work there but also became involved in the medical education of Chinese students. In the Brisbane Courier it was reported that Edward had withdrawn his application for exemption to serve in WWI but had applied for a three month exemption on the 1st November 1916.

Stuckey enlisted in the RAMC in 1916 as a 2nd lieutenant in charge of one of the Chinese Labour Battalions. At the time of enlistment his address was Walnut House, Long Sutton, Longport, Somerset, England. He served in France and Flanders and was promoted to temporary captain in 1918 and temporary major in 1919. He was Mentioned in Despatches and appointed OBE for his services as an ophthalmic surgeon in Noyelle. He was issued with the British War Medal and Victory Medal with Oak Leaves.

Stuckey returned to Australia after the war and was given a farewell in Stow Church before returning to China in 1920. He was accompanied by his wife and three children. He was greatly assisted by his wife. He was reported as being a missionary along with many others associated with the University of Adelaide in 1936. He died in Kew, Victoria on 19th August 1952. He was survived by his wife and five children.

Sources:
http://www.forces-war-records.co.uk
South Australian Register 21st March 1893,
1st December 1899, 31st July 1905, 23rd January 1926
The Advertiser 23rd February 1904
Brisbane Courier 1st November 1916
Northern Argus 26th June 1936
Royal Adelaide Hospital archives

Royal Navy Medical Service [RN]

Surgeons for temporary service in the Royal Navy are required. They will be paid 32s a day, *plus* allowances and equipment allowance for uniform. Their age must not exceed 40 years...

Uniform

Each Surgeon to provide himself as follows:

- Frock coat, waistcoat and trousers
- Undress coat
- Uniform cap
- Mess jacket and waistcoat
- Sword and undress belt
- All as specified in the Uniform regulations.
- To cover the above each officer accepted for service will receive an Equipment allowance of £20, payable on the officer's being called up for active service.
- The following instruments must be provided by the Surgeon

  A Pocket Case of Instruments

  A Stethoscope

  Three clinical thermometers.

BMJ, 8 August 1914, p. 317

STUMP Claude Witherington

FRS(Ed) DSc MD

1891 - 1971

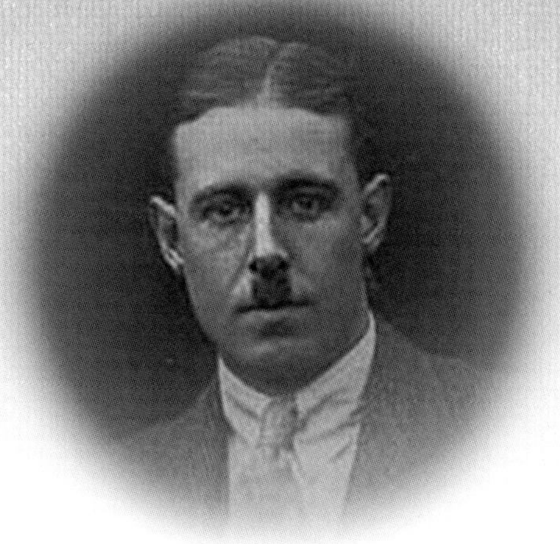

Claude Witherington Stump was born on 28th November 1891 at Malvern, South Australia. He was the second son of Alfred Augustus Stump, a photographer from Tasmania, and his second wife Rosa Ada, nee Potter from South Australia. Their address was "Stonehenge" Austral Terrace, Malvern. He was educated at Kyre College, Unley, South Australia. He travelled to Scotland and enrolled in medicine at Edinburgh University in 1909. Before completing his studies, he served from 1912 to 1913, with a British Red Cross Society unit, which was attached to the Serbian Army during the Balkan War. On return to Edinburgh and at the outbreak of WW1 he served as a lieutenant in the King's Own Scottish Borderers and served in France from 1914 to 1916 at Loos and the Somme. He returned to Edinburgh and completed his medical degree and graduated MB ChB in 1917. He was a house officer and then resident surgeon for Mr Miles in the Royal Infirmary in Edinburgh from late 1916 until his return to Adelaide.

Stump enlisted as a captain in the AIF on 4th November 1917 and was posted to AAMC reinforcements at Mitcham Camp, Adelaide. He was 26 years of age 5ft 9ins, tall 154 lbs. He was proficient in both the German and Serbian language. He embarked in 4 MD on the *Borda* on the 5th January 1918 disembarking in Plymouth on 4th March 1918. After periods with training units in Grantham and Parkhouse he embarked for France at Southampton on 1st of June 1918. He was posted to the 2 AGH until the 4th June 1918 when he proceeded to the 3rd Australian Division joining the 11 FdAmb with a temporary attachment to the 9 FdAmb. He had leave in the United Kingdom from 9th to 23rd November 1918. He returned to England in anticipation of return to Australia on 15th April 1919. He had leave to attend the Royal Infirmary, Edinburgh from 26th April to 26th July for medical education purposes. Following further short leave periods he joined the *Plassy* for return to Australia, classed as fit with no disability. He disembarked in Australia on 23rd October 1919. His appointment to the AIF was terminated on the 22nd November 1919. He was issued with the British War Medal and Victory Medal.

Stump took up a research fellowship in anatomy in Edinburgh from 1920 to 1922 working also as a house physician and surgeon, as well as lecturer and demonstrator in anatomy. During this time he gained his MD and was awarded the FRS(Ed). He married Christina Margaret Calder Urquhart on 30th November 1920. He was appointed to the Chair of Anatomy at Chulalongkorn University, Thailand in 1924. He was subsequently appointed an Associate Professor at Sydney University in 1926. He was responsible for developing his discipline of histology and embryology by gaining two important endowments from George Bosch and the Rockefeller Foundation. This led to the building of the Blackburn Building of the Sydney University's medical school. Stump continued as the Bosch Professor of histology and embryology until he retired in 1956. He was passionate about the independence of the disciplines of histology and embryology and was known to be quite demanding in his relationships with students and colleagues. His address in 1939 was given as Elva Avenue, Killara, New South Wales. His wife Christina died in 1965 and Claude Witherington Stump died on 23rd December 1971 at Mona Vale. He was survived by his daughter and two sons.

Sources:
National Archives of Australia
http://recordsearch.naa.gov.au/NameSearch/Interface/ItemDetail.aspx?Barcode=8095718
Stone J., Australian Dictionary of Biography, Vol. 16, 2002.
http://adb.anu.edu.au/biography/stump-claude-witherington-11797
Photo: Winter 1916-1917. Royal Infirmary Edinburgh
LOTHIAN HEALTH SERVICES Archive

SWEENEY James Gladstone

MB BS

1894 - 1977

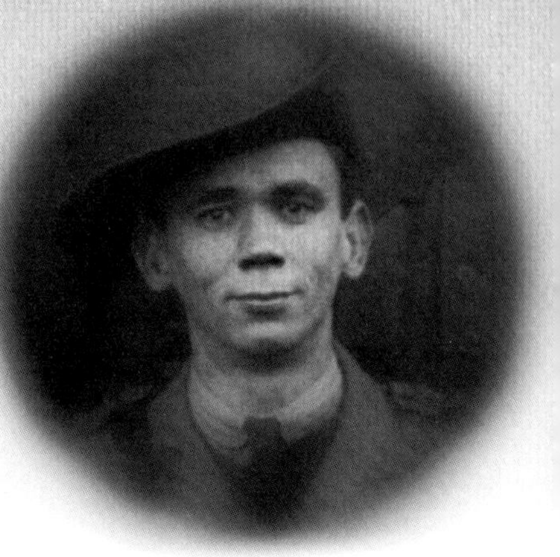

James Gladstone Sweeney was born on the 9th January 1894 at Springbank, Clarence Park, Adelaide. He was the son of John and Isabella Sweeney of Albert Park, SA. Sweeney had three brothers and two sisters. He was educated at Adelaide High School where he won a Bursary to the University of Adelaide where he studied medicine and graduated in 1915.

Sweeney enlisted in the AIF on the 8th October 1915 as a captain, aged 22 years, single, with three weeks experience as a resident at the Adelaide Hospital. His father, then of Nottingham Terrace, Glandore, was recorded as his next of kin. Previously he was a senior cadet for 1 year and in the Citizen Forces as Corporal in 19 AAMC for 4 years. He was 5ft 10ins, weighed 11st 4lbs, and could ride. He was allocated to 11 FdAmb with Michael Henry Downey as the CO. He embarked on the 31st May 1916 and arrived at Devonport, England and after 4 months proceeded to France on the 24th November 1916. He returned to England to hospital with bronchitis and after two weeks re-joined the unit as OC. He was transferred to 10 FdAmb in France on the 25th May 1917 but was wounded in action with a gunshot wound to the right loin on the 7th June 1917. He was taken to England for treatment and returned to duty with 11 FdAmb, in France, on the 6th October 1917. Sweeney was posted in the field to be the CO of 3 ADAC until the end of hostilities. He was recommended for a Military Cross for *"coolness and gallantry under fire and set a splendid example to his men"*, however, it was not awarded. He was granted leave in England for 3 months and returned to Australia on the *Zealand* on the 3rd July 1919 on duty as ships staff. He arrived in 4 MD in September 1919 with his appointment terminated on the 14th October 1919. Sweeney was issued with the British War Medal and the Victory Medal.

Following discharge from the Army he completed his residency at the Adelaide Hospital and then moved to Orroroo as a general practitioner in 1920 where Dr Ray Last (later Professor) was a partner. He married Mina Kathleen Ballantyne, the Matron of the Orroroo Hospital, on the 14th April 1926. They had five children, three of whom became doctors and two nurses. The family moved to Adelaide in 1935 where he practiced at Croydon until he retired. During the WW2 he served as a reserve medical officer at Warradale. In 1969 his address was 9 Sturt Place, Beaumont, South Australia. He was the President of the 11th Field Ambulance Returned Soldiers Club for 25 years. James Gladstone Sweeney died on the 22nd April 1977. The 11th Field Ambulance Returned Soldiers Club disbanded after his death and at their final meeting they allocated £20.00 to the War Veterans Home at Myrtle Bank and all matters of historical interest were handed to the RSL, Adelaide.

Sources

http://recordsearch.naa.gov.au/scripts/Imagine.asp?B=8097384
Photo; AWM
Personal family story from son Dr Don Sweeney
The register Adelaide 24th September 1915

SWIFT Sir Brian Herbert

MC MD MA FRCS(Ed) FRACS FRCOG

1893 - 1969

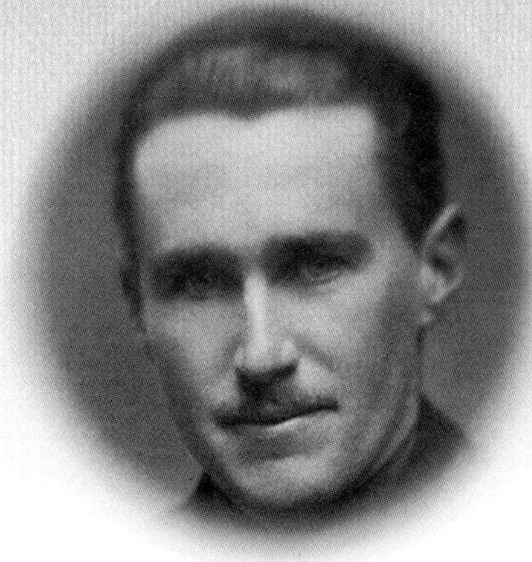

Brian Herbert Swift was born on 2nd February 1893 in Adelaide. He was the second son of Harry Swift, a medical practitioner from England, and his South Australian-born wife Kate Marion Lilian, nee Peacock. He was educated at St Peter's College. Swift studied science for a year in 1907 at the University of Adelaide before going to England to study medicine at Caius College, Cambridge.

Swift joined the RAMC on 2nd August 1916 and was promoted from lieutenant to captain within a year. After a brief period at Leith, near Edinburgh, Swift went to the Western Front. He was awarded the Military Cross in 1918 for his *'splendid example of courage and determination'* under enemy fire. Swift transferred to the Royal Air Force in September 1918. Swift's younger brother Neville Swift DSO MC also went to England after the outbreak of WWI and was commissioned in the East Lancashire Regiment on 26 June 1915. During the fighting in December 1917 he was awarded the Military Cross. In January 1918 he won a Bar to his MC and was promoted acting major. Two months later he was wounded and died next day. He was awarded the DSO and Mentioned in Despatches.

Swift returned to Adelaide where he entered general practice and took up appointments as an anaesthetist at the Adelaide Children's Hospital, as senior obstetrician at the Queen's Home and as a lecturer in obstetrics at the University of Adelaide. He was winner of the South Australian Amateur Golf Championship in 1924, and later captain and president of the Royal Adelaide Golf Club. Swift travelled to Britain in 1925 to study obstetrics and gain his Fellowship of the Royal College of Surgeons, Edinburgh. He also studied obstetrics in Vienna. He returned to Adelaide in 1928, and continued his consultant position in public hospitals and obstetrics and gynaecology in particular. He was made a fellow of the Royal Australasian College of Surgeons in 1931. Swift married Joan Royal Tennant on 5th April 1934 at the St Peter's College Chapel; they had a son and daughter. He visited Cambridge in 1936 to successfully present his doctoral thesis. He continued to go overseas to progress his professional career and, in 1937, he was elected a Fellow of the RCOG. Swift served in the AAMC in WW2 and, on 1st November 1940, Swift was promoted to major. He served from 1941 to 1942 in the Middle East. He transferred to the Reserve of Officers list on 24 July 1943, when he became the consultant gynaecologist to the Royal Australian Air Force until 1945. He was knighted in 1954 for his service to public hospitals and the University of Adelaide. His son, Brian T Swift, aged 19 years, a second year medical student, was killed in a road accident in England in 1958. Sir Brian Herbert Swift died on 19th May 1969 at his Medindie home and was buried in the North Road cemetery. He was survived by his wife and their daughter.

Sources:

Harford J., Hicks N., 'Swift, Sir Brian Herbert (1893–1969)', Australian Dictionary of Biography.

Medical Journal of Australia, 20 Sept 1969.

Photo: from Family

The Register Adelaide 15th December 1906The Chronicle Adelaide 11 December 1920

The Adelaide Advertiser 10th December 1936

The Broken Hill Barrier 2nd January 1954

Open-Air Hospitals in War-Time

Robert Saundby, MD FRCP

Why have we been so slow to recognize that fresh air is the best tonic, the best antiseptic? It is cheaper, pleasanter, and undoubtedly more efficient than drugs.

BMJ, 19 September 1914, p. 493

SYMONS Eric Lindsay

MB BS

1893 - 1971

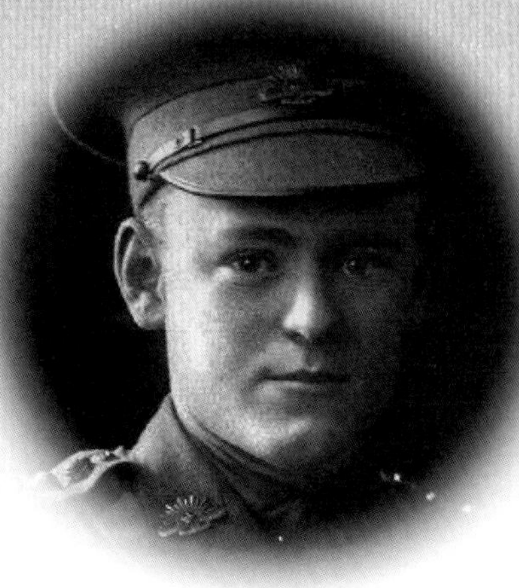

Eric (Brickie) Lindsay Symons was born on 16th June 1893 in Port Augusta the son of William Symons and Alice Anderson, nee Westwood the daughter of David Westwood. He was educated at St Peter's College and he studied medicine at the University of Adelaide, graduating in July 1917. He was the cox of the eight for the University of Adelaide team which finished second in 1914, in what was to be the last Universities Rowing Championship until after the war.

Symons joined the AIF on 7th August 1917 within a month of his medical registration. He had previously served in the cadets. He was 5ft 3½ins tall, and weighed 124lbs. Following training at Mitcham Camp he embarked on the *Borda* in Adelaide on 5th January 1918 and disembarked in Plymouth on 4th March 1918. He was attached to the 5th Training Battalion. He was admitted to Fovant Military Hospital on 15th April 1918 and discharged on 20th April. He proceeded to France on the 31st May 1918 via Folkstone and he was attached to 2 AGH. He was attached to the 22nd Corps Mounted Troops on 22nd June. He was posted to 13 LHR on 14th December 1918 and subsequently on 21st December to 2 FdAmb. Following leave in England from 4th January to 18th January 1919 he was attached to the 2nd Division and marched out to England for return to Australia. He joined the embarkation group from Devonport on the *Ulysses* on 12th July 1919 disembarking in Perth on 20th August 1919. His appointment was terminated on the 24th September 1919. He was issued with the British War Medal and the Victory Medal.

After the war Symons spent a year in Kapunda with Dr James Riddell, followed by a short period at Broken Hill Hospital and in 1921 he commenced practice in Yankalilla. He was married on 14th March 1922 at the St Peter's College Chapel to Meta Gertrude Ker daughter of Archibald Gordon Ker. He replaced Dr Peter Gorrie in Port Augusta in 1923 as the sole practitioner undertaking both obstetrics and surgery and remained there for 18 years. At that time patients were referred from surrounding towns including Whyalla and Iron Knob because it was the only hospital in the region and it was a very busy practice. He was made a Serving Brother of St. John Ambulance in 1940. Eric Lindsay Symons died in Adelaide on 29th December 1971.

Sources:

National Archives of Australia
http://recordsearch.naa.gov.au/NameSearch/Interface/ItemDetail.aspx?Barcode=4780514
Guerin Foster History of Australian Rowing
McEachern A. C., 'Obituary' Medical Journal of Australia, 1972
South Australian Indexes of Births, Marriages and Deaths
Photo: Adelaide University Archives. Medical Graduates 1917.
The Register Adelaide 8th October 1908
The Adelaide Advertiser 11 July 1917

TASSIE Leslie Gemmell

DSO MB BS

1890 - 1959

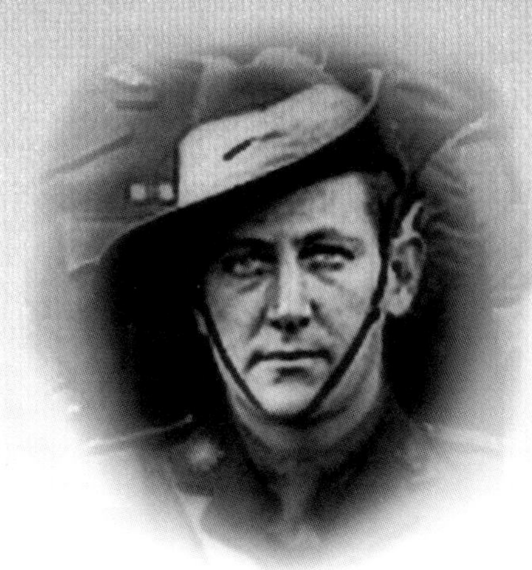

Leslie Gemmell Tassie was born in Kent Town, South Australia on 21st April 1890. He was the second of four children of Thomas Wilson Tassie and Jemima Reid, nee Wilson. He was educated at Norwood School and Prince Alfred College and studied medicine at the University of Adelaide graduating in 1912. After graduation he was a resident surgeon at the Adelaide Hospital in 1913 and then an honorary medical officer at Port Pirie Hospital and deputy quarantine officer at Port Pirie. He married Doris Stirling Howell on 14th August 1915 at St Cuthbert's Church, Prospect, South Australia. She was the daughter of Mr and Mrs H. Howell of Prospect.

Tassie enlisted in the AIF as a captain on 2nd December 1916. His previous military experience was as an area medical officer from July 1915. He was 5ft 11ins, weighed 162lbs, of medium complexion with blue eyes and fair hair. His wife was named as his next of kin and they lived at *Indoota*, Highbury Street, Prospect. He embarked on the *Orontes* in Melbourne on the 23rd December 1916 and disembarked in Plymouth on 17th February 1917. He proceeded to France on the 4th May 1917 and was briefly on the strength of the 2 AGH. He was posted to 4 FdAmb on 12th June 1917 and subsequently was appointed RMO of the 52 Bn on 15th June 1917. He was in hospital sick with a 'debility' from 12th August to 1st September 1917. He re-joined his Battalion on 1st November. He was promoted major on 1st of February 1918 and, on the 21st April, was posted to 13 FdAmb. Tassie was awarded the DSO on 18th June 1918 for his actions during operations near Villers-Bretonneux, the citation read: *"For conspicuous gallantry and devotion to duty. This officer set a fine example of coolness in going about amongst his stretcher-bearers directing and encouraging them. Day and night he visited the regimental aid post, and loading posts, re-arranging bearer relays, and supervising the evacuation of wounded. Hearing there were several wounded in a village which was being heavily shelled, he organised parties and cleared the village".* Tassie was then Mentioned in Despatches on the 31st December 1918. He assumed temporary command of 12 FdAmb on 16th March 1919 before leaving France for education leave in England on 7th April 1919. He returned to Australia embarking on the *Boonah* on 20th April 1919 disembarking in Melbourne and arrived in 4 MD on 10th June 1919. His appointment to the AIF was terminated on 18th July 1919. He was issued with the British War Medal and the Victory Medal with Oak Leaves.

Tassie and his wife returned to Port Pirie after the war. When he was acting superintendent of the Port Pirie Hospital in 1925, he gave evidence to the Royal Commission into lead poisoning in Port Pirie, an issue that has continued throughout the 20th Century. He continued to be a leading citizen of Port Pirie and in the 1940s lived in Florence Street, Port Pirie. During WW2 Tassie was placed on the Reserve of Officers. In 1944 whilst driving from Crystal Brook to Port Pirie with two nurses he was involved in a vehicle accident but no injuries were sustained. Leslie Gemmell Tassie died on 3rd March 1959 and his wife Doris died on the 16th August in 1959. At the time they lived in Toorak Gardens, Adelaide.

Sources:

National Archives of Australia
http://recordsearch.naa.gov.au/NameSearch/Interface/ItemDetail.aspx?Barcode=8098514
Family Search Community Trees
The Advertiser Adelaide 18th December 1905
The Advertiser Adelaide 20th December 1907
The Advertiser Adelaide 13th November 1939
The Recorder Port Pirie 9th January 1944
www.ww1sa.gravesecrets.net/ta.html

THOMAS Edward Brooke
MB BS

1887 - 1949

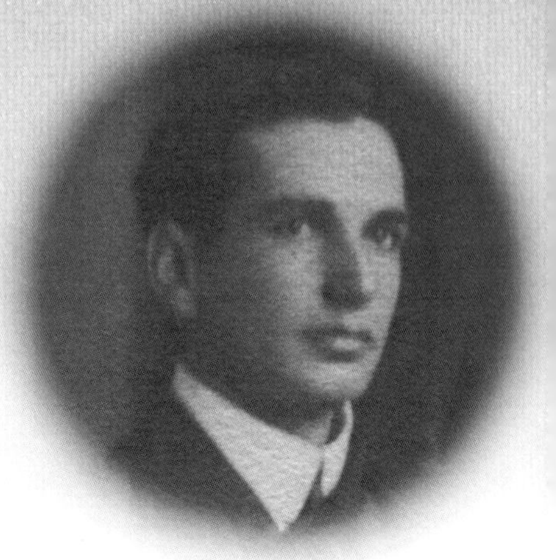

Edward Brooke Thomas was born in Perth, Western Australia on 30th July 1887. His father was the Reverend P. C. Thomas and prior to Edward's birth was the minister of the Wesley Church in Port Adelaide. The Reverend Thomas was appointed to the Wesley Church in Perth in 1887. Reverend Thomas returned to Adelaide to take up an appointment at the Draper Memorial Church, Adelaide in 1890 when Edward was three years old. Thomas was educated at Prince Alfred College. He studied medicine at the University of Adelaide and graduated in 1911.

Thomas enlisted as a captain in the AIF Adelaide on 17th January 1916 and was posted to 12 FdAmb. He was described as single and aged 28 years old, 5ft 7½ins tall, weighed 141lbs of dark complexion with brown eyes and black hair. His father was given as his next of kin and they lived at *Kalimna* 24 Marlborough Street, College Park, South Australia. He embarked on the *Orsova* from Melbourne on 16th March 1916 and he joined his unit, 12 FdAmb, on 22nd April 1916 in Egypt and moved from Alexandria to Marseilles on 4th June 1916 disembarking on 11th June 1916. He was detached to three of the Battalions during September and October 1916. He was posted to the 46 Bn as RMO on 16th December 1916. He suffered gunshot wounds to the left elbow and right knee on 10th July 1917 at Messines. He was hospitalised in 14th General Hospital in Boulogne and later transferred to England. He was discharged to duty on 13th of August 1917. He was first sent to 2nd Convalescent Depot and on 20th October 1918 to Cambridge Military Hospital He was *"brought to the notice of the Secretary of State for War for the valuable services he had rendered"*, on 27th March 1919. He apparently suffered no permanent disability from his wounds. He was appointed as medical officer on 16th June 1919 for the Transport *Ormonde* returning to Australia and disembarked on 30th July 1919 in 4MD. His appointment in the AIF was terminated on 21st September 1919. He was issued with the British War Medal and the Victory Medal.

Thomas was appointed as the Deputy Officer of Health for the district of English in 1920. He married Ida Florence Kingston Annells, the daughter of Edward Thomas Annells and Mary Crossman, nee Brown, on the 6th December 1922 in the Methodist Church, Woodville, South Australia. He was appointed as Deputy Officer of Health for the District of Julia. He spent most of his working life in Eudunda as a general practitioner. Edward Brooke Thomas, died on 28th July 1949 in Eudunda.

Sources:
National Archives of Australia
http://recordsearch.naa.gov.au/NameSearch/Interface/ItemDetail.aspx?Barcode=3001461
Returned Services League Last Post
South Australian Marriage - Index of Registrations 1917-1937
Biographical Index of South Australians 1836-1885
http://www.gould.com.au/Biographical-Index-of-South-Australians-1836-85-p/au5044.htm
Photo; Adelaide University Archives, Medical graduates 1911

TURNER Charles Trevor

MC MB BS

1889 - 1977

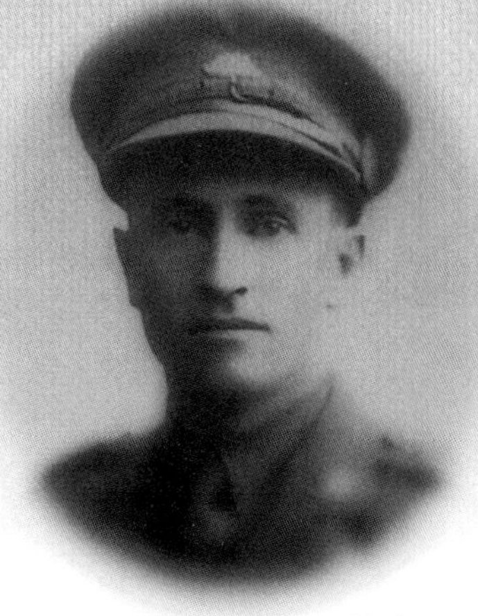

Charles Trevor Turner was born in Morgan, SA on 2nd January 1889, the second son of Charles John Turner and Agnes Sarah Matilda, nee Street. He was educated at Perth Technical School, Western Australia. He studied medicine at the University of Adelaide and graduated MB BS in 1914.

Turner enlisted in World War I on 14th July 1915, at which time he was working at the Adelaide Hospital, and was posted to 2 AGH. He was single and his mother, of 113 Rundle Street, Kent Town, named as next of kin. He was 5ft 5ins tall, and weighed 13st. He was appointed RMO to the newly formed 1st Pioneer Battalion in Egypt on 15th March 1916. He was awarded the Military Cross on 5th June 1917 for *distinguished service in the Field* during action at Poziers, France. He was promoted major on 7th September 1917. He was posted to the 3rd AGH on 9th January 1918. He was Mentioned in Despatches. He returned to England on 8th January 1919 for return to Australia. He returned to Australia on the *Ceramic* as part of the staff on 25th January 1919. He disembarked in the Fourth Military District on 14th March 1919. His appointment was terminated on 6th May 1919. He was issued with the 1914-15 Star, the British War Medal and Victory Medal with Oak Leaves.

He continued in the Militia after the war. He became engaged to Katherine Rooke Page in 1919, the daughter of Seymour Rooke Page and Effie Fisher nee Beard born in Moonta on 23rd July 1896. They were married in St John's Church, Adelaide on 19th April 1922 and had four children. He was appointed as Medical Superintendent of the Adelaide Hospital and was frequently called to give evidence in court or at coroner's inquiries. He was acting honorary assistant gynaecologist for 9 months whilst Dr Harold Powell was away in 1925. He was practising in Unley, South Australia in 1931. He enlisted in WW2 in Mount Gambier, South Australia and was called up for full time duty on 28th September 1942. After World War II he continued in the AAMC Reserve. Later he was practising in Mount Gambier. Turner's wife Katherine died on 1st March 1949 in Elsternwick, Victoria at the age of 52 years. Charles Trevor Turner died in Mitcham, Victoria in 1977 aged 89 years.

Sources:

National Archives of Australia
http://recordsearch.naa.gov.au/NameSearch/Interface/ItemDetail.aspx?Barcode=1919959
The South Australian Government Gazette 11th January 1915
Adelaide Advertiser 23rd December 1909
News 6th January 1931
Register 11th July 1922
South Australian Indexes of births deaths and Marriages
Ancestry.com
RAH Heritage Office

VERCO Joseph Stanley
MB BS FRCRA

1889 - 1971

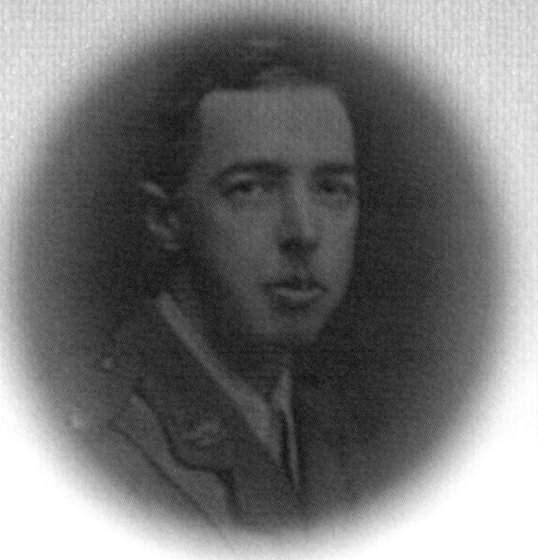

Joseph Stanley (Stan) Verco, was born on the 5th November 1889 in North Adelaide, the youngest of ten children, of William James Verco, a miller, and his wife Elizabeth. His father, died aged 49, in an influenza epidemic when Stan was just two years old. He was educated at Prince Alfred College. Although he failed his first year at Adelaide University his subsequent university career saw him top each year of the medical course, obtain a half blue for lacrosse and, as top student in his final year (1913), the Everard Scholarship. He undertook his resident medical officer training at the Adelaide Hospital. His lifelong passions included sailing and photography.

Verco joined 1ASH on 7th October 1914; he was 5ft 11ins tall and weighed 146lbs. He sailed to Alexandria on the *Kyarra* arriving on 14th January 1915. Half of the unit, which included Verco and Henry Newland, were sent, with two of the motor ambulances, to Ismailia on 27th January 1915 during the first Turkish attack on the Suez Canal. They were commended in the despatches of the General Officer Commanding. They returned to Cairo on 27th February 1915. Verco arrived in Mudros with 1 ASH on 5th March 1915. Subsequently he was to go to Gallipoli with 1 ACCS, and on hospital ships, including the *Aquitania,* which took the wounded back to Alexandria. He was evacuated from Lemnos in October 1915 with dysentery. He arrived in London in October and after a relatively short convalescence at 3 LGH he joined 6 AAH (Moreton Gardens) and, later, as he was only fit for home service, promoted major and joined 1 AAH, Harefield in May 1916. He married one of the Australian VADs, Dorothy Elise Willis, in South Kensington in 1917. He was posted to 1 AGH, Rouen, in July 1917 and his interest in Radiology, initially stimulated on Lemnos and Gallipoli, was greatly enhanced. He was again evacuated October 1918 and returned to Australia with his wife and eldest daughter in 1919.

Verco entered general practice with his older brother, William Alfred Verco, and was a surgical registrar at the Adelaide Children's Hospital. He lived in North Adelaide and had two children. He embarked on a career in radiology in 1921. He had rooms in Verco Buildings on North Terrace and later Harley Chambers in North Adelaide. He was joined in his practice by Colin Gurner and later, Bronte Creagh Smeaton. He was appointed radiologist in charge of X-Ray services for the Army during WW2. He commenced full time service on 16th March 1942, as a major, when 101 AGH was established and later DADMS and President of the Military Medical Board, South Australia. He was promoted lieutenant colonel in 1944. His various hospital appointments included honorary radiologist at the Adelaide and Adelaide Children's Hospitals. He was the advisor to the South Australian Government on the Mass Chest X-Ray Health Survey from 1942. He was the first president of the College of Radiologists (Australia and New Zealand) now the RANZCR and described *"his friendly, anxious, kindly manner must endear itself to all. Furthermore, his definite opinions and wise decisions when in the chair have shown members their first president is a man of wide knowledge and untold experience. The College was indeed fortunate to be initiated with him in command".* After Smeaton's death in 1950, the practice became Verco and Gurner: they were joined by their radiologist sons, Peter Verco and Colin Gurner junior. Joseph Stanley Verco continued to practise until shortly before his death in 26th July 1971. Predeceased by his wife he was survived by his son Peter, who was also to follow his father as President of the RACR, and his two daughters. All served in the Army in WW2. His grandsons have all served in the ADF, two in the RAADC and one in the RAAF.

Sources:
Ryan J, Sutton K, Baigent M, 1996" Australian Radiology A history" McGraw-Hill Sydney 74-81

VERCO Reginald John

MB BS FRACS

1885 - 1950

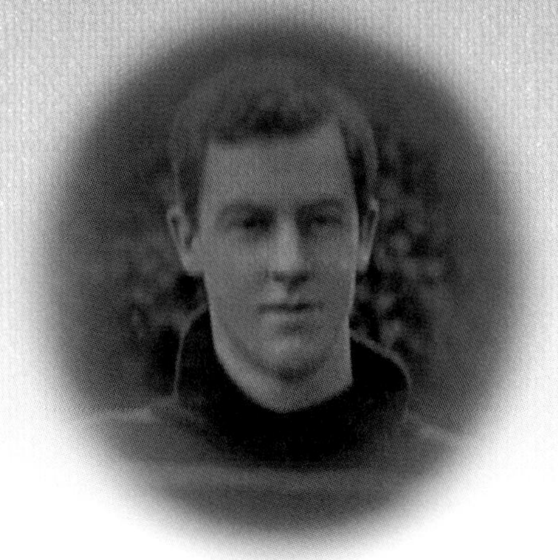

Reginald John Verco was born on 27th September 1885 at Mills Terrace, North Adelaide. He was the youngest son of John Verco, a merchant, and Caroline Blisset, nee Webb. He was educated at Prince Alfred College where he was somewhat impish but always a most unselfish and delightful companion, possessing a keen sense of humour and spontaneous dry wit. He studied medicine at the University of Adelaide and topped first year winning the Davies Thomas Scholarship. He later topped final year MB BS in 1907 and was awarded the Everard Scholarship. During his student days he played intervarsity lacrosse gaining his Blue. He married Phoebe Francis Hawkes in 1909. He established a general practice at 98 Payneham Road, St Peters where he was to live for the rest of his life.

Verco joined the AIF in March 1918 as a captain. He was 32 years old, father of two, and 5′ 11½ins tall, weighing 189lbs. He indicated that he had served for one month with the AAMC at 7AGH. He embarked on the *City of Karachi* on 30th November 1918 and arrived in London on 30th January 1919. He served in southern England before returning, on the *Mahana*, to Australia. He was struck off strength on 25th September 1919. He was not issued with any medals. Verco returned to continue with his general practice. He was the traditional family doctor on whom so many of his patients could lean and obtain solace from his advice. When unable to keep an appointment punctually he would say, *"Here comes the late Dr Verco".* He was the state president of the South Australian branch of the BMA from 1940-1943 and a member of the SA Council of Australian Trained Nurses Association. Reginald John Verco died on 5th June 1950 after a heart attack at the age of 64. His son, Major Geoffrey Webb Verco, a doctor, served in the AAMC in WW2.

Sources:
MJA August 1950 19:2(8) 309-310
http://recordsearch.naa.gov.au/NameSearch/Interface/ItemDetail.aspx?Barcode=8397841

From the diary of Major John Corbin

Friday, 28th May [1915]

Got some fresh eggs from Newland at Mudross [sic] also figs and raisins. Very acceptable after bully beef and biscuit.

WALKER William Delano

MB BS BSc(Hons)

1897 - 1938

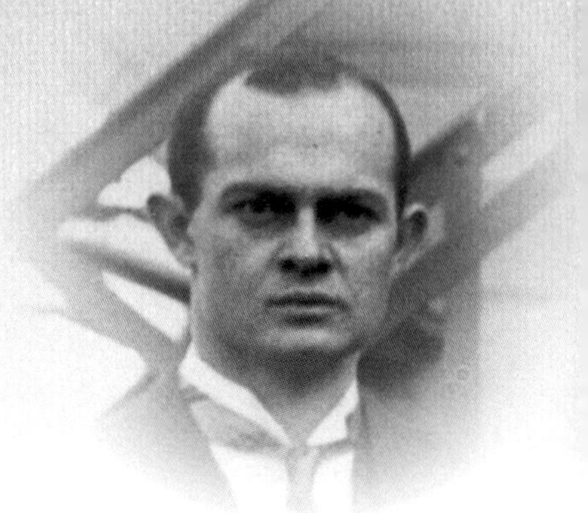

William Delano Walker was born in Port Pirie, SA, on 30th October 1897, the son of Dr William John Walker and Mary, nee Delano. His father was a well-known figure in Port Pirie and died of 'consumption' in 1903 when Walker was five years old. Two years later, in 1905, his mother drowned at Port Pirie when he was seven years old. He was brought up by his aunt Elizabeth Mary Thow. He was educated at the Victor Harbor High School and St Peter's College. He studied medicine at the University of Adelaide obtaining a BSc(Hons) in 1923 and graduated with MB BS in 1925.

Prior to enlistment in the AIF, Walker served for four years in the senior cadets and then the AAMC of the Citizen Military Force. He was a third year medical student when he enlisted on 3rd July 1918 at the Mitcham Camp as a private in the AAMC. He was described as single, 5ft 6ins tall weighed 149lbs, of medium complexion, with brown eyes and dark hair. His aunt, of Port Elliot, was named as his next of kin. He made a statutory declaration that both his parents were dead. He embarked on the *Gaika* on 6th August 1918 and disembarked in London on 13th October 1918 and marched in to AAMC Training Depot. He was admitted to hospital with influenza on 23rd October 1918 and with measles on 5th December 1918. He was charged with being absent without leave from 11th to 22nd January 1919 and admonished and lost 11 days' pay. He was granted leave from 8th August 1919 to 31st October 1919, on full pay, to go to Scotland to further his medical training. He embarked on *Ypiranga* on 15th November 1919 for return to Australia disembarking in 4 MD on 1st January 1920. He was discharged on 25th January 1920. He was issued with the British War Medal.

Walker applied for a Rhodes scholarship in 1923 and cited medical training provided to him in Glasgow and Edinburgh by Lieutenant Colonel T R Marsden DSO. It would appear he was not successful in his application. He married Mary (Mollie) Vera Alexander, a teacher, on 11th May 1927 at the St Peters' College Chapel. His life following graduating in medicine is well documented. He and his wife travelled widely in Australia and abroad, motoring 8500 miles in a model T Ford. They took many photographs and recorded their experiences in diaries from 1915 to 1938. The subject matter included the condition of Aborigines, nature and commented on life and society of both the middle and upper classes. He gave lectures in the United Kingdom with his own lantern slides. These diaries are now held in the South Australian Museum. He was awarded the Medal of the Royal Photographic Society in September 1931 for a series of photos illustrating the life cycle of the kangaroo. He also provided locum medical services in outback Australia. Walker and his wife were both musicians, often critiquing performances of others. He became a medical officer in the Royal Air Force and gained his licence to fly in 1936. William Delano Walker was killed in a Royal Air Force plane crash on 16th August 1938 at Catterick Flying Camp, Yorkshire, England. Following his death, his wife had to file an affidavit for his will which was mailed to London in November 1938 but the Empire Flying Boat *Calpurnia* crashed in the Middle East killing the pilot and the crew and all the post was lost. Mollie Walker served as an executive of the South Australian Country Women's Association for many years and chaired the University of Adelaide Adult Education Committee. She was awarded an OBE and died in the Adelaide Home for Incurables on 22 June 1975 following an extended illness.

Sources:
http://www.nzstamps.org.uk/air/empire/calpurnia.html
http://recordsearch.naa.gov.au/NameSearch/Interface/ItemDetail.aspx?Barcode=3005379
SA Museum AA357
http://archives.samuseum.sa.gov.au/aa357/provlist.htm
British Photographic History
Photo Adelaide University Archives Graduates 1924

WALL Frederick Lawrence

MC CdeG MB BS

1892 - 1958

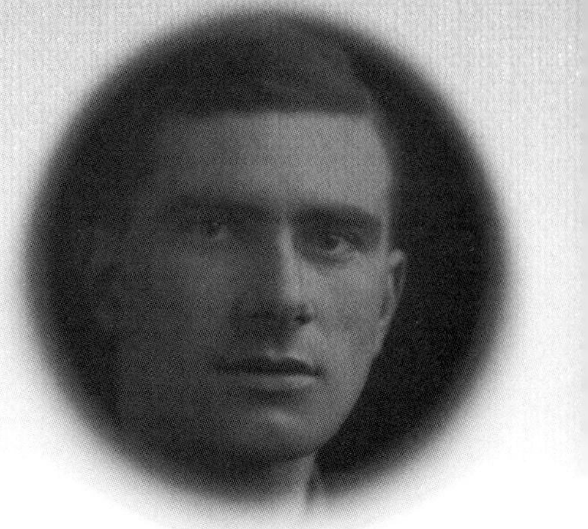

Frederick Lawrence Wall was born at Norwood, South Australia, on the 16th February 1892. He was the son of George Lawrence Wall, later Manager of Harris Scarfe Ltd, and his wife Charlotte Elizabeth, nee Elliott of Brougham Place, North Adelaide. He was educated at Prince Alfred College, where at the age of 14 he won a prize for excellence in Latin. He was a lieutenant in the school cadets. He studied medicine at the University of Adelaide and graduated in 1914.

Wall enlisted in the AIF in 1914, whilst he was a resident at the Adelaide Hospital. He applied for a commission on the 19th May 1915. He was a 23 years old, single, stood 5ft 10ins, and weighed 145lbs. His father was named as his next of kin. He embarked with reinforcements for 1 AGH at Melbourne in June 1915, but on arrival in Egypt was promptly sent to Gallipoli and posted to 3 FdAmb. He arrived at the height of the Lone Pine attacks in August 1915, and manned the unit's forward ADS. A month later he was evacuated to Egypt with typhoid and dysentery, but returned to Gallipoli in October. After his return he was attached to 6 Bn which moved to France in the spring of 1916, and went into the line to the south of Armentieres. The Australians, from the beginning of June, undertook a series of raids on the German trenches. 6 Bn carried out such a raid west of Le Bridoux on 13 June. The Bn was again in action at Pozières and at Mouquet Farm. At this time Wall wrote to his brother praising the wonderful bravery and devotion to duty of the men he served with. He was recommended for a Military Cross for his actions in the field but he was only Mentioned in Despatches. However, he was awarded a Military Cross in June 1917 for his devotion to his men in action and in the prevention of illness. He was promoted to major on the 29th June 1917. After a respite posting in England, Wall returned to France in November 1917 to join 7 FdAmb and 7 Brigade. Wall was appointed DADMS of 2 Division after the Battle of Passchendaele and the battle of Hamel. He occupied this position for the advance of the Australian Corps, the capture of Mt St Quentin, and the breaking of the Hindenburg Line. He was again Mentioned in Despatches, and awarded the Croix de Guerre which was cited: *'A assuré avec beaucoup de zèle et une grande bravoure l'evacuation des blessés pendant l'offensive victorieuse d'Aout 1918'.* Wall returned to Australia in March 1919, with his appointment terminated on the 27th June 1919. He was issued with the 1914-15 Star, the British War Medal and the Victory Medal with Oak Leaves.

Wall returned to the Adelaide Hospital for 6 months before taking a locum at Wallaroo for a year. He married Dr Winifred Clark in 1924 of Georgetown near Pt Pirie. He then established a practice and residence at 179 Magill Road where he remained for 30 years. It was a large practice and later included his son in law Dr Frank Riddell. In 1938 he took a year off to further his obstetrics and gynaecology training in England. He was generous to a fault for the benefit of his children and compassionate to the general community. He was a member of the Royal Adelaide Golf Club and purchased a cottage adjoining the Mount Lofty Links. He again volunteered for duty in WW2 in 1940 aged 48 years, and was appointed DADMS at HQ 4 MD, served overseas in Command of 10 CCS in New Guinea and retired in 1946 with the rank of honorary colonel. It is reported that he took his No 2 Iron to Milne Bay in WW2. He was a strong supporter of the SA Branch of the BMA and its President in 1947. Wall remained on the Reserve of Officers List. Frederick Lawrence Wall died on the 25th September 1958 and was survived by his widow Dr Winnie Wall, son Gordon Elliott Wall and three daughters, Margaret, Kathleen and Ellen.

Sources:

NAA:
http://recordsearch.naa.gov.au/NameSearch/Interface/ItemDetail.aspx?Barcode=6257050
Person interview and photo from grandson, Dr Geoff Wall and daughter Margaret Riddell.
MJA March 7th 1959, p 342.
Likeman R., "Gallipoli Doctors" Slouch Hat Publications, 2010
Letter to the University of Adelaide dated 6th December 1916
The Register Adelaide 15 December 1906

WALLMAN Douglas Robson

MB BS

1896 - 1969

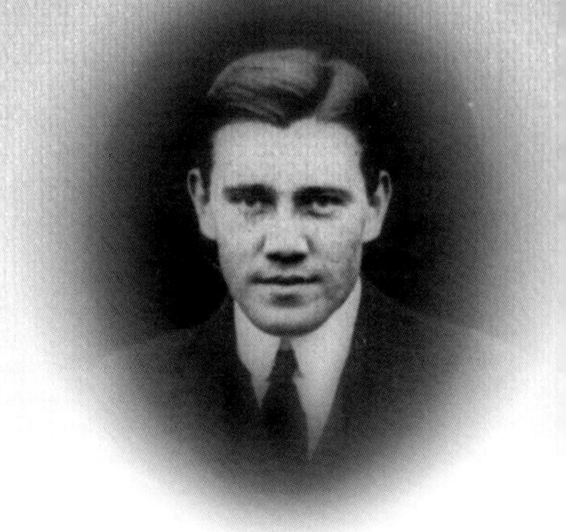

Douglas Robson Wallman was born in North Adelaide, South Australia on 4th March 1896 the son of August Gustav Wallmann and Louisa Haynes, nee Davis. He studied medicine at the University of Adelaide. He was single at the time of enlistment and still a medical student living with his parents at 26 Strangways Terrace, North Adelaide. He had served in the cadets and the citizen forces for a number of years.

Wallman enlisted with the agreement of his parents on 18th June 1915 at Keswick as a private soldier in the AAMC. He was discharged on 30th July 1915 to complete his medical degree. He enlisted again on 17th June 1918 at Keswick with the rank of temporary captain. He was 5ft 9ins tall, weighed 145lbs, of fair complexion, grey eyes and light brown hair. He was not called up for duty and was discharged on the 18th November 1918. He enlisted in World War II at Wayville on 1st November 1940 and served until 13th January 1944. At the time of his discharge he was posted to 3 FdAmb.

After the war Wallman married Miss Florence Maya Wood on 10th April 1920 in Sydney. She was the daughter of Mr and Mrs JR Wood who at the time were living in Drummoyne, but were previously from Woodville, South Australia. Wallman and his wife lived on Grange Road, West Hindmarsh, SA. Douglas Robson Wallman died on 16th June 1969 at Walkerville; he was survived by his wife Florence.

Sources:

Photo Adelaide University Archives, Medical graduates 1918.
http://recordsearch.naa.gov.au/NameSearch/Interface/ItemDetail.aspx?Barcode=8366441
The Mail Adelaide 17 April 1920
The News Adelaide 4 August 1947
http://www.ww2roll.gov.au/veteran.aspx?ServiceID=R&VeteranID=690147

South Australia
From our Special Correspondent

There are yet more demands being made upon the ranks of our profession for service in England, in Egypt, and on transport steamers. Dr J.A.G. Hamilton, the lecturer on gynaecology at the university; Dr Smeaton, a clinical lecturer at the Adelaide Hospital; Dr Gilbert, a surgeon of the Children's Hospital;–all have gone, and still more recently Dr W.T. Hayward, who is to be attached to a military hospital in England. Meanwhile many of the juniors have silently disappeared; we see them in brand new uniforms one day, and hear of them at Lemnos shortly afterwards. We others, whom on account of age or infirmity the fates have left behind, naturally admire the pluck and self-denial of those who have gone as such sacrifice to their own interests, and notice with pride that Drs H.A. Powell and John Corbin have been mentioned in dispatches. As the result of an inquiry into the management of the No. 1 Australian General Hospital at Heliopolis, Lieutenant Colonel Ramsay Smith has relinquished its command. The Director of Medical Services in Australia (Colonel Fetherston) has left for Egypt to straighten out matters and Colonel Shepherd of Adelaide is now filling his post.

BMJ, 6 November 1915, p. 690-691

WATSON Arthur Harrison Edward

MB BS

1896 - 1954

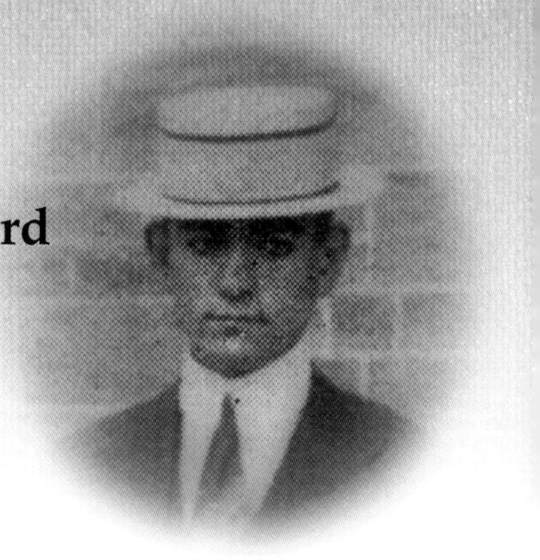

Arthur Harrison Edward Watson was born on 5th July 1896 at Plympton, South Australia. He was the son of Harry Watson and Adelaide Elizabeth, nee Menz. He was educated at Adelaide High School and in 1913 was awarded The Thomas Price Scholarship which was awarded for the first time. The award of £75 was for four years to pursue studies at university. It is only awarded to a student from a government school. Watson studied medicine at the University of Adelaide and graduated in 1920.

Watson enlisted in the AIF on 17th June 1918 in Adelaide, South Australia when he was a fourth year medical student. He was single and living with his parents at the Bay Road, Plympton, SA. He had served four years in the senior cadets before transferring to the Citizen Force. He was 5ft 7ins tall, weighed 131lbs, and of medium complexion with grey eyes and brown hair. He had an appendicectomy scar and a mole over his right clavicle. He was not called up and was discharged on 18th November 1918.

Watson was first registered with the Medical Board of South Australia in January 1921. He married Florence Dulcie Mobbs on 11th April 1923 at Stow Memorial Church, Adelaide. While living in the Quorn area he stood for council but was defeated in 1929. Watson and his wife had a collision with a lorry and trailer near Two Wells, South Australia in 1940, and subsequently sued for damages. This later led to an appeal to the High Court which resulted in award of damages to both of them. They were living in Yorketown, South Australia at the time. Arthur Harrison Edward Watson died on 12th February 1954, while a resident of North Adelaide, and was survived by his wife and three sons John, Graham and Richard. John was to become the Lord Mayor of the City of Adelaide.

Sources:
http://recordsearch.naa.gov.au/NameSearch/Interface/ItemDetail.aspx?Barcode=1912851
South Australian Indexes of Birth, Deaths and Marriages
The Register Adelaide 1st February 1913
The Chronicle Adelaide 27 June 1940
The Chronicle Adelaide 18 February 1954
Photo AHS Magazine Prefects, 1913

Larrey at Waterloo

When Napoleon returned from Elba in 1815 he almost at once sent for Larrey and discussed with him the organization of the ambulances for the forthcoming campaign...He [Larrey] was left for dead on the field, but recovering consciousness tried to make his way to the frontier...he was again surrounded by a corps of Prussian Cavalry and taken prisoner. The description of the ruthlessness with which the Prussians slaughtered prisoners and wounded alike reads like a letter from the front at the present day....Larrey, who was held in high esteem by the King of Prussia, and who was well known to many German officers, was stripped of his clothes, robbed of his money, his watch, a ring given to him as a talisman by a dying Mameluke after the battle of the Pyramids, a sabre presented to him at Aboukir by Napoleon, and even his boots... That officer...would listen to no explanations, and ordered Larrey to be shot. Fortunately, a military surgeon, who went to blindfold him as he was standing before the firing squad, recognized Larrey and insisted that the execution should be put off. After some difficulty Larrey was brought before Bluecher, whose son he had saved when wounded and a prisoner in 1813. The old soldier apologized, ordered that Larrey's clothes and money should be restored to him, [and] invited him to dinner.

BMJ, 19 June 1915, p. 1056-1057

WATSON Archibald

MD(Gottingen) MD(Paris) MD FRCS LSA

1849 - 1940

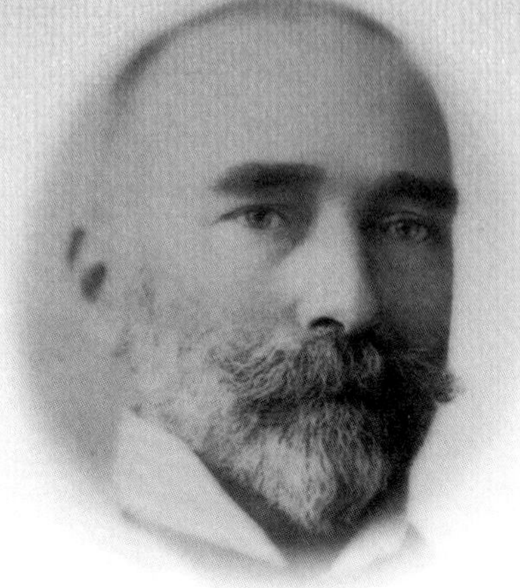

Archibald Watson, was born on 27th July 1849 in Tarcutta NSW. He was the eldest son of Sidney Grandison Watson, a wealthy pioneer pastoralist of the Upper Murray who had settled in Walwa in 1840. His mother died from a ruptured ectopic pregnancy. He was educated at the National School in Sydney and Scotch College, Melbourne. Leaving school he travelled to Fiji on the brig *Carl* in what has subsequently been alleged to be a blackbirding mission. He was arrested on piracy charges and later released on bail, he returned briefly to Australia before setting off to Europe to study medicine. He distinguished himself with his MD theses Gottingen (1878) and Paris (1880) before travelling to London where he took the LSA and FRCS in 1882 and 1884. He was a Demonstrator in Anatomy at Charing Cross Hospital when he applied, successfully, for the inaugural Elder Chair of Anatomy at the University of Adelaide. He was later to be appointed lecturer in surgery, pathologist and finally surgeon at the Adelaide Hospital. He became involved in the 'Adelaide Hospital Row' which closed the medical school for over 3 years. During this time the Boer War took place and Watson joined the Natal Field Force in 1900 as consulting surgeon and later the Johannesburg Volunteers in 1900-1901. He wrote" *I was surprised at the number of soldiers with hammer toes, flat feet, varicose veins, visceral pthisis, skeletal syphilis, mental aberration, hernia and defective dentition and the absence of the means of treating it"* He was awarded the Queens South African Medal with the Natal clasp. Watson became the consulting surgeon to the Military Forces of the Commonwealth in 1906. It was said that Watson had a *'puckish sense of humour and a passionate dislike of pretension and insincerity. His condemnation of ineptitude was like a roll of thunder; when ineptitude was coupled with pomposity, the lightning of his wit struck.'* He was well loved however-even by those who understood him least and his knowledge was well respected. He was a surgical anatomist whose surgical ideal was the gentle handling of tissues, the knowledge of and use of anatomical planes in the surgical approach, and control or prevention of haemorrhage by ligation of the feeding vessels. He was fluent in 7 languages and had a passion for motor bikes, some with an attached wicker passenger sidecar. His professional and personal diaries are with the RACS and the National Library respectively. The professional diaries contain many original observations and superb anatomical and pathological drawings. The personal are reputed to contain details of his private relationships.

Watson, at the age of 65, joined the AIF at the rank of major and was posted to 1ASH in November 1914 as a surgeon. He travelled to Egypt on the *Kyarra*. At some point he transferred to 1AGH and saw service in Egypt, Lemnos and Gallipoli. He performed post mortem examinations as required although the details of a lot of these have been lost over time. It is likely that he acquired the Nubian mummy now in the South Australian Museum during this time; the mummy is interesting for a number of reasons not least the Australian bayonet wound to the abdomen. He returned home having completed his service in 1916 and was discharged on 7th March 1916. He was issued with the 1914-15 Star, the British War Medal and the Victory Medal. The Director of Medical Services, Colonel Neville Howse VC, discouraged Watson returning to overseas service as; *"He is a very charming man but his presence has a very bad influence on the younger men of any unit".*

Watson returned to the University of Adelaide. He later retired to Darwin where he did much to improve the standards of surgical care in the tropics. He made the Federal Hotel, Thursday Island his home from 1936. Archibald Watson died on the 30th July 1940 on the veranda of the Federal Hotel three days after his 91st birthday. He never married and had no known children.

Sources:

Elmslie R. Nance S, 'Watson, Archibald (1849–1940) Australian Dictionary of Biography, National Centre of Biography, Australian National University.

The Australian Medical Gazette, 10Aug1901, p318

http://recordsearch.naa.gov.au/NameSearch/Interface/ItemDetail.aspx?Barcode=1912809

WEBB John Newton

MB BS DPH

1893 - 1980

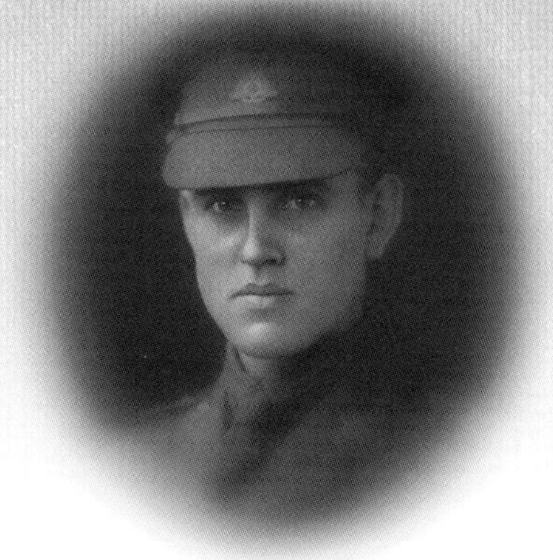

John Newton Webb was born in Melbourne, Victoria on 20th September 1893. He was the second son of Reverend Frederick and Emma Jane Webb; he had two brothers and two sisters. His brother Walter Frederick Swanton Webb also served in WW1. The Reverend Webb was appointed to the Holy Trinity Church, the first church in South Australia, on North Terrace, Adelaide in June 1895, when Webb was two years old. Reverend Webb's previous post was in Armadale, Victoria. Webb's father became prominent in Anglican circles in Adelaide until his death in March 1925 one month after the death of his wife. Webb was educated at St Peter's College and studied medicine at the University of Adelaide, graduating on 17th July 1917. He was a keen member of the Holy Trinity Church and taught in the Sunday school there. After graduation he was a house surgeon at the Adelaide Hospital before enlisting in the AIF five months later.

Webb joined the AAMC Reserve on 1st August 1917, following his medical registration and was posted to 7 AGH. He enlisted into the AIF on 12th January 1918 as a captain; he was single and living with his parents in Trinity Rectory, North Terrace Adelaide, South Australia. His mother was nominated as his next of kin. Military records incorrectly recorded his father as Frank Webb. He was described as 24 years and five months old, 5 feet 11 inches tall, weighed 140lbs, with fair complexion, blue eyes and brown hair and limited French. He embarked on *Persic* in Sydney on 21st March 1918 and disembarked in London on 24th May 1918. Webb proceeded to France via Folkestone on 12th Jun 1918. He was attached to 2 AGH initially but subsequently in June 1918 proceeded to 9 FdAmb. He was posted to 3 Div Engineers on 23rd November 1918 before returning to 9 FdAmb on 21st December 1918 and on to 11 FdAmb on 23rd March 1919. He left France on 28th April 1919. After periods of leave with and without pay he resigned his appointment on 5th June 1920 in England to undertake the Diploma of Public Health at University College, London. He gave his address as 279 Goldhawk Road, Shepherds Bush. He was required to return to Australia no later than 31st Dec 1921. Resignation of Australian's from the military in countries other than Australia was not accepted lightly and he made several declarations confirming that he would return to South Australia after his course was completed. He was issued with the British War Medal and the Victory Medal.

Webb was living in Melbourne with his sister when his father died in 1925. He was resident at 226 North Road, Brighton, Victoria, in 1939 when he wrote to the War Office saying that he had lost his medals and his Returned Soldiers Badge, and had them replaced at his expense for 13 shillings and nine pence. He did not appear to have married. John Newton Webb died in Alphington, Victoria in 1980, aged 86 years.

Sources:

Photo: SRSA; GRG26_5_4_0_846

http://recordsearch.naa.gov.au/NameSearch/Interface/ItemDetail.aspx?Barcode=8377386

South Australian Register 1st June 1895

The Mail Adelaide 7 July 1917

The Register Adelaide 7 July 1917

The Chronicle Adelaide 28 March 1925

Ancestry.com

WEBB Walter Frederick Swanton

LRCP&S Edin LRCP&S Glas

1888 - 1963

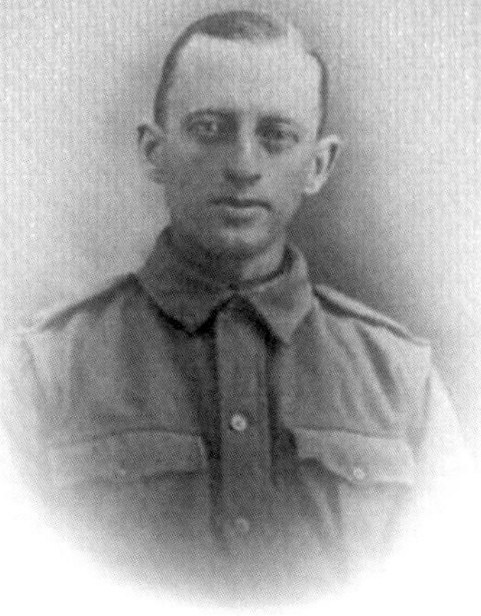

Walter Frederick Swanton Webb was born in Armidale, NSW, in 1888. He was the son of Reverend Frederick and Emma Jane Webb and was the brother of John Newton Webb. His family moved to South Australia for his father to take up a post at Holy Trinity Church, North Terrace Adelaide.

Webb enlisted in the AIF on 23rd November 1914 at Keswick, South Australia after passing his third year medical degree examinations. He was 5ft 7ins tall, weighed 128lbs of fair complexion, blue eyes and fair hair. His next of kin was given as Frederick Webb, his father, of Trinity Church, North Terrace Adelaide. He embarked from Melbourne on the *Kyarra* on 5th December 1914 as a Private to join 1 AGH in Egypt. He returned from Egypt and was discharged on 31st July 1915, at his own request, to complete his medical degree. He was issued with the 1914-15 Star, the British War Medal and the Victory Medal. He had completed 242 days service.

He was registered with the Medical Board of South Australia in 1920 with the qualifications of LRCP and S Edinburgh and LRCP and S Glasgow 1920. He married Winifred Myrtle Western, who was the 30 year old daughter of George Western and Caroline nee Shearing, on 4th August 1920, at Holy Trinity Church, Adelaide. Walter Frederick Swanton Webb died on 29th September 1963 at Eastwood, South Australia.

Letter from Helen Bollen in response to request by the University of Adelaide

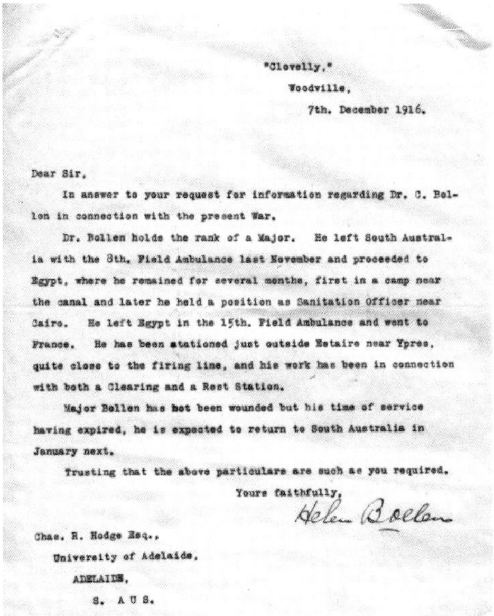

"Clovelly,"
Woodville,
7th. December 1916.

Dear Sir,

In answer to your request for information regarding Dr. C. Bollen in connection with the present War.

Dr. Bollen holds the rank of a Major. He left South Australia with the 8th. Field Ambulance last November and proceeded to Egypt, where he remained for several months, first in a camp near the canal and later he held a position as Sanitation Officer near Cairo. He left Egypt in the 15th. Field Ambulance and went to France. He has been stationed just outside Estaire near Ypres, quite close to the firing line, and his work has been in connection with both a Clearing and a Rest Station.

Major Bollen has hot been wounded but his time of service having expired, he is expected to return to South Australia in January next.

Trusting that the above particulars are such as you required.

Yours faithfully,
Helen Bollen

Chas. R. Hodge Esq.,
University of Adelaide,
ADELAIDE,
S. A U S.

University of Adelaide Archives

Sources:

National Archives of Australia
http://recordsearch.naa.gov.au/NameSearch/Interface/ItemDetail.aspx?Barcode=8377461
World War I Pictorial Honour Roll of South Australia
Adelaide Advertiser 1920
South Australian Indexes of Births Deaths and Marriages

WIEN-SMITH Geoffrey

MB BS

1892 - 1973

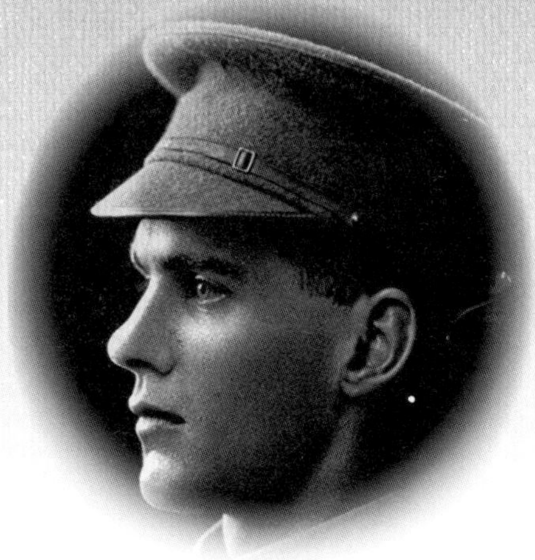

Geoffrey Wien-Smith and his twin sister, Clair Winifred, were born on 19th April 1892 in Clare, South Australia. They were the children of Otto Wien-Smith, a medical practitioner, and his wife Blanche Isabel, nee Richardson. Otto travelled to Australia as a ship's doctor arriving in 1878; he and his wife had four other children all born in Australia. Wien-Smith was educated at St Peter's College and the University of Adelaide, graduating MB BS in 1915.

Wien-Smith had served one year in the Cadets in 1908 and enlisted in the AIF on 8th October 1915 in Adelaide and was posted into the 11 FdAmb. He was described as 5ft 8ins tall, weighed 146lbs, of dark complexion, with black hair and blue eyes. It was also noted that he had 4 lozenge shaped vaccination marks on his left arm. After early training at Mitcham camp he embarked on *Beltana* in Sydney on 15th May 1916, disembarking in Devonport on 10th July 1916. He went to France to join 11 FdAmb on 24th November 1916. He was admitted to hospital with "debility" and "trench fever" in July 1917 and returned to duty on 28th July 1917. Wien-Smith was again hospitalised on 29th December 1917 and eventually transferred to hospital in England in March 1918. There appeared to be considerable concern for his health expressed by two hand written comments; one by Charlton Yeatman and the other by Otto's brother Russell, the latter writing from Australia dated 27th December 1917. He was eventually admitted to Queen's Hospital, Sidcup, England on 3rd July 1918 with influenza and cystitis and when recovered he was posted as a medical officer to that hospital. He embarked on the *Nevasa* for return to Australia on 5th March 1919 disembarking to the 4 MD on 25th April 1919. His illness was deemed to be caused by his military service which would enable him to claim a pension. His appointment was terminated on 3rd August 1919. He was issued with the British War Medal and Victory Medal.

After the war Wien-Smith continued a medical practice in Clare. He married thirty year old Roma Elsa Wadey, the daughter of Alfred Ernest Wadey and Elsa Hansie, nee Mueller, on 29th July 1936 in St the Peter's College Chapel. He and his wife became well known identities in the Clare and Burra area of South Australia. They had one daughter Susan. Roma Wien-Smith died in 1950 and Geoffrey Wien-Smith died on 24th December 1973. He is buried in Clare with his parents and wife.

Sources:

South Australian Biographical Index 1836-1885
South Australian Genealogical and Heraldry Society
Ancestry.com
http://www.awm.gov.au/research/people/nominal_rolls/first_world_war_embarkation/person.asp?p=257213
http://recordsearch.naa.gov.au/NameSearch/Interface/ItemDetail.aspx?Barcode=8389044
http://www.appletree.com/Roma_Elsa_Wadey_1

Medical Notes in Parliament

Lord Robert Cecil congratulated the Army Medical Service on having in the earliest stages initiated the reform of allowing nurses to go to clearing stations and hoped that system would be continued and extended, as two were not enough.

BMJ, 13th February 1915, p. 304

† WELLS John Clarence

MB BS

1889 - 1918

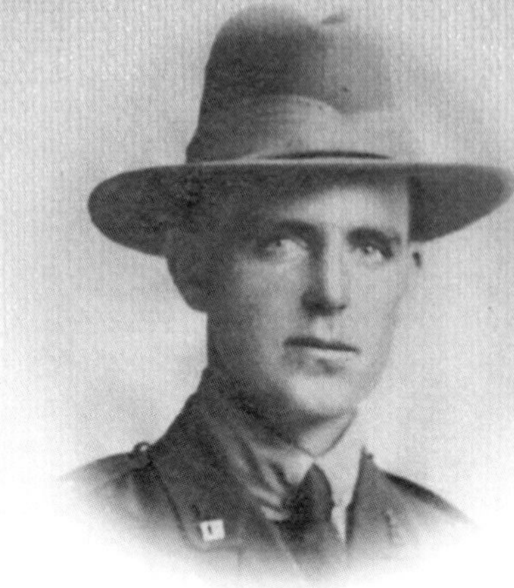

John Clarence Wells was born at Hawthorn on 28th March 1889, the youngest son of Clement Victor Wells JP MB BS LRCP, (1845-1926) for many years an alderman of the City of Adelaide, and an unsuccessful candidate for Mayor in 1901. His father was successful in the Victorian gold fields and ran a large joinery business in Adelaide on his return. Wells was educated at St Peter's College Adelaide and a volunteer cadet. He studied medicine at the University of Adelaide and graduated in 1912. He was working at Gawler, South Australia in 1914.

Wells enlisted in the AIF soon after the outbreak of war and was commissioned on the 1st January 1915. He was described as 29 years old, single and his father of 72 and 112 South Terrace, Adelaide was named as his next of kin. He was 5ft 11ins and weighed 182lbs, He was attached to 1 AGH and sent to Egypt but was then posted to 1 LHR as RMO. He went to Gallipoli with the unit on 9th May 1915, but soon fell ill with dysentery and was evacuated to Egypt in June for six weeks. He returned to the Peninsula on the 1st August 1915 and remained until the evacuation. He was attached to the Western Frontier Force in January 1916 and took part in the campaign against the Senussi. Wells remained with 1 LHR which now became part of the ANZAC Mounted Division. He was present at the Battle of Romani, and was recommended to be Mentioned in Despatches *'for good work just behind the firing line'* but was not confirmed. Immediately after the capture of Rafa in February 1917 he was promoted to major. After the Battles of Gaza, Wells was sent back to Egypt with recurrent attacks of dysentery, and precordial pain. This resulted in his being repatriated to Australia in June 1917 suffering from debility. He worked at 15 AGH in North Adelaide until he was able to convince a medical board that he was again fit for overseas service. He sailed from Sydney for Liverpool in January 1918, and in April joined 1 AGH at Rouen. During the next month Wells had short detachments to both 15 and 8 FdAmb on the Somme, before being posted as RMO of 30 Bn in May. During the Battle of Amiens on the 8th August 1918 he was wounded in the head by shrapnel from a shell that burst near Bn HQ, which was situated to the East of Villers Bretonneux. John Clarence Wells died at 3pm on the 10th August 1918 at 53 CCS, and is buried in the Vignacourt British Cemetery, between Amiens and Doullens, in plot 6 row B 18. The sole beneficiary of his will was his fiancée, Miss B O Bennett of "Kumara" 107 Barton Terrace, North Adelaide. John Clarence Wells' name is located at panel 184 in the Commemorative Area at the Australian War Memorial

His father Dr Clement Victor Wells received the Memorial Scroll in 1922, and in 1923 the Memorial Plaque and Kings Message. He also received the 1914-15 Star, the British War Medal and the Victory Medal. It is also reported that Wells' father embarked in the *Takada* as surgeon captain, AAMC in 1918. However his name does not appear in the National Archive records of WW1.

Sources:

Likeman R, "Gallipoli Doctors" Slouch Hat Publications, 2010

http://recordsearch.naa.gov.au/scripts/Imagine.asp?B=8380687

Photo

https://www.google.com.au/search?q=John+clarence+Wells&tbm=isch&tbo=u&source=univ&sa=X&ei=tZ9tUuv_LMSPrQfk64GQAg&ved=0CFoQsAQ&biw=1536&bih=747

Letter to the University of Adelaide undated 1916

The Register Adelaide 15 December 1906

The Advertiser Adelaide 11 august 1919

Recorder Port Pirie SA 3 August 1926

German Army Surgeons

The Berlin Society of Military Surgeons celebrated the fiftieth anniversary of its foundation on February 20th. The Society has a membership of 300.

BMJ, 14 March 1914, p. 610

WHITE Alan Hubert

MB BS

1896 - 1950

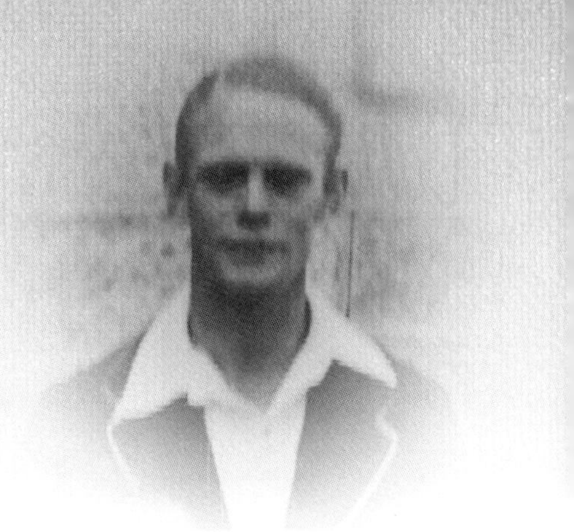

Alan Hubert White was born in Kent Town, South Australia on 28th May 1896. He was the fourth son of John White and Helen Georgina, nee Nicholson of "Conara" George Street, Unley Park, South Australia. He was educated at Prince Alfred College, where he excelled in all sports especially athletics. He studied medicine at the Adelaide University commencing in 1916 and continued his love of athletics at University.

White enlisted on 11th September 1918 in Adelaide when he was a third year medical student aged 22 years and single. He gave his father as next of kin; he was still living with his parents. He had served four years with the senior cadets and had transferred to the Citizen Forces. He was 5ft 7ins tall, weighed 140lbs, of fair complexion with blue eyes and fair hair. He stated his religion as Baptist. He was not called up for duty and was discharged on 18th November 1918. He had a scar on his left index finger, a small left varicocele and moles on his lower abdomen and both shoulders. He also had an apical murmur in his heart.

White graduated with his medical degree in 1921 and was registered with the Medical Board of South Australia in December 1921. He was a resident medical officer at the Adelaide Hospital in 1922. He married Aileen Peachey on the 22nd July 1922 in the Holy Trinity Church, North Terrace, Adelaide. White took up general practice Lameroo, in May 1922, where his first child, a daughter, was born. He moved to Snowtown in 1925, and was a very active member of the town community. He continued his love of sport and became the inaugural president of the Snowtown golf club. White and his family moved back to Adelaide in 1937, and took up a practice on Napier Terrace, (now Cross Road). He was an honorary medical assistant at the Adelaide Hospital from 1937 to 1939. White was involved in a serious accident with his car and a train on the Hawthorn railway crossing. After months of recuperation he returned to his general practice. He had to defend himself against a claim for damages arising out his accident, but this was eventually dismissed, following an appeal to the High Court. He was also an honorary clinical assistant to the surgical section at the Adelaide Hospital, from 1941 until his resignation on 12th November 1945. White re-enlisted in WW2 and it is presumed he was on the Reserve of Officers as he maintained his employment at the Adelaide Hospital during this time. Alan Hubert White died on 8th April 1950 at his home leaving his wife Aileen and three children Valerie, Maxine and Graham.

Sources:

http://recordsearch.naa.gov.au/NameSearch/Interface/ItemDetail.aspx?Barcode=1846232
South Australian Indexes of Births, Deaths and Marriages
Photo: Adelaide University Archives, Intervarsity Cricket Team 1920.
Royal Adelaide Hospital Heritage Office, records.
Jones Alan, Snowtown the first Century
Family photograph and records provided by Alan G White and Maxine E Rennison.
The Daily Herald Adelaide 17 December 1921
The Register Adelaide 20 October 1922
The News Adelaide 3 March 1942
The Adelaide Advertiser 10 April 1950
The Adelaide Advertiser 9 November 1940

The Nursing Emergency

The nursing profession, like the medical, has responded splendidly to the call of the country in this war, and a very large number of nurses are in the military hospitals in this country and abroad.... The largest number of nurses employed belong to the Territorial Force Nursing Service and are serving in the Territorial general hospitals. There are over 3,000 serving now....All these nurses are fully trained certificated women.

BMJ, 1 May 1915, p.771

WIBBERLEY Brian William

MC MB BS BSc

1891 - 1973

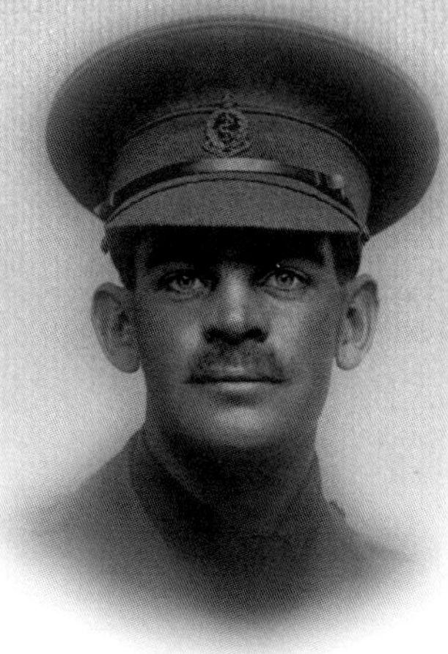

Brian William Wibberley was born in Brighton, Victoria on 12th January 1891. He was the son of Brian Wibberley, a Methodist minister, and his wife Marie Anne, nee Hunt. He had a sister, Nancy. The Reverend Brian Wibberley moved to South Australia in 1898, serving in Moonta and Kent Town before travelling to serve in the Wesley Church in Perth. They returned to Adelaide where the Reverend Wibberley remained until his death in 1944. Wibberley went to school in Moonta before his secondary education, which was aided by a scholarship, at Prince Alfred College. At the University of Adelaide he gained a BSc (1911) and later MB BS (1914). He served in the cadets and was appointed as lieutenant in 1908.

He joined the British Army in May 1915; after training at the Torquay and Salisbury Plain Training Schools he joined the RAMC as a temporary lieutenant. He was posted to 56th Field Ambulance which was attached to 7 Bn, Loyal North Lancashire Regiment (Mounted). He was decorated with the Military Cross for his conspicuous service during the first battle of the Somme (1915), later he served at Cambrai; these were regarded as two of the bloodiest of battles during the war. Later he served with the 88th Field Ambulance at Passchendaele and as part of the occupation army. He had served in France, Belgium and Germany during WW1. He was promoted to temporary captain on 26th March 1916 and later, acting major from 23rd December 1918.

Wibberley returned to Australia, took a refresher course at the Adelaide Hospital, and married Margery Rebecca Godlee in 1919. He became a Justice of the Peace in January 1921. He was to visit Tumby Bay after a locum in Streaky Bay and it was here that he remained for 37 years. His palatial new home was erected in 1939. He had two sons and two daughters. He was a significant member of the local community. Wibberley unveiled the Tumby Bay Soldiers Memorial in June 1926 to those from the area who enlisted. He lectured on "Greece in the Time of Socrates" on 22nd June 1934. He joined the 5 Bn Volunteer Defence Corps in 1943 and remained with them until discharged on 25th November 1945. At the end of WW2 he again unveiled an Honour Roll at Port Neill on 29th September 1945 and laid the foundation stone for the new Port Neill kindergarten hall on 13th February 1948. He returned to his practice in Tumby Bay from which he retired in 1957, handing over the practice to his youngest son, Dr David Wibberley. He did not fully retire and continued to work for the Red Cross Blood Bank and as a school Medical officer for the Department of Education. He also undertook locums for his son in Tumby Bay. Brian William Wibberley died of a heart attack at the age of 83 in September 1973.

Sources:

District Council of Tumby Bay Community News March 2009 p4
Photo: PAC Collection
The Adelaide Advertiser 19 May 1908
The Adelaide Advertiser 13 December 1905

WILLCOX Frank Mayes

MD MS DPH

1873 - 1946

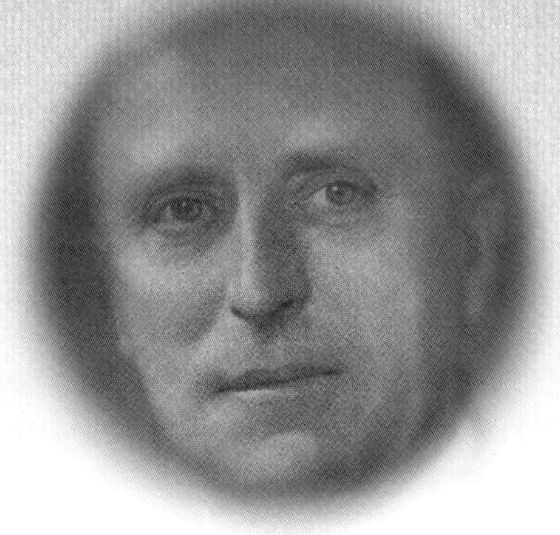

Frank Mayes Willcox was born in North Adelaide, South Australia on 1st January 1873. He was the son of Charles Willcox, later Sir Charles, Mayor of Adelaide and a Member of Parliament, and his first wife Coralie Rose. He was educated at Winham and Hahndorf Colleges and later St Peter's College. He studied medicine at Edinburgh University and graduated MB BCh (1898) and MD (1908). He later studied at the University of Adelaide and was awarded a MS in December 1919. He also had a DPH. He had worked as a house surgeon and clinical assistant at the Edinburgh Royal Infirmary before returning to Adelaide in 1913 and gaining a position as assistant gynaecologist at the Adelaide Hospital. He had a medical practice on North Terrace, Adelaide. Willcox married Mary Veitch in Edinburgh and on return to Australia they resided at 18 Magill Road, Norwood, at the time of his enlistment.

Prior to his enlistment in the AIF Willcox had previously served with the Edinburgh Medical Staff Corps, later known as the Officer Training Corps, from 1893-1896. During that time he had training with regular army units at Aldershot. He enlisted in the AIF as a captain AAMC on 11th September 1918 in Adelaide at the age of 45 years and 9 months. He was described as 5ft 7ins tall and weighed 143lbs of fair complexion, blue eyes and brown hair. His records noted that he seemed *"capable and keen"*. His next of kin was recorded as his wife Mary. He was also noted to be able to ride both horse and cycle and spoke limited German. Following initial training at Mitcham he embarked in Sydney on 16th October 1918 on the *Malta* disembarking in Suez on 22nd November 1918. He was immediately admitted to 31st General Hospital with influenza and discharged from hospital on 10th December 1918 and attached to 14 AGH on 12th December 1918. He joined the 5 LH FdAmb in February 1919 and on 5th April 1919 was transferred to the 2nd Sig Sqn. On 22nd July 1919 he embarked on the *Tagus* for the United Kingdom. On arriving in the UK he was granted leave without pay and allowances from 7th August 1919. He returned to Australia on the *Ascanius* disembarking on 7th November 1919. His appointment in the AIF was terminated on 22nd November 1919. He was issued with the British War Medal.

On his return as well as continuing to practise in South Australia he spent a considerable amount of time in the England and on the continent. Later in life he lived at 35 Hawkers Road, Medindie, South Australia. Frank Mayes Willcox died on 6th September 1946 aged 73 years. He was survived by his wife Mary.

Sources:

Advertiser Newspaper 9th sep1946
http://recordsearch.naa.gov.au/NameSearch/Interface/ItemDetail.aspx?Barcode=8389749
Photo: Adelaide Whose Who 1936
The Adelaide Advertiser 18 December 1919
The Adelaide Advertiser 9 September 1946

WILSON Laurence Algernon

MB BS FRACS

1896 - 1989

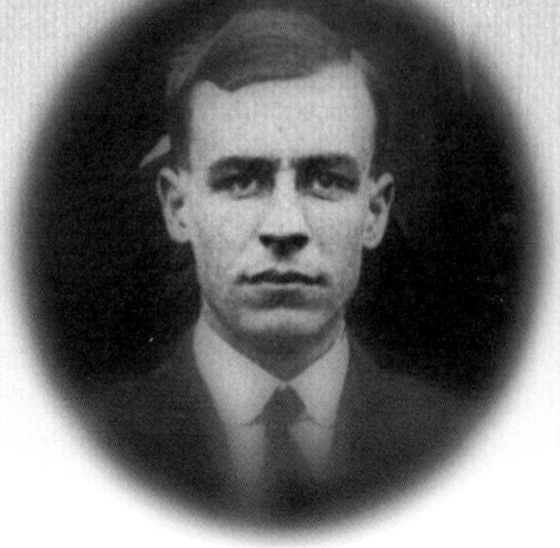

Laurence Algernon Wilson was born on 3rd September 1896 at Norwood, South Australia. He was the son of Algernon Theodore Wilson and Lillian Charlotte, nee Laurence. He was the grandson of Charles Algernon Wilson whose extensive diary, in the South Australian State Library, documented his journey from England to South Australia in 1838. Wilson was educated at St Peter's College and studied medicine at the University of Adelaide, graduating MB BS in 1918.

Wilson enlisted in the AIF on 18th June 1918 when he was a 5th year medical student. Prior to enlistment he had served four years as a senior cadet. He was 21 years and 9 months of age 5ft 11ins tall and weighed 152lbs of fair complexion with blue eyes and fair hair. His father was named as next of kin and they lived at 6th Avenue, St Peters, South Australia. Wilson completed his medical degree at the end of the 1918 academic year and was granted the rank of captain on 25th November 1918. His appointment was terminated on 1st February 1919 and it was recorded that he had 50 days of war service in the AIF home service.

Wilson married Nance Mildred Lamphee on 30th August 1924 at the St Peter's College Chapel. Nance was the sister of Alan Dunstone Lamphee. He was elected a Fellow of the Royal Australasian College of Surgeons in 1932. At the beginning of WW2 after recruit training at Wayville in November 1939 he moved into Woodside Camp in South Australia as an honorary captain. Laurence Algernon Wilson died in 1989.

Sources:

http://www.slsa.sa.gov.au/archivaldocs/PRG/PRG1399_3_1_WilsonDiary_transcript.pdf
http://recordsearch.naa.gov.au/NameSearch/Interface/ItemDetail.aspx?Barcode=2013278
The Daily Herald Adelaide 13 December 1918
The Adelaide Advertiser 25 January 1913
The Register Adelaide 31 October 1924
http://www.genealogysa.org.au/resources/online-databases.html?option=com_search&ref=search

The German Medical Congress in Warsaw

The much advertised German Medical Congress was held on May 1st to 3rd in Warsaw, where over one thousand medical delegates from the Central Powers and their allies met to discuss the medical experiences and achievements of the past year... and the time table of the Congress was so full and the sense of duty of the delegates was so strong that we are told time was permitted for only one "Bier abend"...Professor V Schjerning said that more than 24,000 medical men were serving, two-thirds being engaged in the field and one-third at home...There were 238 hospital trains and trains for slight cases taking wounded and sick back to Germany from the field hospitals.

BMJ, 1 July 1916, p. 27

WILSON Sir Thomas George

CMG MD (Syd) MD FRCS(Ed)
FRACS FRCOG FACS

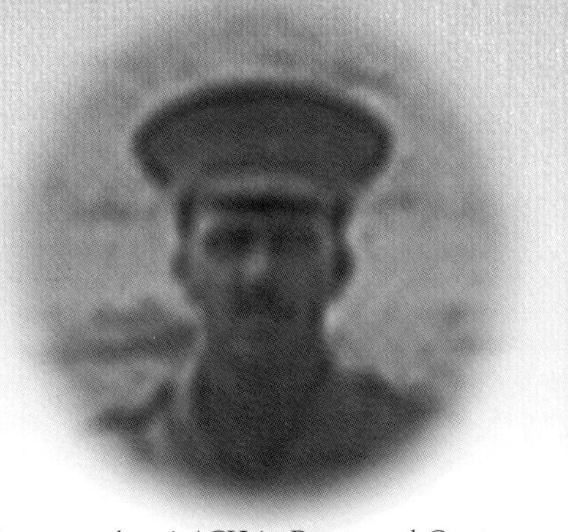

1876 - 1958

Thomas George Wilson was born on 27th March 1876 in Armidale NSW. He was the 4th child of six children of Charles Graham and Annie Jane, nee McBride. He was educated at the New England Grammar School and Sydney University. At university he rowed for Sydney University and played tennis for NSW. He graduated MB BS in 1899 and MD in 1904. He undertook post graduate study in London, Dublin and Vienna. He took the FRCS Edinburgh in 1901. Returning to Australia he moved to Adelaide and practised first as a physician and later as a surgeon. He married Alice May, daughter of Sir George Brookman at Christ Church in North Adelaide in 1902, but they later divorced. He was the honorary gynaecologist at the Adelaide Hospital from 1902 to 1927 and honorary Obstetrician at the Queen's Home from 1903 to 1946. He established the first antenatal clinic at the Adelaide Hospital in 1910. He was one of a group of doctors who helped found the Ru Rua Hospital on Barton Terrace in North Adelaide in 1910.

Wilson enlisted in the AIF on 19th October 1914. He was 6ft 1ins and weighed 14st 4lb. He was appointed to the 1ASH and embarked for Egypt on the *Kyarra*. He served in Egypt, on the island of Lemnos and off the shore at Gallipoli when the unit was deployed on the *Clan McGillivray* and subsequently the *Alaunia*. He contracted enteric fever and was admitted to 1 ASH, transferred to 19th General Hospital in Alexandria with the added complications of pleurisy and a left leg thrombosis. He was admitted to 3rd London General Hospital in Wandsworth on 23rd August 1915 before repatriation to Adelaide to the 7 AGH at Keswick Barracks, where he was discharged medically unfit on 21st January 1916. Wilson continued in the army and was promoted lieutenant colonel and allotted as OC of the hospital ship *Karoola* on 12th May 1916; an appointment he continued to hold until early 1918. He was then appointed staff officer to Major General RHJ Fetherston DGMS Australian Military Forces. He accompanied him on a tour through Canada, USA, UK, France, Switzerland, Italy Greece and Salonika. He was then posted to 1 AGH in Rouen and Great Britain before returning to Adelaide and discharge early in 1919. He was issued with the 1914-15 Star, the British War Medal and the Victory Medal.

Wilson married Elsa May Cuzens in 1923 and they had two sons, one of whom became a surgeon and the other a diplomat. After the war Wilson returned to his clinical career and recommenced the antenatal clinic which was moved to the Queen's Home in 1927 and named after him in 1932. He exerted a strong influence on the Queen's Home policy and development; he was on the committee of management from 1908 and its president from 1935-1950. He was generous with his resources and contributed funds for teaching and equipment for the Queen's Home. He endowed the TG Wilson travelling scholarship in obstetrics at the University of Adelaide; many have benefitted from this. He examined ways of reducing maternal mortality during an overseas tour in 1935 and, when he returned, lobbied for better medical training in obstetrics and gynaecology; to this end a full time director of obstetrics and gynaecology was appointed at the University of Adelaide in 1940 and ultimately the Chair in Obstetrics and Gynaecology was established. He recognised the importance of nurse education and in 1905 was the founder of the SA branch of the Australasian Trained Nurses Association and was later their president and patron. A keen golfer, he was captain and later president of the Royal Adelaide Golf Club. He was a founding fellow of the RACS and RCOG (London). He was decorated with the CMG in 1942 and knighted in 1950. Sir Thomas George Wilson died on 15th March 1958 at his North Adelaide home. He was survived by his wife and two sons.

Sources:

Love J. H., 'Wilson, Sir Thomas George (1876–1958)', Australian Dictionary of Biography, National Centre of Biography, Australian National University, http://adb.anu.edu.au/biography/wilson-sir-thomas-george-12051/text21615.

http://recordsearch.naa.gov.au/NameSearch/Interface/ItemDetail.aspx?Barcode=2015707

WILTON Alexander Cockburn

MB BS

1888 - 1954

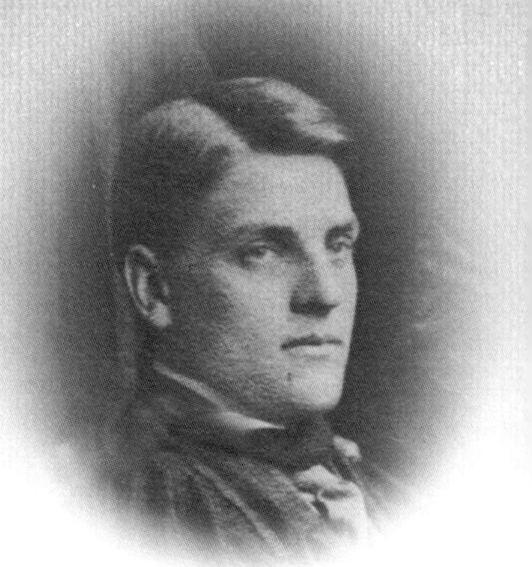

Alexander Cockburn Wilton was born at Port Fairy, Victoria, on 22 April 1888, although other sources suggest he was born in Adelaide. He was the son of Charles Richard Wilton and Annie Isabel, nee Gladstone. He was educated at Prince Alfred College and he undertook his medical studies at the University of Adelaide. Wilton was registered with the Medical Board of South Australia on 14 December 1911. He was a resident medical officer at the Adelaide Hospital in 1912. He subsequently had a medical practice in Redhill, South Australia. He married Shylie Kathleen Mathews the daughter of Mr and Mrs Llandaff Mathews of Wayville on 15th July 1914. Wilton then lived at 102 Kent Street, Kent Town.

Prior to WW1 Wilton was a 2nd lieutenant in Cadets and in 1912 Wilton joined the AAMC Reserve with John Le Messurier Kneebone and Cyril Frederick Pitcher. He enlisted in the AIF on 16 March 1918 aged 29 years 11 months; he was described as 5ft 10ins and weighed 13st and had a limited proficiency in German language. His next of kin was given as his wife Shylie Kathleen Wilton. Wilton embarked on the *Persic* in Sydney on 21 March 1918. He was initially appointed as a captain to the 9th Trg Bn. He was posted to 3 AGH on 11th September 1918 and then to the 1 FdAmb on 20th September 1918. He was detached to 1st Fd Artillery Bde and 1st Australian Division Engineers before returning to the 1 FdAmb. He was admitted to the 2 FdAmb with tonsillitis in April 1918 and on 26th May 1919 he was admitted the 3rd London General hospital with laryngitis. He returned to Australia on the *Kanowna* disembarking in 4 MD on 20 October 1919 and discharged on 12th November 1919 at which time he was described as being well. He was issued with the British War Medal and the Victory Medal.

Wilton had a medical practice in Clarendon after the war. Alexander Cockburn Wilton died in Clarendon on 6th June 1954. He was survived by his wife and son Geoffrey Cockburn Wilton who was born in 1915 and died in 1967.

Sources:

http://recordsearch.naa.gov.au/NameSearch/Interface/ItemDetail.aspx?Barcode=8846280
My Heritage Family Trees
The Mail Adelaide 4 July 1914
The Advertiser Adelaide 7 June 1954
Photo; Adelaide University Medical graduates 1911.

Two Score and Five to Three Score and Ten

The duty of medical men of military age and capacity – that is to say, those under 45 and physically fit – is now well defined.... What are the duties of medical men over 45 years of age at this crisis in their country's need? .... If he is between the ages of 45 and 55 and physically fit, if he can be easily spared from the work in which he is engaged, and wishes to take uniformed service, it is open to him to apply for a commission in the RAMC for home service only.

BMJ, 22 January 1916, p. 135

WYLLIE Hugh Alexander

MC MB BS

1893 - 1931

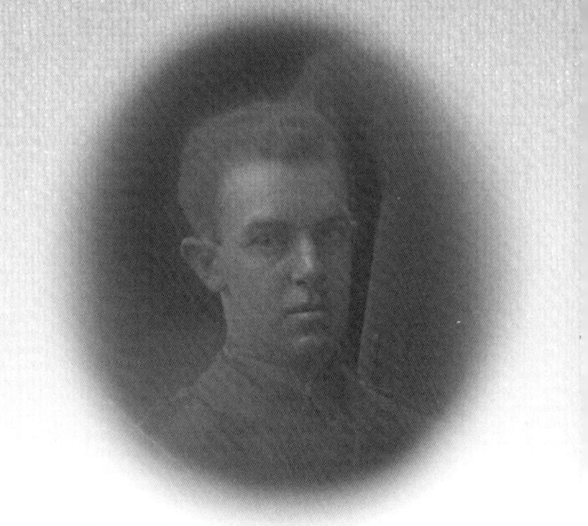

Hugh Alexander Wyllie was born in Kent Town, South Australia on 17th September 1893. He was the youngest son of Robert James Wyllie and Clara Ann,nee Green. He was educated at Norwood Public School and studied medicine at the University of Adelaide, graduating in 1915. After graduation he was a house surgeon at the Adelaide Hospital for one month before enlisting in the AIF.

Wyllie was still a medical student in his fifth year when he first enlisted in the AIF at Oakland's Camp on 3rd December 1914. He was 5ft 9ins tall and weighed 140lb, of sallow complexion with blue eyes and red hair. His next of kin was his father of Victoria Avenue, Unley Park, South Australia. However, all communication was to be made to Davenport Chambers, Currie Street, Adelaide. He was posted to the AAMC Base Depot at Mitcham. The PMO 4 MD intervened and ordered his discharge on 7th March 1915 to complete his degree. After completing his degree, on 8th December 1915, he re-enlisted at the rank of captain. He was posted to 3rd Reinforcements for the 4 FdAmb. He departed by train for Sydney on 20th December 1915 and embarked on the *Kanowna* on 22nd December 1915 disembarking in Egypt on 16th February 1916 where he was posted to the 55th Battalion. The unit moved to Marseilles on 20th June 1916 on the *Caledonian*. He was admitted to the Military Hospital, Chatham with paratyphoid in September. He was awarded the Military Cross on 19th June 1917. The citation read *for conspicuous gallantry and devotion to duty. He treated the wounded continuously for 2 days under heavy fire. He set a splendid example of courage and determination.* He was posted to 3 AGH on 8th March 1918 and promoted to major on 20th September 1918. He was sent to the 3rd Australian Division on 21st December 1918. He took a year's leave without pay to work at the Prince of Wales Hospital on 17th April 1919. Following a further short period of leave he embarked for Australia on the *Kigoma*. His appointment was terminated on 15th September 1920. He was issued with the British War Medal and Victory Medal. His older brother Kenneth also enlisted in 1915 and was an officer with the 10 Bn. Hugh Alexander Wyllie died on 27th December 1931 at York Gate, London.

Sources:

University of Adelaide Archives photo Graduates Medical School 1915

The Adelaide Advertiser 1st June 1906

The Adelaide Advertiser 7th October 1915

http://recordsearch.naa.gov.au/NameSearch/Interface/ItemDetail.aspx?Barcode=3453132

Some Notes from the Battle Front in Northern France

The three most important elements of success in treating wounds we had there in abundance – sunlight, fresh air, and pure water – and we made use of them all to the fullest extent. Every bed in the hospital was carried out of doors at 10 am and the patients remained out until sundown.

BMJ, 22 April 1916, p. 581

YEATMAN Charleton

OBE MB BS MRACP

1887 - 1959

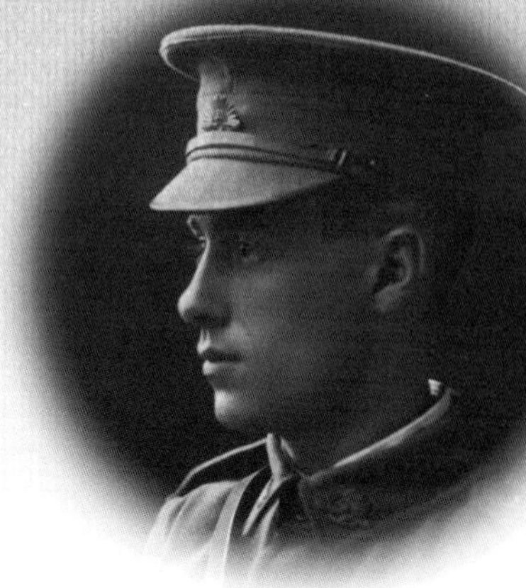

Charleton Yeatman was born in Auburn, SA, on 27th July 1887, the son of Dr John Walter Yeatman, who practised in Auburn and later in Brighton, and his wife Katherine Maud, nee Browne. He was one of eight children; three sons and five daughters. He was educated at St Peter's College and studied medicine at the University of Adelaide, graduating in 1910. Yeatman married Mignonette Des Vignes Jacob, one of four daughters of Mr and Mrs JW Jacob. He was serving in the Reserve Forces in 1913. During his time overseas in WW1 his wife followed him to England with their son John Charleton Yeatman. Yeatman succeeded Sir Trent Champion de Crespigney as Medical Superintendent of the Adelaide Hospital.

Yeatman enlisted as a captain in the AIF on 1st May 1915. He was 27 years old, 5ft 10ins tall, of dark complexion with brown eyes and dark brown hair. His wife was named as his next of kin and his address was Penzance Street, Glenelg but gave his postal address as the Bank of Adelaide in London. He embarked on the *Mooltan* on 20th May 1915. He was promoted major on 1st January 1916 and reported to 2 AGH in Egypt on the 8th February 1916. He embarked from Alexandria on 26th March 1916 and disembarked in Marseilles on 4th April. He proceeded to duty with 3rd Auxiliary Hospital on 29th March 1916. He was ill from 15th to 20th April 1916 with bronchitis and laryngitis. He was transferred from 2 AGH at Wimereux to 1 CCS on 21st August 1916 and on 22nd August he was transferred back to 2 AGH. He had severe influenza and was transferred to England on sick leave on 24th October. He was promoted to temporary lieutenant colonel on 20th February 1917 which was confirmed on 19th September 1919. He was again sick on 11th September 1917 and admitted to 3rd London General Hospital before being transferred to the 6th Auxiliary Hospital. He assumed command of the 1 AAH at Harefield on 29th September. He had two months leave in England from 5th Jan 1919. Yeatman was awarded the OBE for his conspicuous and valuable services rendered in connection to the war on 23rd May 1919. He embarked on the *Osterley* for return to Australia on 21st May 1919 arriving in 4MD on 3rd July 1919. His appointment was terminated on 2nd September 1919. He was issued with the 1914-15 Star, the British War Medal and the Victory Medal. Three of his brothers and one sister served in WW I.

Yeatman first practised in Port Pirie where he was Officer of Health on his return to Australia. At the time of his wife's mother's death in 1930 they were living in Mount Gambier. However, when Yeatman had an incident with his car in King William Road in 1935 he was reported to be living at 188 Cross Road, Malvern, South Australia. He enlisted for services in WW2 at Wayville on 28th May 1942, where he served on full time service until, on 23rd Jan 1946 he was transferred from the Reserve of Officers and appointed as Commanding Officer 130 AGH with the BCOF in Japan. His memorabilia, including his medals, are held in the Army Museum of South Australia at Keswick Barracks Adelaide. His son, Dr John Charleton Yeatman, also served in WW2. Charleton Yeatman died on 4th February 1971. An extensive amount of material of the Yeatman family is held by the University of Adelaide.

Sources:
National Archives of Australia
http://recordsearch.naa.gov.au/NameSearch/Interface/ItemDetail.aspx?Barcode=3454611 and
http://recordsearch.naa.gov.au/NameSearch/Interface/ItemDetail.aspx?Barcode=6346295
University of Adelaide Library MS0040
Northern Argus 7July 1933, 10OCT1946
The Advertiser 13Dec1917
South Australian Indexes Births, Deaths and Marriages

YOUNG Warren Hastings
MB ChB

1892 - 1957

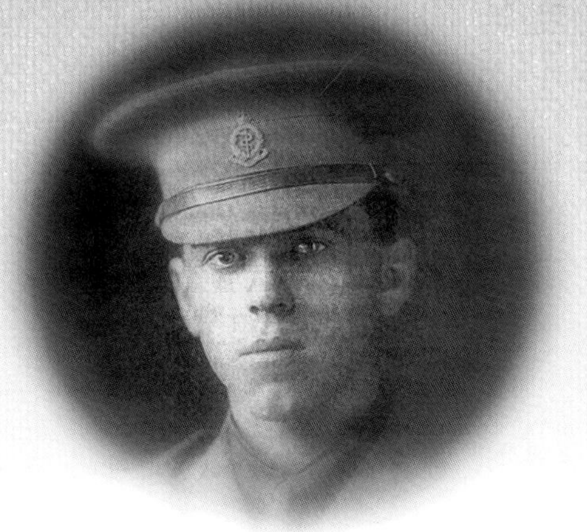

Warren Hastings Young was born in Snowtown, South Australia, on 17 November 1892, the son of Dr David Hastings Young MB, ChM (Edin), MB (Adel.) ad eundem gradum and Elizabeth, nee Mumford. When Warren was 14 months old his mother died of pulmonary tuberculosis, and his care was taken over by his maternal aunt, Ellen Mumford, (later Hamlin), in Adelaide, a city for which he retained fond memories. His father re-married, and, in 1904, Warren went with his father and step-mother to the South Island of New Zealand. He completed his secondary education at Southland Boys High School, Invercargill and studied medicine at Otago University, Dunedin, graduating MB ChB in 1915. He began practice next year in Greytown, in the North Island of New Zealand. He married Daisy Clare Chapman in Te Puke on 2 January 1917.

Young, a member of the New Zealand Territorial Army, enlisted as a lieutenant in the New Zealand Medical Corps in January 1917 and embarked for Egypt in February 1917. En route to the Middle East, he was able to visit his South Australian cousins in Adelaide. Whilst serving with the New Zealand Mounted Field Ambulance he was promoted to captain in September 1917. After detachment to the School of Instruction at Moascar, he was posted to the 27th General Hospital in Cairo and then to the Australian Mounted Rifles in Palestine, under General Allenby. Young returned to New Zealand, in January 1919, on the *Malta*.

Following the war, Young was the Medical Superintendent of the Greytown Hospital, the Tauranga Hospital, and then Honorary Anaesthetist to the Auckland Hospital. He subsequently entered general practice at Carterton before moving to Papakura in 1937. He was joined in his practice at Papakura by one of his sons, Dr Gordon Hastings Young in 1952. Young was much admired by the communities in which he worked. He had a good singing voice, and was one of the inaugural Vice-Presidents of the Carterton Choral Society. Warren Hastings Young died of coronary sclerosis in Papakura on 20 July 1957. He was survived by his three sons, two daughters and six grandchildren. His wife Daisy predeceased him in 1946.

Sources:

The Register, Adelaide, 1st October 1921
Biography and photo courtesy Dr Richard Travers 2014 whose sources were Barbara Hendry (nee Young) and Mary Nitz.

ZWAR Bernard Traugott

CMG MD MS FRACS

1876 - 1947

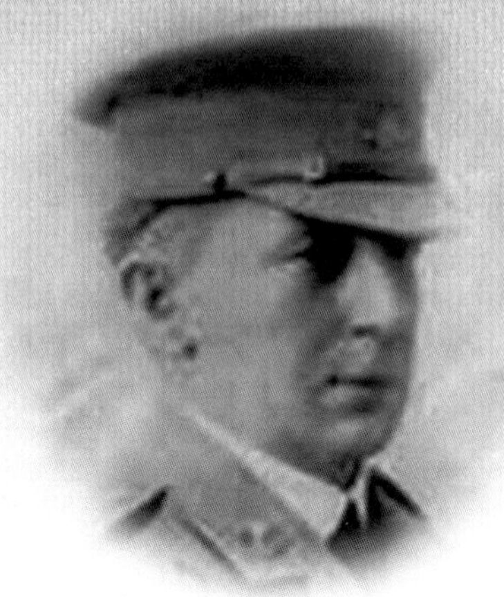

Bernard Traugott Zwar was born on the 20th June 1876 at Ebenezer, near Stockwell in the Barossa Valley. He was the youngest of 10 children of Johann Zwar and Anna, nee Kaiser, who had migrated to Australia in 1851. Zwar attended the state school at Stockwell and then went on to an English High School in the Barossa Valley, where he excelled in German, and finally to Prince Alfred College, Adelaide. He hoped to become a Lutheran Pastor, but as this would have meant studying in Europe he decided to study medicine, like his older brother Hermann, at the University of Adelaide. He began his medical studies in March 1895. Due to the 'Adelaide Hospital Row' the two brothers moved to Ormond College, Melbourne and completed their medical studies at the Melbourne University where they both graduated. Zwar graduated MB (1899), ChB (1901) and MD (1902). Zwar topped the class, won the Exhibition in Medicine, and was placed first on the list for the seven resident positions at the Melbourne Hospital. At the age of 28 in 1904, Zwar went overseas for post-graduate studies. He had a special interest in Neurology and Tuberculosis. He met and conversed with the world famous bacteriologist Dr Robert Koch and worked at various hospitals in London. For a time he was clinical clerk to Sir William Gowers at the National Hospital, Queen Square. Bernard returned to Melbourne early in 1906 and went on to build a distinguished career as a surgeon and administrator.

Zwar was a captain in the AAMC reserve in 14 FdAmb from July 1912. He enlisted in the AIF on the 28th November 1914, at the age of 38 years. He was 5ft 10ins, and weighed 12st. He was attached to the 2 ASH with the rank of major. He embarked on the 14th December 1914 and served in Egypt and Gallipoli in 2 ASH. Whilst in Egypt, at Wazza, he was the senior AIF specialist in venereal disease, he lamented the wastage that this caused. Early in 1915, 1000 AIF men were infected at any one time. He was transferred from Lemnos on 3rd July 1915 via Cairo to London with a festering appendicitis. He returned to Egypt on 25th September 1915 but did not return to duty. He returned to Australia with his appointment terminated on 19th February 1916. He was issued with the 1914-15 Star, British War Medal and the Victory Medal.

Early in his career with the armed forces Zwar was advised that he would not have a career future if he remained a member of the Lutheran Church. He joined the Presbyterian Church, became an elder and remained a faithful member for the rest of his life. Bernard had travelled to the Middle East on the same troopship as a young nurse, Essy Craig, whom he had met at the Melbourne Hospital. They renewed their acquaintance and were married on the 4th May 1916 and lived in Collins Street, on his return to Melbourne, next to The Melbourne Club. Zwar was an honorary surgeon to the Melbourne Hospital from 1919 and an honorary consulting surgeon from 1935. He was a founder of the RACS in 1927 and was on the Medical Board of Victoria, the advisory committee of the Repatriation Board and the Anti-Cancer Council. When Don Bradman was in Melbourne and needed medical attention it was Zwar who treated him. He was appointed CMG in January 1941. A portrait of Zwar hangs in the main entrance to the Royal Melbourne Hospital as a tribute to his outstanding service to the Hospital over a period of 46 years. It was unveiled by the Lieutenant Governor, Sir Edmund Herring, just before he died. Bernard Traugott Zwar died at his home in Melbourne on 16th January 1947. He was survived by his wife and son.

Sources:

http://recordsearch.naa.gov.au/scripts/Imagine.asp?B=3457930
The Adelaide Advertiser 15 December 1908
The Argus Melbourne 1st January 1941
The Argus Melbourne 17 Jan 1947
Rank B. K., 'Zwar, Traugott Bernhard (1876–1947)', Australian Dictionary of Biography, National Centre of Biography, Australian National University,.
www.becker-zwar.com
Photo: Zwar Family